D0619630

Oncology Nursing
Clinical Reference

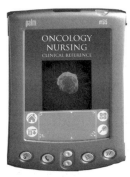

Oncology Nursing Clinical Reference

SHIRLEY E. OTTO, MSN, CRNI, AOCN
Oncology Consultant
Formerly Oncology Clinical Nurse Specialist
Via Christi Regional Medical Center
St. Francis Campus
Wichita, Kansas

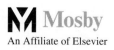 Mosby
An Affiliate of Elsevier

Mosby

An Affiliate of Elsevier

11830 Westline Industrial Drive
St. Louis, Missouri 63146

ONCOLOGY NURSING ISBN 0-323-02517-X
CLINICAL REFERENCE
Copyright © 2004, Mosby, Inc. All rights reserved.

Notice

Nursing is an ever-changing field. Standard safety precautions must
be followed, but as new research and clinical experience broaden
our knowledge, changes in treatment and drug therapy may
become necessary or appropriate. Readers are advised to check the
most current production information provided by the manufacturer
of each drug to be administered to verify the recommended dose,
the method and duration of administration, and contraindications.
It is the responsibility of the appropriately licensed health provider,
relying on experience and knowledge of the patient, to determine
dosages and the best treatment of each individual patient. Neither
the publisher nor the editor assumes any liability for any injury
and/or damage to persons or property arising from this
publication.

International Standard Book Number 0-323-02517-X

Vice President, Publishing Director: Sally Schrefer
Editor: Sandra Clark Brown
Developmental Editor: Sophia Oh Gray
Editorial Assistant: Brooke Bagwill
Publishing Services Manager: Melissa Lastarria
Associate Project Manager: Bonnie Spinola
Design Manager: Gail Morey Hudson
Cover Design: Liz Rohne Rudder

Printed in the United States of America.
Last digit is the print number: 9   8   7   6   5   4   3   2   1

To

Donna Sweet, Sharon Sullivan, and
Marian Martin Scott,

who have supported and encouraged me before,
during and through all my publications.

Contributors

Barbara B. Hodgson, RN, OCN
Cancer Institute
St. Joseph's Hospital
Tampa, Florida

Robert J. Kizior, BS, RPh
Education Coordinator
Department of Pharmacy
Alexian Brothers Medical Center
Elk Grove Village, Illinois

Reviewers

Carmencita C. Mercado-Poe, EdD, APN, CS, OCN, CHPN
Oncology Clinical Nurse Manager
De Paul Medical Center
Norfolk, Virginia

Phyllis G. Peterson, RN, MN, AOCN
Assistant Professor of Nursing
Our Lady of Holy Cross College
New Orleans, Louisiana

Preface

Caring for the patient and family with cancer is personally and professionally rewarding but also challenging. Oncology is an ever-changing field, and keeping abreast of the innovative technologies, pharmaceutical developments, and cancer disease discoveries requires a theoretical and clinical commitment. Multiple opportunities exist to meet these challenges and enable the oncology professional to be competent and conscientious in his or her respective practice setting.

Oncology Nursing Clinical Reference is a succinct text resource that contains the comprehensive topics for oncology nursing practice applicable for the novice to expert nurse. The book may be used as a "clinical quick reference," a study source for oncology education or certification exams, and/or a clinical practice resource for multiple oncology professionals. All the essentials of oncology nursing practice are included, such as disease pathology, diagnostics, clinical trials, 2003 ACS prevention, screening and detection guidelines, cancer diseases, cancer treatments and therapies, pharmaceutical drugs, infusion therapy, oncologic emergencies, symptom management, and cancer resources.

Oncology Nursing Clinical Reference is divided into five major sections for user ease in seeking specific oncology information. *Unit I – General Cancer Principles and Concepts* contains the oncology foundation chapters such as pathophysiology, genetics, epidemiology, prevention, screening and detection, diagnosis and staging, and cancer clinical trials.

Unit II – Cancer Types contains the major cancer disease groups (brain, breast, colorectal and gastrointestinal, genitourinary, gynecological, head and neck, HIV and related cancers, leukemia, lymphoma, lung, multiple myeloma, skin and melanoma, and pediatric cancers).

Cancer treatment, therapies, and symptom management are the significant topics in Unit III. Cancer treatments include surgical oncology, radiation therapy, chemotherapy, biotherapy, and bone marrow and peripheral stem cell transplantation. The pharmaceutical drugs section covers all the major drug categories used in oncology clinical practice, such as analgesics, antiemetics, antimicrobials, chemotherapy, and multiple symptom management drugs, all presented in an easy-to-use table format. Infusion therapies include blood and blood products and vascular access devices. The supportive therapy topics include complementary and alternative therapies and herbal medicines. An additional table contains an extensive list of the most common herbal therapies with potential interactions. Hormonal therapies and nutrition complete the therapy portion of this unit. An extensive symptom management section with assessment and intervention strategies and an end-of-life section containing hospice and palliative care with grief and bereavement issues complete Unit III.

Unit IV covers the most common oncologic emergencies, including the topics of definition and pathology, patient population at risk, and clinical features, with medical and nursing interventions. Unit V contains multiple cancer professional, patient/family, pharmaceutical, and product resources.

The last section of *Oncology Nursing Clinical Reference* is an appendix containing multiple drug categories, enteral and parenteral nutrition products, and herbal therapies with interactions in a user-friendly table format.

Shirley Otto

Contents

UNIT I

GENERAL CANCER PRINCIPLES AND CONCEPTS

1

Pathophysiology

I. THE NORMAL CELL

The basic unit of structure and function in all living things is the cell. Approximately 60 billion cells are in the adult human body. Although there are many different types of cells, all of them have certain common characteristics. Whenever cells are destroyed, the remaining cells of the same type reproduce until those that were destroyed are replaced. This orderly replacement of cells is governed by a control mechanism that stops when the loss or damage has been corrected. Dynamic, active, and orderly, the healthy cell is a small powerhouse, laboratory, factory, and duplicating machine—perfectly copying itself over and over.

II. PROLIFERATIVE GROWTH PATTERNS

Cancer cells are not subject to the usual restrictions placed by the host on cell proliferation. However, proliferation is not always indicative of cancer. Abnormal cellular growth is classified as *nonneoplastic* or *neoplastic* growth.

A. Nonneoplastic Growth Patterns—

   1. **Hypertrophy** is an increase in the cell size, usually resulting from an increased workload, hormonal stimulation, or compensation directly related to the functional loss of other tissue.

   2. **Hyperplasia** is a reversible increase in the number of cells of a certain tissue type, resulting in increased tissue mass such as in adolescence and pregnancy.

   3. **Metaplasia** is the process in which one adult type cell is substituted for another type not usually found in the involved tissue (glandular for squamous). This process is reversible if the stimulus is removed, or metaplasia may progress to dysplasia

3

if the stimulus persists. A common site for meta-plasia to occur is in the uterine cervix.

4. *Dysplasia* is characterized by an alteration in healthy adult cells in which the cell varies from its normal size, shape, or organization or one mature cell type is replaced with a less mature cell type such as with inflammation (e.g., chronic irritation from exposure to toxic substances). Dysplasia is possibly reversible if the stimulus is removed.

B. Neoplastic Growth Patterns—

1. *Anaplasia* (without form) is an irreversible change in which the structure of adult cells regresses to more primitive levels. These cells lose their capacity for specialized functions and are positionally and cytologically disorganized. Anaplasia is a hallmark of cancer.

2. *Neoplasia* (new growth) describes an abnormal tissue that extends beyond the boundaries of healthy tissue, failing to fulfill the normal function of cells in that tissue. Uncontrolled functioning, unregulated division and growth, and abnormal motility characterize neoplasms.

III. CHARACTERISTICS OF CANCER CELLS

A. Microscopic Properties—

The microscopic examination of cancer cells shows certain structural changes that are described in pathologic terms:

1. *Pleomorphism*—Cancer cells vary in size and shape and may be either too small or too large, and multiple nuclei are usually present.

2. *Hyperchromatism*—Nuclear chromatin, the major component of genes, is more pronounced with staining.

3. *Polymorphism*—The nucleus is larger and varies in shape.

4. *Aneuploidy*—Unusual number of chromosomes are seen.

5. *Abnormal Chromosome Arrangements*—A variety exists, such as translocations, exchange of material between chromosomes, loss of or weak chromosome sections, deletions, additions, or extra chromosomes.

B. **Kinetic Properties—**
   Cancer cells possess certain kinetic characteristics as follows:
   1. *Loss of Proliferative Control*—Cell production stops when the stimulus is gone, producing a balance between cell production and cell loss.
   2. *Loss of Capacity to Differentiate*—This is the extent to which cancer cells resemble comparable healthy cells—well differentiated, undifferentiated, and dedifferentiated—a process in which cells (cancer) lose characteristics of healthy cells. The more undifferentiated a malignant cell, the more virulent it is believed to be and the less likely to respond to chemotherapeutic drugs.
   3. *Altered Biochemical Properties*—Certain biochemical properties may be missing because of a cell's new immature state, or a cell may acquire new properties because of enzyme pattern changes or alterations in the DNA. Examples of these properties include production of tumor-associated antigens marking the cancer cell as "nonself," loss of cell-to-cell cohesiveness and adhesiveness, and continued or abnormal production of hormones. Cancer cells may inappropriately release or produce a hormone that results in signs and symptoms not directly related to the local effects of the tumor (such as parathyroid hormone–related peptide in breast or renal cancer–related hypercalcemia).
   4. *Chromosomal Instability*—Cancer cells are less genetically stable than healthy cells because of the development of abnormal chromosome arrangements.
   5. *Capacity to Metastasize*—Metastasis is the spread of cancer cells from a primary (parent) site to distant secondary sites. Cancer cells become increasingly malignant with each mutation, and an association exists between a cell's degree of malignancy and its ability to metastasize.

IV. CELLULAR KINETICS
Cellular kinetics is the study of the quantitative growth and division of cells. The cell cycle is the sequence of events involved in replication and distribution of DNA to the daughter cells produced by cell division. All cells,

nonmalignant and malignant, progress through the five phases of the cell cycle. Cancer cells are able to complete the cell cycle quicker by decreasing the length of time spent in the G1 phase, and are less likely to enter or remain in the G0 phase of the cell cycle than are healthy cells.

A. **G0 (or Postmitotic Resting) Phase—**
    The G0 phase encompasses that period of the cycle when healthy renewable tissue, including nondividing and resting cells, is not actively proliferating.

B. **G1 Phase Growth (or Postmitotic Presynthesis Period)—**
    The G1 phase is 18 to 30 hours in duration, extending from the completion of the previous cell division to the beginning of chromosome replication.

C. **S Phase—**
    The S phase is approximately 16 to 20 hours in duration. RNA is synthesized, which is essential for the synthesis of DNA.

D. **G2 Phase (or Postsynthetic/Premitotic Phase)—**
    The G2 phase is 2 to 10 hours in duration and involves relative hypoactivity while the cells await entry into the mitotic phase.

E. **M Phase Mitosis—**
    Mitosis and cell division occur during the M phase, which is 30 minutes to 1 hour in duration.

V. TUMOR GROWTH

In normal cell proliferation, cell birth approximates cell death. The human body's demand for an increase in the number of cells and for cell replacement is initiated by loss of cells of the same type or by extra tissue function demands.

In general, cancer cells possess the following properties:

A. **Tumor Growth Properties—**
    1. *Immortality of Transformed Cells*—Cancer cells are capable of passing through an infinite number of population doublings if sufficient nutrition and growth factors are available.
    2. *Decreased Contact Inhibition of Movement*—Healthy cells adjust to the proximity of neighboring cells by halting growth. Cancer cells invade other cells without respect to these constraints.
    3. *Decreased Contact Inhibition of Cell Division*—Cancer cells lack or exhibit decreased contact

inhibition of growth, continuing to divide, even piling atop one another.

4. ***Decreased Adhesiveness***—Cancer cells are less adhesive, resulting in increased cell mobility.
5. ***Loss of Anchorage Dependence***—Cancer cells do not need a surface on which to attach and proliferate. This property affects cell shape and adhesiveness.
6. ***Loss of Restrictive Point Control***—Cancer cells lose this stringent restriction of point control and continue to proliferate despite suboptimal nutrition and high cell density.

B. **Tumor Growth Concepts—**
   Healthy cells are divided into three major categories of cell growth: static (nondividing), expanding (resting), and renewing (continuously dividing). Static cells (e.g., nerve and brain cells) do not continue to divide after the postembryonic period. If these cells are damaged or destroyed they cannot be replaced. Expanding cells (e.g., liver, kidney, and endocrine gland cells) temporarily stop reproduction on reaching normal size, but they can reenter the cell cycle and divide during times of physiologic need. Renewing cells (e.g., germ cells, blood cells, and epithelial cells of the gastrointestinal mucosa) have the highest level of reproductive activity. These cells have a finite life span and continuously replicate to replace dying cells.

   The growth rate of tumors is expressed in *doubling time* (DT). Tumor volume DT is the time needed for a tumor mass to double its volume. Tumor cells undergo a series of doublings while the tumor increases in size. The average DT of most primary tumors is approximately 2 to 3 months, with a range of 11 to 90 weeks. In general, a tumor must progress through approximately *30 doublings before becoming palpable.* The minimum clinically detectable body burden of tumor (tumor volume) is 10 billion cells (1 g). Tumor masses are usually 100 billion cells, or 10 g, at detection.

   Because not all tumor cells divide simultaneously, growth fraction (GF) is an important concept in the determination of DT. GF is the ratio of the total number of cells to the number of proliferating cells. Tumors with larger GFs increase their tumor mass more quickly. As tumor volume increases, GF decreases. The rapid proliferation of tumor cells followed by continuous but slowed proliferation is called the Gompertz function. The initial exponential growth of cancer cells followed by a steady and progressive decrease in GF is caused by the decrease in the fraction of proliferating cells and an increase in the rate of cell death.

VI. CARCINOGENESIS

Carcinogenesis is the process by which healthy cells are transformed into cancer cells. The *Berenblum theory* states that cancer occurs as the result of two distinct events: initiation and promotion. Initiation occurs first and is usually believed to be rapid and mutational. An initiating agent (e.g., virus, chemical substance) brings about the change. The second event involves a promoting agent, and changes occur in cell growth, transport, and metabolism. Without promotion, initiation will not result in a truly transformed cell. Promotion may occur shortly after initiation or much later in an individual's life. Initiation produces a change in the cell, but cancer will not develop until one or several promoting agents affect the cell. The following terms clearly explain the process of carcinogenesis:

A. **Initiating Agent (Carcinogen)—**

This is a chemical, biologic, or physical agent capable of permanently, directly, and irreversibly changing the molecular structure of the genetic component (DNA) of a cell. Viral, environmental, lifestyle, and genetic factors have all been identified as initiators of carcinogenesis.

B. **Promoting Agent (Cocarcinogen)—**

This agent alters the expression of genetic information of the cell, thereby enhancing cellular transformation. It includes hormones, plant products, and drugs. Hormones promote the carcinogenic process by sensitizing a cell to the carcinogenic insult or modifying the growth of an established tumor. The main types of cancers that have hormone-responsive tissue are prostate, breast, cervical, colon, endometrial, and ovarian cancers.

C. **Complete Carcinogen—**

Complete carcinogens possess both initiating and promoting properties and are capable of inducing cancer on their own, (e.g., radiation). Radiation appears to initiate carcinogenesis by damaging susceptible DNA, which produces changes in the DNA structure. Factors that influence the risk for carcinogenesis by ionizing radiation include host characteristics (e.g., genetic makeup, age), cell cycle phase (cells in G2 are more sensitive than cells in S or G1 phase), degree of differentiation (immature cells are most vulnerable), cellular proliferation rate (cells with high mitotic rates), tissue type (gastrointestinal and hematopoietic), radiation rate, and total dose (the higher the dose and total dose, the greater the chance for mutation to occur).

D. Reversing Agents—
Reversing agents inhibit the effects of promoting agents by stimulating metabolic pathways in the cell that destroy carcinogens or by altering the initiating potency of chemical carcinogens, (e.g., drugs, enzymes, and vitamins).

E. Oncogene—
This gene has evolved to control growth and repair of tissues. It includes proto-oncogenes, the portion of the DNA that regulates normal cell proliferation and repair, and antioncogenes, the portion of the DNA that stops cell division.

F. Progression—
Progression is the change in a tumor from a preneoplastic state, or low degree of malignancy, to a rapidly growing, virulent tumor, characterized by changes in growth rate, invasive potential, metastatic frequency, morphologic traits, and responsiveness to therapy.

G. Heterogeneity—
Heterogeneity refers to the differences among individual cells within a tumor (e.g., genetic composition, growth rate, metastastic potential, and susceptibility to antineoplastic or radiation therapy). The degree of heterogeneity increases as the tumor increases in size.

H. Transformation—
Transformation is a multistep process by which cells become progressively dedifferentiated after exposure to an initiating agent (e.g., virus). Transformation results from a genetic alteration in the cell, which deregulates the control of cell proliferation.

I. Immune System—
The immune system usually controls the proliferation of potential cancer cells. Human immunity to

cancer cells is a function of humoral factors (tumor-specific antibodies) and cellular factors (sensitized lymphocytes). Cancer cells often possess antigens that differ from the patient's own antigens and therefore are recognized as foreign cells by the immune system and are destroyed.

J. Genetics—

It is estimated that approximately 5% to 10% of all cancers result from hereditary predisposition. A hereditary cancer predisposition may be characterized by diagnosis of the same cancer in multiple family members, an earlier age of onset, unique tumor site combinations, an increased number of bilateral cancers in paired organs, and the presence of precancerous syndromes or rare cancers.

VII. HISTOGENETIC TUMOR CLASSIFICATION SYSTEM

A. Solid Tumor Malignancies—

Tumors are grouped according to the tissue from which they originate and are described by the histogenetic classification system (Table 1-1). Benign tumors usually end in the suffix *-oma*. Malignant tumors also use the suffix *-oma*, but are also designated by the root word *carcin.* Carcinomas compose about 90% of human cancers. Certain prefixes are used to describe the type of epithelial tissue from which carcinomas originate (*adeno-*, glandular columnar epithelium; *squamous-*, squamous epithelial tissue). *Blastoma* is a suffix used for neoplasms with histologic features suggesting origin in embryonic tissue. *Sarcomas* compose about 10% of human cancers, and prefixes that describe their specific connective tissue include the following:

1. *Osteo:* Sarcomas arising in the bone
2. *Chondro:* Sarcomas arising from cartilage
3. *Lipo:* Sarcomas arising from fat
4. *Rhabdo:* Sarcomas arising from skeletal muscle
5. *Leiomyo:* Sarcomas arising from smooth muscle

B. Hematologic Malignancies—

Abnormal proliferation and release of white blood cell precursors (leukocytes) characterize leukemia, a cancer of the hematologic system. It is classified as either lymphoid or myeloid according to the predominant cell type and as acute or chronic according

Table 1-1 CLASSIFICATION OF NEOPLASMS

Parent Tissue	Benign Tumor	Malignant Tumor
Epithelium		
Skin and mucous membrane	Papilloma	Squamous cell carcinoma
	Polyp	Basal cell carcinoma
		Transitional cell carcinoma
Glands	Adenoma	Adenocarcinoma
	Cystadenoma	
Endothelium		
Blood vessels	Hemangioma	Hemangiosarcoma
		Angiosarcoma
Lymph vessels	Lymphangioma	Lymphangiosarcoma
Bone marrow		Multiple myeloma
		Ewing's sarcoma
		Leukemia
		Lymphosarcoma
		Lymphangioendothelioma

Continued

Table 1-1   CLASSIFICATION OF NEOPLASMS—cont'd

Parent Tissue	Benign Tumor	Malignant Tumor
Endothelium—cont'd		
Lymphoid tissue		Reticular cell sarcoma (difficult to classify because of cell embryology)
		Lymphatic leukemia
		Malignant lymphoma
Connective tissue		
Embryonic fibrous tissue	Myxoma	Myxosarcoma
Fibrous tissue	Fibroma	Fibrosarcoma
Adipose tissue	Lipoma	Liposarcoma
Cartilage	Chondroma	Chondrosarcoma
Bone	Osteoma	Osteogenic sarcoma
Synovial membrane	Synovioma	Synovial sarcoma
Muscle tissue		
Smooth muscle	Leiomyoma	Leiomyosarcoma
Striated muscle	Rhabdomyoma	Rhabdomyosarcoma

Nerve tissue		
Nerve fibers and sheaths	Neuroma	Neurogenic sarcoma
	Neurinoma (neurilemoma)	
	Neurofibroma	Neurofibrosarcoma
Ganglion cells	Ganglioneuroma	Neuroblastoma
Glial cells	Glioma	Glioblastoma
		Spongioblastoma
Meninges	Meningioma	
Pigmented neoplasms		
Melanoblasts	Pigmented nevus	Malignant melanoma
		Melanocarcinoma
Miscellaneous		
Placenta	Hydatidiform mole	Chorion-epithelioma (choriocarcinoma)
	Dermoid cyst	Embryonal carcinoma
		Embryonal sarcoma
		Teratocarcinoma

From Phipps WJ, Sands JK, Marek JF, editors: Medical-surgical nursing; concepts and clinical practice, ed 6, St Louis, 2003, Mosby.

to the maturity level shown by the predominant cell. The prefix *myelo-* or *granulo-* describes leukemia of myeloid bone marrow origin, and the prefix *lympho-* describes leukemia of lymphoid origin. Malignant lymphoma is a cancer of the lymphoid tissue. Both non–Hodgkin's lymphoma and Hodgkin's disease are classified according to four primary features: cell type, degree of differentiation, type of reaction elicited by tumor cells, and growth patterns. If a nodular growth pattern is observed, the term *nodular* is used after the cell type. If no mention of growth pattern is made, the lymphoma is of a diffuse type. Multiple myeloma is a cancerous proliferation of plasma cells (B lymphocytes) characterized by bone marrow involvement, bone destruction, and the presence of a homogeneous immunoglobulin.

VIII. ROUTES OF TUMOR SPREAD

Cancer may remain a locally invasive process, or it may spread to nonadjacent areas by hematogenous or lymphatic channels. The cancer may exhibit an orderly pattern or progress. Initially tumors grow locally, and as the tumor grows, the cells spread to and colonize regional nodes. Finally, distant metastasis occurs. Other tumors metastasize to distant organs before or with their spread to regional nodes.

A. **Direct Spread—**
   Direct spread is the ability of a tumor to penetrate and destroy adjoining tissue. This occurs by:
   1. ***Tumor Angiogenesis Factor—***This factor stimulates new capillary formation and becomes vascularized, resulting in growth rate increase and ability to invade local tissue.
   2. ***Mechanical Pressure and Rate of Tumor Growth—*** Uncontrolled replication produces densely packed and expanding tumor masses that exert pressure on adjacent tissue.
   3. ***Cell Mobility and Loss of Cellular Adhesiveness—*** This process promotes tumor cell dispersion.
   4. ***Tumor-Secreted Enzymes—***Enzymes have a major role in the destruction of healthy tissue barriers, which allows the invasion of cancer.
   5. ***Serosal Seeding—***Cells spread locally into tissue and penetrate body cavities (e.g., lung, ovarian, pleural, and peritoneal cavities).

General Principles

6. *Surgical Instrumentation*—Tumor cells may be seeded by needles as they are removed, or manipulation of the tumor during surgery may release cells into the circulation.

B. Metastatic Spread—

Metastasis permits the release of cells from the primary site and subsequent spread and attachment to structures in distant sites. The sequence of events in the metastasis process by hematogenous channels (dissemination through veins or arteries) is as follows:

1. *Growth and Progression of Primary Tumor*—Most tumors reach 10 billion cells or 1 cm in size before metastasis is possible.

2. *Angiogenesis at the Primary Site*—Angiogenesis stimulates new capillary formation and promotes tissue vascularization.

3. *Detachment*—Cancer cells are more motile than healthy cells, thus enabling the detachment process with the potential to enter the bloodstream.

4. *Arrest of Tumor Cells on Vascular Endothelium*—Tumor cells aggregate with lymphocytes, platelets, or other tumor cells and form a fibrin-platelet clot, offering a protection factor to the tumor cells in a hostile environment.

5. *Site Predilection*—The site and survival of disseminated tumor cells depend on the qualities and properties unique to the tumor cell itself.

6. *Escape from the Circulation (Extravasation)*—Tumor cells appear to damage the intact endothelium of the blood vessel by compression, then escape through the vessel wall.

7. *Angiogenesis of Metastatic Implant*—New blood vessels induced by the tumor's release of tumor angiogenesis factor is needed for the continued growth of new metastatic lesions.

8. *Lymphatic Spread*—This occurs when the cancer cells penetrate lymphatic channels draining the affected site.

Bibliography

Berenblum I: Established principles and unresolved problem in carcinogenesis, *J Natl Cancer Inst* 60:723, 1978.

Brown HK, Healey JH: Metastatic cancer to the bone. In DeVita VT Jr, Hellman S, Rosenberg SA, editors: *Cancer principles and practice of oncology,* ed 6, Philadelphia, 2001, Lippincott Williams & Wilkins.

Chu E, DeVita VT Jr: Principles of cancer management: chemotherapy. In DeVita VT Jr, Hellman S, Rosenberg SA, editors: *Cancer principles and practice of oncology,* ed 6, Philadelphia, 2001, Lippincott Williams & Wilkins.

Cotran RS, Kumar V, Collins T: *Pathologic basis of disease,* ed 6, Philadelphia, 1999, WB Saunders.

Goedegebuure PS, Eberlein TJ: Tumor biology and tumor markers. In Townsend CM Jr, Beauchamp RD, Evers BM, et al, editors: *Textbook of surgery: the biological basis of modern surgical practice,* ed 16, Philadelphia, 2001, WB Saunders.

Groenwald SL, Goodman M, Frogge M, et al: *Cancer nursing: principles and practice,* ed 4, Boston, 1999, Jones and Bartlett.

Hawkins R: Mastering the intricate maze of metastasis, *Oncol Nurs Forum* 28:959, 2001.

Holland JF, Frei E III, Bast RC Jr, et al, editors: *Cancer medicine,* ed 5, American Cancer Society, Hamilton, London, 2000, BC Decker.

Karayalcin G: Hodgkin's disease. In Lanzkowsky P, editor: *Manual of pediatric hematology and oncology,* ed 3, San Diego, 2000, Academic Press.

Lyndon J: Metastasis: Part I. Biology and prevention, *Oncol Nurs* 2:1, 1995.

Marx J: Cell growth control takes balance, *Science* 239:975, 1988.

Pfeifer K: Pathophysiology. In Otto SE, editor: *Oncology nursing,* ed 4, St. Louis, 2001, Mosby.

2 | Genetics

I. OVERVIEW

Understanding genetics and correlating the relationship between genetics and cancer can be a challenge. Following is a list of terms and corresponding definitions that should assist in the understanding of this concept.

A. Allele—
One of two or more DNA sequences occurring at a particular gene locus; typically one allele (normal DNA sequence) is common, and other alleles (mutations) are rare.

B. Chromosome—
A linear thread in the nucleus of a cell containing the DNA that transmits the genetic information. Humans have 46 chromosomes, arranged in 23 pairs, with one copy inherited from each parent.

C. Aneuploidy—
Condition of having an abnormal number of chromosomes; cancer conditions associated with aneuploidy such as leukemia are detected by flow cytometry and cytogenetic analysis and have prognostic implications.

D. Genes—
The fundamental unit of heredity. Approximately 50,000 to 100,000 genes are in the human genome. Each gene is composed of DNA that carries instructions for protein formation.

E. Oncogene—
One type of regulatory gene associated with cancer development.

F. Proto-oncogenes—
Activated oncogenes that lead to uncontrolled cell growth.

G. **Knudson "Two Hit" Hypothesis**—
   The inactivation of both copies of a given regulatory gene; individuals are born with two copies of almost every gene, and both copies of a regulatory gene must be inactivated for cancer to occur.

H. **Tumor Suppressor Genes**—
   A second class of genes that function as regulators of cell growth; when inactivated, this regulation of cell growth is affected.

I. **Mutation**—
   A change in the usual DNA sequence of a particular gene. Mutations can have harmful, beneficial, or neutral effects on health and may be inherited as autosomal-dominant (AD), autosomal-recessive (AR), or X-linked traits. Many cancer-predisposing mutations are AD, meaning the cancer susceptibility occurs when only one copy of the mutation is inherited. For AD conditions, the term *carrier* is often used in a different way; that is, to denote people who have inherited the genetic predisposition conferred by the mutation. *Germline* mutations are inherited and *somatic* mutations are acquired.

J. **Autosomal Dominant**—
   AD inheritance refers to genetic conditions that occur when a mutation is present in *one copy* of a given gene; only one parent is needed to donate a copy of a mutated gene for a disease to be expressed.

K. **Autosomal Recessive**—
   AR inheritance refers to genetic conditions that occur when mutations are present in *both copies* of a given gene. It occurs when both parents carry a single gene mutation; therefore their offspring have a 50% chance of inheriting a single copy of the mutated gene and thus becoming a carrier.

L. **X-linked Recessive**—
   X-linked recessive inheritance refers to genetic conditions associated with mutations in genes on the X chromosome. The mutations are passed through the mother and can be either dominant or recessive. With the X-linked dominant inheritance, both sexes have a 50% chance of inheriting a copy of the mutated gene and expressing the disease and a 50% chance of not inheriting the mutation or the disease. In X-linked recessive inheritance there is a 50% chance of

passing a mutation to a son who would express the disease or a daughter who would be a carrier, and a 50% chance of passing a normal copy to the gene of her offspring.

M. Inherited Cancer Syndrome—
This syndrome is used to describe the clinical manifestations associated with a mutation conferring a cancer susceptibility.

N. Sporadic Cancer—
Sporadic cancers develop in people who do not carry a high-risk mutation. They are cancers seen in the general population and make up the majority of all cancers diagnosed.

Cancer is a genetic disorder and occurs because of mutations in the genes and chromosomes. *Harmful genetic mutations*, the hallmark of some malignant disorders, are acquired during life and cause sporadic cancers, whereas the *initial mutation is inherited* and causes hereditary cancers. This inheritance of a cancer susceptibility follows a certain transmission pattern (Mendelian, AD). When a tumor-suppressor gene is involved, the normal copy initially allows cells to function normally. Cancer usually arises sometime during adulthood, when the normal allele acquires a somatic, cancer-inducing mutation.

II. CANCER GENETIC RISK ASSESSMENT

Genetic information including information from family history and from DNA-based testing provides a means to identify people who have an increased risk for cancer. Family medical history often identifies people with a moderately increased risk for cancer, and in some cases identifies indicators that influence cancer susceptibility. Identifying a person with an increased risk for cancer can reduce the occurrence of cancer through clinical management strategies, such as tamoxifen for breast cancer prevention and colonoscopy for colon cancer, and can improve the patient's prognosis with improved knowledge about cancer risk.

A cancer susceptibility syndrome present in families is based on a family history pedigree (pictorial representation of family members and cancer history) and evidence of certain physical findings. This family history should detail three generations, including both affected and unaffected relatives, age of diagnosis, and death if applicable.

General features of hereditary cancer syndromes include:

- Multiple cancers in close relatives, particularly in multiple generations
- Early age of onset, younger than age 40 to 50 years for adult-onset cancers
- Multiple cancers in a single individual
- Bilateral cancer in paired organs (breast, kidney)
- Recognition of the known association between the etiologic factors (cause) of related cancers in the family
- Presence of congenital anomalies or precursor lesions that are known to be associated with an increased cancer risk (presence of atypical nevi and risk for malignant melanoma)
- Recognizable Mendelian inheritance pattern (transmission from one generation to another)

III. CANCER GENETICS RISK COUNSELING

Genetic counseling has been defined by the American Society of Human Genetics as "a communication process" that deals with the human problems associated with the occurrence or risk for occurrence of a genetic disorder in a family. The process involves an attempt by one or more appropriately trained professionals to assist the individual or family in the following:

- Comprehending the medical facts, including the diagnosis, probable course of the disorder, and the available management
- Appreciating the way that heredity contributes to the disorder and to the risk for recurrence in specific relatives
- Understanding the alternatives for dealing with the risk for recurrence
- Choosing a course of action that seems appropriate in view of their risk, their family goals, and their ethical and religious standards and acting in accordance with that decision
- Making the best possible adjustment to the disorder in an affected family member or to the risk for recurrence of that disorder, or both

The cancer genetic counseling experience begins by addressing each individual's needs, worries, questions, and concerns and giving some indication of what to expect. Early in the session, it is essential to establish trust, a sense of safety, and rapport. Other tasks during the early phase include eliciting beliefs about cancer, understanding questions, and negotiating a mutually agreeable agenda. Later in the process, the focus should be promoting autonomy in decision-making, recommending active coping strategies, and assisting the individual in dealing with practical and other emotional issues.

IV. GENETIC PREDISPOSITION TESTING

Genetic predisposition testing in individuals with a family history of cancer refers to the detection of genetic mutation or variation in the sequence of DNA in a cancer-susceptible gene. Several professional organizations have issued position statements regarding the clinical application of genetic predisposition testing and include the following:

- A confirmed family history of cancer or very early-onset disease exists.
- The test can be interpreted once performed.
- The results will influence medical management.
- Cancer predisposition genetic testing requires informed consent.
- Efforts should be made to include family members in the counseling process.
- The genetic counseling process should occur in a manner consistent with individual cultural and healthcare beliefs.

V. BREAST AND OVARIAN CANCER RISK PREDICTION MODELS

A number of models (see later) are available to assess the breast and ovarian cancer risk among individuals based on their family and personal medical histories. These models are used to predict the risk for developing breast and ovarian cancer and the risk for having a mutation in a breast cancer–susceptible gene. These models were developed from epidemiology studies in families with high risk for breast and ovarian cancer. The following models are used most often when the cancer mutation carrier is unknown.

A. Gail—

Calculates a 5-year and a lifetime risk for breast cancer in a woman with risk factors compared with another woman of the same age without the same risk factors.

B. **Claus—**
Considers maternal and paternal breast cancers and calculates a 10-year and a lifetime risk for breast cancer.

C. **Couch/Weber—**
Calculates risk when the family history includes any of the following: breast cancer only with a relative with breast or ovarian cancer; different family members with breast or ovarian cancer; consideration of non-Jewish and Ashkenazi Jewish families' risk for *BRCA1* mutations.

D. **Frank—**
Calculates mutation detection risks based on various ages of onset of breast cancer; risks are calculated for both *BRCA1* and *BRCA2* mutations.

E. **Shattuck-Eldens—**
Calculates risks for *BRCA1* mutations.

VI. SELECTED HEREDITARY CANCERS AND GENE MUTATIONS

A. **Breast Cancer—**
Approximately 5% to 10% of all breast cancer cases in the United States are the result of genetic mutations, and these genetic mutations cause as many as 80% of the breast cancer cases among women younger than 50 years. The most common known mutations occur in the *BRCA1*, *BRCA2*, *p53*, and *PTEN* genes. In women who do not carry such a genetic mutation but who have breast cancer, the disease usually develops after age 50, and the risk increases with age. Women who carry a *BRCA1* gene mutation and have a family history of breast cancer have a 56% to 85% lifetime risk for developing the disease, compared with a 12% lifetime risk for women who do not. The lifetime risk for breast cancer developing in a woman with a *BRCA2* mutation is 50% to 85%. Women who carry a *BCRA* mutation and are diagnosed with breast cancer also have a higher risk for cancer developing in the contralateral breast.

A mutation of either the *BRCA1* or the *BRCA2* gene increases the risks for developing breast, ovarian, colon, and prostate cancers, and these mutations can be passed down from either parent. If a parent tests positive for the genetic mutation, his or her child has a 50% chance of having that same genetic mutation. Men who have inherited the mutation can pass it on to their daughters.

B. Ovarian Cancer—

Mutations of the *BRCA1* gene are associated with breast and ovarian cancers; those of the *BRCA2* gene are associated with cancers of the breast, ovaries, prostate, head and neck, and pancreas, as well as malignant melanoma. Presence of either of these mutations may increase a woman's lifetime risk for ovarian cancer to as high as 60%.

When there is a family history of ovarian cancer, the benefits of genetic testing are clear, and screening for ovarian cancer should be initiated because an early diagnosis promotes a better prognosis. In addition, the testing provides information that can illuminate treatment and lifestyle choices. For example, a woman in her childbearing years may decide to start having a family, whereas an older woman may elect to have prophylactic oophorectomy to minimize her risk for ovarian cancer.

C. Colon Cancer—

Hereditary colorectal cancers are the result of germ-line mutations in specific cancer-susceptible genes and include hereditary nonpolyposis colorectal cancer (HNPCC), familial adenopolyposis (FAP), juvenile polyposis, Peutz-Jeghers syndrome, Muir-Torre syndrome, and Turçot syndrome. An individual with a mutation in the mismatch repair genes that leads to HNPCC has an 80% lifetime risk for colorectal cancer, and the lifetime risk for those with FAP is more than 95%.

Clinical features of HNPCC include early age of onset, with an average age at diagnosis of 45 years. The affected individuals have no polyps and only one to two adenomas. Additional classification for HNPCC includes the "Amsterdam criteria" for identification of HNPCC families. This criterion includes the following: three or more relatives have colorectal cancer, one case being a first-degree relative, cancers occur within two or more generations, and patients have one diagnosis by 50 years of age. This information is useful in targeting certain families for early prevention, screening, and detection measures.

Familial adenomatous polyposis is a hereditary colorectal cancer syndrome that is responsible for approximately 1% of all colorectal cancers, and the lifetime risk in FAP families is greater than 95% compared with the general population risk of about 5%. Approximately one third of patients with FAP syndrome has no family history and probably represents new mutations. A unique identifying clinical feature associated with FAP is the hundreds to thousands of adenomatous polyps found in the colon of affected individuals as young as 10 years of age. The diagnosis of FAP is made on the basis of having at least 100 adenomatous polyps throughout the colon. Another clinical feature associated with FAP is congenital hypertrophy of the retinal pigment epithelium, which was used as a benign marker for FAP before the availability of genetic testing.

Variants of FAP known as Gardner's syndrome exhibit the same clinical features, including epidermal cysts, osteomas, desmoid tumors, and more than the usual number of teeth. Attenuated FAP is another variation of FAP characterized by smaller numbers of adenomas in the colon, and usually occurs in patients older than 50 years, but it is associated with a high risk for colon cancer.

D. **Multiple Endocrine Neoplasia—**
Multiple endocrine neoplasia (MEN) is a hereditary disorder characterized by the occurrence of tumors involving the endocrine glands. MEN is further divided into clinically and genetically distinct syndromes known as MEN1 and MEN2.

1. *MEN1,* known as Wermer's syndrome, is associated with germline mutations characterized by tumors of the pituitary and parathyroid glands and the pancreatic islet cells. Tumors can also involve the adrenal cortex and the thyroid gland.

2. *MEN2* is an AD inherited syndrome associated with germline mutations associated with medullary thyroid cancer.

E. **Malignant Melanoma—**
Inherited risk factors account for 5% to 7% of melanoma, but the gene and mutation frequencies are unknown. Melanoma syndromes have been described as dysplastic nevus syndrome, familial atypical multiple mole–malignant melanoma syndrome (FAMMM), and melanoma-astrocytoma syndrome.

Hereditary predisposition to melanoma should be suspected in a patient with invasive melanoma in at least two first-degree relatives. Early age at diagnosis and multiple primary melanomas are typical of melanoma-prone families. FAMMM is associated with pancreatic cancer, and astrocytomas occur in excess in some melanoma-prone families.

F. **Retinoblastoma—**

Retinoblastoma is the most common intraocular cancer in children, with an incidence between 1/13,500 and 1/25,000 births; male and female children are equally effected. The tumors may be unilateral (20% are hereditary) or bilateral (almost all are hereditary), and most (90%) retinoblastomas are diagnosed when the patient is younger than 3 years.

G. **Von Hippel-Lindau Disease—**

Von Hippel-Lindau disease is inherited as AD, with an incidence of 1/36,000. Multiple cysts in kidney, liver, and pancreas; retinal and cerebellar hemangioblastoma; and increased risk for renal cell carcinoma and pheochromocytoma characterize von Hippel-Lindau disease. Angiomas and cysts of the spleen are occasionally described. Renal cell carcinoma occurs in as many as 75% of affected individuals, with an average age at diagnosis of 40 to 45 years.

H. *p53* **Gene—**

The *p53* gene is the most commonly mutated tumor-suppressor gene, with mutations found in at least half of all cancer types. Abnormal p53 protein is associated with a decreased cancer survival. Li-Fraumeni syndrome is a rare genetic condition caused by a germline mutation in the *p53* gene and is responsible for cancer of the breast and brain, soft tissue sarcomas, leukemias, and adrenocortical cancers, all within the same family. This gene is located on chromosome 17 and encodes for a protein that stops cell division when the DNA damage is detected and allows the DNA to repair. Thus a *p53* gene mutation will allow cell division to continue without repairing the damaged DNA. Persons with *p53* mutations have a 50% risk for cancer development by age 35, with 30% of these cancers occurring before age 15.

I. *PTEN*—

Cowden disease is a rare condition caused by germline mutations in the *PTEN* gene. It is located on chromosome 10 and is associated with the following clinical conditions: mucocutaneous lesions, breast and thyroid cancer, fibrocystic disease, macrocephaly, and gastrointestinal benign growths. Women with a *PTEN* mutation have a 25% to 50% lifetime risk for developing breast cancer before age 40 years, and they frequently have bilateral breast cancers.

VII. HUMAN GENOME PROJECT

The human genome is the total genetic information found in most human cells. The Human Genome Project (HGP), an international effort, began in 1990 and was completed in June 2000. HGP's mission was to identify the full set of genetic instructions (genes) contained in human cells and to construct and sequence genetic maps. The National Institutes of Health and the U.S. Department of Energy coordinated the HGP.

The following is a list of goals that were completed by the HGP:

- Develop a genetic map
- Develop a physical map
- Sequence the entire genome
- Develop technologies
- Investigate the ethical, legal, and social implications of the project

This information generated by HGP will be the source book for biomedical science in the twenty-first century and will be of immense benefit to the entire healthcare field.

Knowledge gained from the HGP will have enormous implications for cancer practice, such as designing and implementing chemoprevention studies; developing models for cancer risk profiles; providing cancer genetic testing and counseling; and prevention, screening, and detection measures for targeting high-risk individuals or families at risk for cancer disease.

VIII. WEBSITES

American College of Medical Genetics:
www. acmg.net

Genetic Alliance:
www.geneticalliance.org

National Cancer Institute:
www.nci.nih.gov

National Coalition for Health Professional Education in Genetics:
www.nch.peg.org

National Human Genome Research Institute:
www.nhgri.nih.gov

Secretary's Advisory Committee on Genetic Testing:
www.4.od.nih.gov/oba/sacgt.htm

Bibliography

Appel CP: Genetics. In Otto SE, editor: *Oncology nursing*, ed 4, St. Louis, 2001, Mosby.

Baker DL, Shuette JL, Uhlmann WR, editors: *A guide to genetic counseling*, New York, 1998, Wiley-Liss.

Cancer predisposition genetic counseling and risk assessment counseling. Oncology Nursing Society, *Oncol Nurs Forum* 27:1349, 2000.

Giarelli E: Ethical issues in genetic testing, *J Infus Nurs* 24:310, 2001.

Harris LL: Ovarian cancer: screening for early detection, *Am J Nurs* 102:46, 2002.

Held-Warmkessel J: What your patient needs to know about prostate cancer, *Nursing* 32:36, 2002.

Lea DH, Williams JK: Genetic testing and screening, *Am J Nurs* 102:36, 2002.

Lin EM: Laboratory value assessment. In Lin EM, editor: *Advanced practice in oncology nursing*, Philadelphia, 2001, WB Saunders.

National Cancer Institute: Cancer genetics overview, http://cancer.gov/cancerinfo/pdq/genetics/overview. Retrieved 12/18/2002.

Pasacreta JV, Jacobs L, Cataldo JK: Genetic testing for breast and ovarian cancer risk: the psychosocial issues, *Am J Nurs* 102:40, 2002.

Petersen GM: Genetic testing, *Hematol Oncol Clin N Am* 14:939, 2000.

Spahis J: Human genetics: constructing a family pedigree, *Am J Nurs* 102:44, 2002.

Wickham R, McCaffery S: Genetics. In Lin EM, editor: *Advanced practice in oncology nursing*, Philadelphia, 2001, WB Saunders.

Zimmerman VL: BRCA gene mutations and cancer, *Am J Nurs* 102:28, 2002.

General Principles

3

Epidemiology

I. EPIDEMIOLOGY

Epidemiology studies the various disease frequencies among human population groups and the factors influencing those disease variations. The goal of epidemiology is to identify the cause of disease so that the causative agent can be removed and thus the disease is prevented. The focus of epidemiology is on humans as part of study groups or populations rather than as individuals. In the early 1940s epidemiology focused on infectious diseases; however the number of deaths from chronic illnesses (heart, cancer) has increased, and thus the focus has changed. Cancer epidemiology became a refined discipline with committed resources to address the causes of cancer. In 1973, the National Cancer Institute established and funded the Surveillance, Epidemiology, and End-Results Program (SEER), consisting of 11 population-based registries to collect data from individual cancer sites. These registries continuously gather information on cancer incidence, prevalence, mortality, and survival rates.

A. **Incidence—**

The number of newly diagnosed cases of cancer in a specified period of time (e.g., 1 year) within a defined population. **In 2003, approximately 1,334,100 new cancer cases will occur in the United States.**

B. **Prevalence—**

The measurement of all cancer cases, both *old* and *new*, as a designated point in time (e.g., 1 year).

C. **Mortality—**

The number of deaths attributed to cancer in a specified time period (e.g., 1 year) within a defined population. **In 2003, approximately 556,500 cancer deaths will occur in the United States.**

D. **Survival**—
The link between incidence and mortality data is survival analysis. Survival analysis is the observation over time of persons with cancer and the calculation of their probability of dying over several time periods (e.g., 1-, 2-, 5-year periods).

The 5-year survival rates are the most common measure used for reporting survival cancer data. For many cancer diseases the chances of surviving the *second* 5 years are *greater* than surviving the first 5 years after diagnosis.

1. *Event-Free Survival*—The time from a clinically significant event such as diagnosis, treatment, or transplantation until some other survivor type event occurs.
2. *Overall Survival*—The disease-free, progression-free, or local recurrence-free survival and time to identification of distant metastasis.
3. *Relative Survival*—The ratio of the observed (cancer) survival rate to the expected rate for a group of people (noncancer) in the general population similar to the patient group with respect to age, race, and sex.

II. CURRENT TRENDS IN CANCER INCIDENCE, MORTALITY, AND SURVIVAL RATES
A. **Incidence**—
   - Approximately 1,284,900 new cases of invasive cancer were diagnosed in 2002.
   - Since 1990, about 16 million new cancer cases have been diagnosed. (This excludes basal and squamous cell skin cancers and in situ carcinomas, except those in the urinary bladder.)
   - Higher rate of incidence is seen in men than women.
   - Overall incidence is greatest in blacks than for any other racial or ethnic group.
   - Prostate cancer incidence rates are 49% greater for black men than white men.
   - Among men, cancers of the prostate (30%), lung and bronchus (14%), and colon and rectum (11%) compose 55% of all new cancer cases.
   - Among women, the most commonly diagnosed cancers are cancers of the breast (31%), lung and bronchus (12%), and colon and rectum (12%).

- Cutaneous malignant melanoma is the most common cancer diagnosed in whites between the ages of 25 and 29 years, with a median age of onset of 44 years of age.

B. Mortality—
- One in four deaths in the United States is due to cancer.
- More than 555,500 cancer-related deaths occurred in the United States in 2002.
- Lung cancer accounts for 31% of male and 25% of female cancer deaths.
- Risks for death from lung cancer are 22 times greater for current male smokers and 12 times greater for current female smokers than for nonsmokers.
- Leading causes of male death are cancers of the lung, prostate, colon, and pancreas and non–Hodgkin's lymphoma.
- Leading causes of female deaths are cancers of the lung, breast, colon, pancreas, and ovary.
- Overall, blacks are more likely to die from cancer than are persons of any other racial or ethnic group.
- For all ages, cancer is the second most common cause of death, exceeded only by heart disease.
- For children younger than 14 years, cancer is the second most common cause of death.
- After significant increases for the previous 70 years, mortality rates for all cancers combined began to decline in the 1990s.

C. Survival—
- The 5-year survival rate for all cancers combined is 62%.
- The 5-year survival rates for children vary depending on the cancer site: all sites, 77%; bone cancer, 73%; neuroblastoma, 71%; Wilms' tumor, 92%; Hodgkin's disease, 92%; brain and central nervous system, 69%; and acute lymphoblastic leukemia, 85%.

III. ENVIRONMENTAL CAUSES OF HUMAN CANCER

A. Environmental Cancer Risks—
Environmental cancer risks include smoking, diet, infectious disease, and exposure to chemicals and radiation; these risks cause an estimated three quar-

ters of all cancer deaths in the United States. Tobacco use, unhealthy diet, and physical inactivity have a greater effect on individual cancer risk than do trace levels of pollutants in food, drinking water, and air. The *degree of risk* from pollutants depends on the concentration, intensity, and duration of exposure. Substantial increased risks have occurred in work settings where employees have been exposed to high concentrations of ionizing radiation, certain chemicals, metals, and other substances. In addition, patients treated with drugs or therapies known or later found to be carcinogens have increased risks for ill health.

B. Risk Assessment—
This process evaluates both the cancer-causing potential of a substance, as well as the levels of this substance in the environment, and the extent to which people are exposed.

C. Chemicals—
Various chemicals (e.g., benzene, asbestos, vinyl chloride, arsenic, and aflatoxin) show definite evidence of causing cancer in humans. Additional carcinogens based on animal experiments include chloroform, formaldehyde, polycyclic aromatic hydrocarbons (PCBs), and dichlorodiphenyltrichloroethane (DDT).

D. Radiation—
The types of radiation proven to cause human cancer are high-frequency ionizing radiation (IR) and ultraviolet (UV) radiation. Exposure to sunlight (UV radiation) causes almost all of the cases of basal cell and squamous cell skin cancer and is a major contributor to skin melanoma.

E. Unproven Risks—
Unproven risks are those cancer risks in the environment in which known carcinogen exposures are at such low levels that risk is negligible. Examples include:

1. *Pesticides*—Also includes insecticides, that is, herbicides used in agriculture in the production of the food supply.

2. *Nonionizing Radiation*—Electromagnetic radiation (radiowaves, microwaves, radar) and electric and magnetic fields (electric currents, cellular phones, and household appliances).

General Principles

3. *Toxic Wastes*—Many toxic chemicals contained in these wastes can be carcinogenic at high levels, but most community exposures are limited; clean up of toxic waste sites is essential to future healthy living conditions.

4. *Nuclear Power Plants*—The ionizing radiation emissions from nuclear facilities are closely controlled and have limited exposure to the population at large.

Bibliography

American Cancer Society: *Cancer prevention and early detection, facts and figures 2003,* Atlanta, 2003, The Society.

American Cancer Society: *Cancer facts and figures 2003,* Atlanta, 2003, The Society.

Carroll-Johnson RM, Jassak PR, editors: Evidence-based oncology nursing practice: improving patient outcomes in the next millennium, *Oncol Nurs Forum* 28(2 Suppl):3, 2001.

Chu E, Grever MR, Chabner BA: Cancer drug development. In DeVita VT Jr, Hellman S, Rosenberg SA, editors: *Cancer principles and practice of oncology,* ed 6, Philadelphia, 2001, Lippincott Williams & Wilkins.

Cotran RS, Kumar V, Collins T: *Pathologic basis of disease,* ed 6, Philadelphia, 1999, WB Saunders.

Oncology Nursing Society: *Cancer chemotherapy guidelines and recommendations for practice,* Pittsburgh, 2001, Oncology Nursing Press.

Parkin DM, Pisani P, Ferlay J: Global cancer statistics, *CA Cancer J Clin* 49:33, 1999.

Sample D: Cancer vaccines: a new era in cancer management has begun, *Nurse Investigator* 6:6, 2002.

Schulmeister L: Epidemiology. In Otto SE (ed): *Oncology nursing,* ed 4, St. Louis, 2001, Mosby.

Thompson JM, McFarland GK, Hirsch JE, et al: *Mosby's clinical nursing,* ed 5, St. Louis, 2002, Mosby.

Trichopoulous D, Lipworth L, Petridou E, et al: Epidemiology of cancer. In DeVita VT Jr, Hellman S, Rosenberg SA, editors: *Cancer principles and practice of oncology,* ed 6, Philadelphia, 2001, Lippincott Williams & Wilkins.

U.S. Department of Labor, Office of Occupational Medicine, OSHA: Controlling occupational exposure to hazardous, CPL 2-2.20B CH-4, Washington, DC, 1995, U.S. Government Printing Office.

4
Prevention, Screening, and Detection

I. OVERVIEW

The American Cancer Society estimates that more than 1,334,100 new cancer cases will be diagnosed in 2003, and approximately 556,500 of those patients are expected to die from cancer, accounting for about 1 of every 4 deaths in the United States. Cancer is the second leading cause of death, exceeded only by heart disease. Scientific evidence suggests that about one third of the 555,500 cancer deaths expected to occur in 2003 will be related to nutrition, physical inactivity, obesity, and other lifestyle factors that can be changed.

Prevention, screening, and early detection are among the best strategies in the quest to conquer cancer. A healthy lifestyle and a healthy diet are the major factors that contribute to decreasing individual risk for cancer developing. A lifetime risk and a relative risk define an individual's risk for cancer. Lifetime risk refers to the probability that an individual over the course of his or her lifetime will have cancer or will die from it. In the United States, men have a slightly smaller than 1 in 2 lifetime risk and women have about a 1 in 3 lifetime risk for having cancer. Relative risk is a measure of the strength of the relationship between risk factors (e.g., smoking) and the particular cancer (e.g., lung) (Figure 4-1).

II. RISKS FOR DEVELOPING CANCER

Major factors placing humans at risk for cancer include tobacco use, high-fat diet, lifestyle behaviors, and occupational or environmental exposures.

Estimated New Cases

- -

Prostate (33%)	Breast (32%)
Lung and Bronchus (14%)	Lung and Bronchus (12%)
Colon and Rectum (11%)	Colon and Rectum (11%)
Urinary Bladder (6%)	Uterine Corpus (6%)
Melanoma of the Skin (4%)	Ovary (4%)
Non–Hodgkin's Lymphoma (4%)	Non–Hodgkin's Lymphoma (4%)
Kidney (3%)	Melanoma of the Skin (3%)
Oral Cavity (3%)	Thyroid (3%)
Leukemia (3%)	Pancreas (2%)
Pancreas (2%)	Urinary Bladder (2%)
All Other Sites (17%)	All Other Sites (20%)

Estimated Deaths

- -

Lung and Bronchus (31%)	Lung and Bronchus (25%)
Prostate (10%)	Breast (15%)
Colon and Rectum (10%)	Colon and Rectum (11%)
Pancreas (5%)	Pancreas (6%)
Non–Hodgkin's Lymphoma (4%)	Ovary (5%)
Leukemia (4%)	Non–Hodgkin's Lymphoma (4%)
Esophagus (4%)	Leukemia (4%)
Liver (3%)	Uterine Corpus (3%)
Urinary Bladder (3%)	Brain (2%)
Kidney (3%)	Multiple Myeloma (2%)
All Other Sites (22%)	All Other Sites (23%)

*Excludes basal and squamous cell skin cancers and in situ carcinomas except urinary bladder.
Note: Percentages may not total 100 percent due to rounding.

Figure 4-1   Ten leading cancer types for the estimated new cancer cases and deaths by sex in the United States in 2003. (From Jemal A, Murray T, Samuels A, et al: Cancer Statistics, 2003, *CA Cancer J Clin,* 53(1):5-26, 2003.)

General Principles

A. **Tobacco—**
   Tobacco use is a major preventable cause of disease and premature death in the United States. It accounted for an estimated 430,700 premature deaths each year from 1990 to 1994. Approximately 90% of all lung cancer cases are caused by tobacco smoke from pipes, cigarettes, cigars, and sidestream or second-hand smoke. Other cancers that have increased risk from tobacco use include larynx, pharynx, esophagus, pancreas, kidney, bladder, and uterine cervix.

B. **Diet—**
   The diet and nutritional guidelines recommend that adults and adolescents reduce their intake of fat, both saturated and unsaturated, and increase the amount of daily intake of natural fiber in the diet. Estimates report that 30% to 60% of all cancers in men and women are related to diet.

C. **Alcohol—**
   An excessive intake of alcohol can lead to cancers of the head and neck, larynx, liver, and pancreas. The combination of alcohol and tobacco use further increases an individual's risk for these cancers and other medical conditions.

D. **Genetic Predisposition—**
   Cancers with genetic predisposition include breast, ovary, and colorectal and malignant melanoma. Breast and ovarian cancer development has been related to changes in certain genes and mutations. The greatest risk exists when there is a primary relative of a patient with an autosomal dominant inherited cancer.

E. **Socioeconomic Factors—**
   Issues related to barriers to prevention and healthcare access have been reported as major factors in the differences in cancer incidence, delayed diagnosis, poor survival statistics, and increased mortality rates from cancer in minority and socioeconomic poor populations. These factors impact significantly the ability to have work employee health benefits or the resources to purchase healthcare insurance. Approximately 20% of Americans younger than 65 years have no health insurance, and about 26% of older adults have Medicare coverage only; and with current national unemployment status at 6%, these statistics are increasing at alarming rates.

F. **Sunlight—**
   The sun is the primary source of natural ultraviolet (UV) light exposure that is known to cause three types of skin cancers: basal cell, squamous cell, and melanoma. Additional risk factors for melanoma, basal cell, and squamous cell cancers are chronic exposure to the sun, personal or family history of melanoma or skin cancer, and having light-colored skin. Other risk factors for melanoma include severe sunburn occurring early in life, presence of moles and freckles, or both. *Avoidance* of direct exposure to the sun between the hours of 10 AM and 4 PM and use of tanning beds or sun lamps, wearing protective clothing (hats with wide brim to shade face and long sleeves to protect arms), and using sunscreen lotion with sun protection factor of 15 or greater are the most effective measures to prevent skin cancer.

G. **Sexual Lifestyles—**
   Certain cancers are related to infectious exposures—for example, hepatitis B virus, human papillomavirus, human immunodeficiency virus, *Helicobacter,* and others—and could be prevented through behavior changes or with vaccines and antimicrobials. Sexually transmitted diseases, genital cancers, and acquired immune deficiency syndrome have a documented direct relationship to sexual lifestyle and practices (such as cancer of the cervix, vulva, and vagina). See Chapter 3 for additional information on environmental and occupational risks related to cancer diseases.

III. CANCER PREVENTION GUIDELINES

Cancer prevention is commonly discussed by using three different approaches: disease prevention, early detection, and limiting the disease consequences.

A. **Primary Prevention—**
   Focuses on ensuring the disease never develops by eliminating causes of disease or increasing resistance to disease (such as health promotion and immunizations).

B. **Secondary Prevention—**
   Interrupts the disease process before it becomes symptomatic through early detection.

C. **Tertiary Prevention—**
   Limits the physical and social consequences of the disease through varied interventions such as improv-

ing care of the long-term cancer survivors (e.g., prevent osteoporosis in women with hormone-dependent cancers). All three approaches are essential to maximize individual health.

1. *Health Promotion Activities (Table 4-1)*—Health promotion activities (education, change in lifestyle behaviors, and following the recommendations for early cancer detection guidelines) are some of the measures individuals can pursue to prevent cancer, detect early disease, or limit the consequences of cancer. Regular screening examinations by a healthcare professional can result in the detection of cancers of the breast, colon, rectum, cervix, prostate, testis, oral cavity, and skin at earlier stages when treatment is more likely to be successful.

2. *Health Promotion Benefits*—Benefits that have been documented to promote a healthy lifestyle and decrease the risk for many cancers include consuming a diet high in vegetables and fruits, limiting intake of red meats and high-fat dairy products, avoiding tobacco use or exposure, avoiding or limiting alcohol intake to no more that one drink per day, avoiding obesity, staying physically active, performing monthly skin examination, seeking semiannual dental/oral examination, and pursuing prompt follow-up with a clinician with onset of certain signs and symptoms.

IV. HEALTHY PEOPLE 2010

Healthy People 2010 is a national agenda health initiative to improve the health of individuals, communities, and the nation. The significant goals are to increase years of healthy life and eliminate health disparities for all individuals. Emphasis will be on certain topics including improving nutrition, adopting a physically active lifestyle, maintaining a healthful weight throughout life, and limiting tobacco and alcohol use. Following are the recommended guidelines for nutrition and physical activity for adults, adolescents, and children.

A. **Eat a variety of healthful foods with an emphasis on plant sources**—
   - Eat five or more servings of a variety of fruits and vegetables each day.

Table 4-1   AMERICAN CANCER SOCIETY RECOMMENDATIONS FOR THE EARLY DETECTION OF CANCER IN AVERAGE-RISK, ASYMPTOMATIC PEOPLE

Cancer Site	Population	Test or Procedure	Frequency
Breast	Women, age 20+	Breast self-examination	Monthly, starting at age 20
		Clinical breast examination	Every 3 years, ages 20–39
			Annual, starting at age 40*
		Mammography	Annual, starting at age 40
Colorectal	Men and women, age 50+	Fecal occult blood test (FOBT)[†] -or-	Annual, starting at age 50
		Flexible sigmoidoscopy -or-	Every 5 years, starting at age 50
		Fecal occult blood test (FOBT)[†] and flexible sigmoidoscopy[‡] -or-	Annual FOBT and flexible sigmoidoscopy every 5 years starting at age 50
		Double contrast barium enema (DCBE) -or-	DCBE every 5 years starting at age 50
		Colonoscopy	Colonoscopy every 10 years starting at age 50

| Prostate | Men, age 50+ | Digital rectal examination (DRE) and prostate-specific antigen test (PSA) | The PSA test and the DRE should be offered annually, starting at age 50, for men who have a life expectancy of at least 10 years.§ |
| Cervix | Women | Pap test | Cervical cancer screening should begin approximately 3 years after a woman begins having vaginal intercourse, but no later than 21 years of age. Screening should be done every year with conventional Pap tests or every 2 years using liquid-based Pap tests. At or after age 30, women who have had 3 normal test results in a row may get screened every 2 to 3 years. Women 70 years of age and older who have had 3 or more normal Pap tests and no abnormal Pap tests in the last 10 years, and women who have had a total hysterectomy, may choose to stop cervical cancer screening. |

Continued

Table 4-1   AMERICAN CANCER SOCIETY RECOMMENDATIONS FOR THE EARLY DETECTION OF CANCER IN AVERAGE-RISK, ASYMPTOMATIC PEOPLE—cont'd

Cancer Site	Population	Test or Procedure	Frequency
Cancer-related check-up	Men and women, age 20+		On the occasion of a periodic health examination, the cancer-related check-up should include examination for cancers of the thyroid, testicles, ovaries, lymph nodes, oral cavity, and skin, as well as health counseling about tobacco, sun exposure, diet and nutrition, risk factors, sexual practices, and environmental and occupational exposures.

*Beginning at age 40, annual clinical breast examination should be performed prior to mammography.

†FOBT as it is sometimes done in physicians' offices, with the single stool sample collected on the fingertip during a digital rectal examination, is not an adequate substitute for the recommended at-home procedure of collecting two samples from three consecutive specimens. Toilet bowl FOBT tests also are not recommended. In comparison with guaiac-based tests for the detection of occult blood, immunochemical tests are more patient-friendly, and are likely to be equal or better in sensitivity and specificity. There is no justification for repeating FOBT in response to an initial positive finding.

‡Flexible sigmoidoscopy together with FOBT is preferred compared with FOBT or flexible sigmoidoscopy alone.

§Information should be provided to men about the benefits and limitations of testing so that an informed decision about testing can be made with the clinician's assistance.

(From Smith RA, Cokkinides V, Eyre HJ: American Cancer Society guidelines for the early detection of cancer, 2003, *CA Cancer J Clin,* 53(1):27-43, 2003.)

- Choose whole grains in preference to processed grains and sugars.
- Limit consumption of red meats, especially those high in fat and those that are processed.
- Choose foods that help maintain a healthful weight.

B. Adopt a physically active lifestyle—
- Adults: Engage in at least moderate-to-vigorous activity for 30 minutes more than 5 days a week.
- Children and adolescents: Engage in at least 60 minutes per day of moderate-to-vigorous physical activity at least 5 days per week.
- Physical activity suggestions include: Use stairs, walk to and while at work, exercise often via stationary bicycle or treadmill, or join a sports team.

C. Maintain a healthful weight throughout life—
- Balance caloric intake with physical activity.
- Lose weight if currently overweight or obese.
- Reduce the proportion of children, adolescents, and adults who are overweight or obese.

D. Tobacco and Alcohol—
- If you drink alcoholic beverages, limit consumption.
- Reduce the initiation of cigarette smoking among adults and adolescents.

V. AMERICAN CANCER SOCIETY GOALS AND OBJECTIVES

The American Cancer Society is dedicated to eliminating cancer as a major health problem by preventing cancer, saving lives, and diminishing suffering from cancer through research, education, advocacy, and service. To advance this mission, in 1999 the Society set bold challenge goals for the nation that, if met, would significantly decrease cancer incidence and mortality rates by 2015 and would improve the quality of life for all cancer survivors. The goals include the following:

- 50% reduction in age-adjusted cancer mortality rates
- 25% reduction in age-adjusted cancer incidence rates
- A measurable improvement in the quality of life (physical, psychologic, social, and spiritual) from the time of diagnosis and for the balance of life for all cancer survivors

Bibliography

American Cancer Society, *Cancer prevention and early detection, facts and figures 2003*, Atlanta, 2003, The Society.

American Cancer Society, *Cancer facts and figures 2003*, Atlanta, 2003, The Society.

Arceci R, Ettinger A, Forman E, et al: National action plan for childhood cancer: report of the national summit meetings on childhood cancer, *CA Cancer J Clin* 52:377, 2002.

Beyers T, Nestle M, McTiernan A, et al: American Cancer Society Guidelines on nutrition and physical activity for cancer prevention: reducing the risks of cancer with healthy food choices and physical activity, *CA Cancer J Clin* 52:92, 2002.

Davis TC, Williams MV, Marin E, et al: Health literacy and cancer communication, *CA Cancer J Clin* 52:134, 2002.

Gullatte MM: Prevention, screening, and detection. In Otto SE, editor: *Oncology nursing*, ed 4, St. Louis, 2001, Mosby.

Jennings-Dozier K, Mahon SM, editors: *Cancer prevention, detection, and control*, Pittsburgh, 2002, Oncology Nursing Press.

Krebs LU: Malignant melanoma: Etiology, risk factor, sun protection, and the use of sunscreens, *Nurse Investigator* 6:21, 2002.

Phillips KC, Paskett ED: Colorectal cancer screening in primary care: how can nurses facilitate patient compliance, *Nurse Investigator* 6:13, 2002.

Sample D: Cancer vaccines: a new era in cancer management has begun, *Nurse Investigator* 6:6, 2002.

Thompson JM: Health promotion and disease and injury prevention. In Thompson JM, McFarland GK, Hirsch JE, et al, editors: *Mosby's clinical nursing*, ed 5, St. Louis, 2002, Mosby.

U.S. Department of Health and Human Services. *Healthy People 2010: Understanding and improving health*, U.S. Government Printing Office, Washington, DC, No. 012-00-00543-6, ISBN 0-160050260-8. Website: www.health.gov/healthy-people/, January 2000.

General Principles

Diagnosis and Staging

I. OVERVIEW

The diagnosis of cancer involves many aspects of patient care. Physical examinations are a systematic assessment of major body sites: head, ears, nose, throat, cardiovascular system, chest, abdomen, genitourinary system, extremities, lymph nodes, and nervous system. Normal and abnormal findings are documented and evaluated in terms of the patient's medical history. The diagnostic work-up is then planned with the patient's current/ previous complaints, symptoms, history, and physical examination to yield a presumptive malignant diagnosis.

A multidisciplinary team of professionals, including the attending physician, oncologists, radiologists, surgeons, pathologists, radiation oncologists, nuclear medicine physicians, nurses, and technicians, should be involved with all diagnostic procedures. Multiple diagnostic studies are used to obtain critical information, thus enabling clinicians to make an accurate diagnosis. That diagnosis is then confirmed through histologic and cytologic examination.

Following are varied diagnostic data used in the diagnosis and staging process of cancer:

- Selected laboratory studies
- Serum tumor markers
- Diagnostic radiographic, nuclear medicine, and imaging studies
- Staging of tumors
- Tissue analysis and grading of tumors

II. SELECTED LABORATORY STUDIES

Multiple laboratory tests are performed in the diagnostic work-up process for a patient with a cancer diagnosis. In addition, the patient with cancer will have multiple and sequential laboratory tests throughout the disease and treatment process to monitor the patient's response to therapy. It is advised that specimen collections be done in an efficient and effective manner to enhance timely and accurate test results. Refer to Table 5-1 for information regarding selected laboratory tests.

III. SERUM TUMOR MARKERS
Serum tumor markers (hormones, enzymes, antigens) measure the serum level of mucin-like glycoproteins that are shed from the tumor cells into the bloodstream.

A. **Alpha Feto Protein—**
   Liver and germ cell tumors   25 µg/L
B. **Bence Jones Protein—**
   Proteins that occur in the urine of   negative
   persons diagnosed with multiple
   myeloma
C. **Beta HCG—**
   Germ cell tumors (testicular, certain   <1 ng/ml
   types ovarian)
D. **CA 19-9—**
   Pancreatic, colorectal, and gastric cancers   37 U/ml
E. **CA-27.29—**
   Breast and ovarian cancer   <38 U/ml
F. **CA-125—**
   Ovarian cancer response to therapy   0–21 U/ml

IV. DIAGNOSTIC RADIOGRAPHIC, NUCLEAR MEDICINE, AND IMAGING STUDIES
A variety of diagnostic studies are required to obtain clinical information to enable clinicians to make an accurate diagnosis. Following is a list of diagnostic examinations used frequently in the cancer diagnosis work-up:

A. **Angiography—**
   Assesses arterial system to determine vascular patency
B. **Barium Studies—**
   Assesses evidence of anatomic abnormalities; in double contrast air is insufflated into the rectum and colon to enhance imaging of the pathologic lesion
C. **Barium Swallow—**
   Assesses structural abnormalities of the esophagus

Table 5-1   SELECTED LABORATORY TESTS INFORMATION

Test	Values
Blood Chemistries	
Albumin	3.5–5.0 gm/dl
Amylase (total)	20–110 U/L
Bicarbonate	21–29 mEq/L
Bilirubin	Total: 0.1–1.2 mg/dl
	Direct: 0.1–0.3 mg/dl
	Indirect: 0.1–1.0 mg/dl
Blood urea nitrogen	8–21 mg/dl
Calcium	8.5–10.5 mg/dl
Calcium ionized	4.4–5.0 mg/dl
Carbon dioxide	17–31 mEq/L
Chloride	95–110 mEq/L
Creatinine	0.7–1.4 mg/dl
Glucose (fasting)	65–110 mg/dl
Glycohemoglobulin (hemoglobin A)	4.3–6.1%
Lactate dehydrogenase	340–670 U/L
Lipase	56–239 U/L
Magnesium	1.6–2.6 mg/dl
Phosphorus	2.7–4.5 mg/dl
Potassium	3.5–5.0 mEq/L
Prealbumin	18–38 mg/dl
Protein, serum	6.3–8.6 gm/dl
Sodium	135–145 mEq/L
Transaminases	
Alanine aminotransferase (ALT/SGPT)	300 U/ml [5–35 U/ml]
Alkaline phosphatase (AST/SGOT)	250 U/ml [8–20 U/ml]
Uric acid	Male patients: 3.4–7.0 mg/dl
	Female patients: 2.4–5.7 mg/dl
Coagulation Studies	
Bleeding time	3.0–10.0 minutes
Fibrinogen	Male patients: 180–340 mg/dl
	Female patients:
	190–420 mg/dl

Continued

Table 5-1 SELECTED LABORATORY TESTS INFORMATION—cont'd

Test	Values
Coagulation Studies—cont'd	
Partial thromboplastin time	24–36 seconds
Prothrombin time	±2 seconds of control
	Control: 11–16 seconds
Thrombin time	±3 seconds of control
	Control: 15–20 seconds
Template B time (bleeding time)	1 8 minutes
International normalized ratio	0.8–1.2 Ug/ml
Hematology	
Hemoglobin	Male patients: 14–18 g/dl
	Female patients: 12.5–16.0 g/dl
Hematocrit	Male patients: 42–52%
	Female patients: 37–47%
Erythropoietin	Male patients: 17.2 mU/ml
	Female patients: 18.8 mU/ml
Ferritin (measures body's storage of iron)	Male patients: 20–300 ng/ml
	Female patients: 15–120 ng/ml
Iron	Male patients: 75–175 µg/dl
	Female patients: 65–165 µg/dl
Iron binding capacity	250–450 µg/dl
Folate serum	>3.5 µg/L
MCH (indicates the average weight of hemoglobin in each RBC)	78–100 fl
MCV (indicates the average volume or size of a single RBC)	27–31 pg
Platelets	150,000–400,000 mm^3
RBC	4–6 million
Reticulocyte count (measures newly released RBCs)	0.5–1.85% of erythrocytes

General Principles

Continued

Table 5-1 SELECTED LABORATORY TESTS INFORMATION—cont'd

Test	Values
Hematology—cont'd	
Transferrin (regulates iron transport in the blood)	240–480 mg/dl
WBC	
Granulocytes—mature WBCs	1.3–6.0 (40–60%)
Bands—immature WBCs	<1.0 (3%)
Lymphocytes (>viral infection)	1.5–3.5 (20–40%)
Monocytes	<1.0 (4–8%)
Eosinophils	<0.7 (1–3%)
Basophils	<0.1 (0–1%)
Immunoglobulins	
IgA	65–650 mg/dl
IgD	0–30 mg/dl
IgE	0–200 mg/dl
IgG	600–1700 mg/dl
IgM	50–300 mg/dl

MCH, mean corpuscular hemoglobin; MCV, mean corpuscular volume; RBC, red blood cell; WBC, white blood cell.

D. **Biopsy**—
An examination of tissue obtained by a surgical procedure, endoscopic procedure, or during a guided computed tomography scan or mammogram

E. **Bone Densitometry**—
Determines bone mineral content and density

F. **Bone Marrow Biopsy**—
Examines bone marrow for abnormalities; a core biopsy of the bone is obtained during this procedure to determine the marrow cellularity (ratio of hematopoietic tissue to adipose tissue)

1. *Normocellular*—Normal proportions of the hematopoietic cells and adipose cells (normocellular marrow for an adult is 30% to 40% cellularity)

2. *Hypercellular*—Increased number of hematopoietic cells and decreased amount of adipose tissue

3. *Hypocellular*—Reduced number of hematopoietic cells and increased amount of adipose tissue

G. Bronchoscopy—
Assesses interior structure of bronchus and lung

H. Colonoscopy—
Examines left, transverse, and right colon and sigmoid rectum

I. Colposcopy—
Provides direct visualization of vagina, vulva, and cervical epithelium

J. Computerized Tomography Scan—
Analyzes tissues for density; assesses for evidence of disease, inflammation, displacement, or enlargement

   1. Abdomen—Used for suspected liver, kidney, pancreas, spleen, gastrointestinal, and lymph node disease

   2. Bone Scintigram or Bone Scan—Evaluates fractures, degenerative disease, or potential bone metastasis; after an approximate 2- to 4-hour delay of intravenous phosphonate uptake by the osteoblasts, if a correlate imaging does not show a lesion, the assumption is bone metastasis; false negatives can occur in multiple myeloma and renal cell carcinoma.

   3. Brain—Used most often in screening for lesions

   4. Musculoskeletal—Detection of a fracture or general examination of bones

   5. Neck—Good for detection of lesion of the neck

   6. Pelvis—Evaluation of bladder when delayed images might be beneficial

   7. Thorax—Best modality for evaluating the lung parenchyma

K. Cystoscopy—
Permits direct visualization of urethra and bladder for strictures or bleeding sites; remove biopsy specimens of prostate, bladder, and urethra; place urethral catheters

L. Cytology Studies—
Examines cells obtained from tissue scrapings, body fluids, secretions, or washings

M. Flow Cytometry—
Evaluates the aggressiveness of a cancer by analyzing the cellular deoxyribonucleic acid content of the cells; ploidy-increased number of chromosomes, and the percentage of cells in S phase cellular division

N. **Electroencephalography—**
Assesses intracranial pathophysiology and organic brain syndrome and determines presence and type of epilepsy

O. **Endoscopy Ultrasonography—**
Assesses tumor depth and stage of local disease, and detects smaller lymph node involvement

P. **Esophagoscopy—**
Permits direct visualization of esophagus and stomach; obtains biopsy specimens, brushings, or washings

Q. **Fecal Occult Blood Test—**
Determines presence of blood in stool not seen by naked eye

R. **Intravenous Pyelogram—**
Permits visualization of kidneys, ureters, and bladder to determine abnormalities, obstruction, or hematoma

S. **Immunoscintigraphy—**
A form of nuclear imaging that uses monoclonal antibodies specific to tumor antigens; the antibodies are tagged with tracer doses of radioisotopes (e.g., imaging of non–small-cell lung cancer) and detect prostate cancer lymph node metastasis; detection of recurrence in colorectal and ovarian cancers (scinti-mammography radioisotope technetium-99m ses-tamibi is used for detection of breast malignancy and metastasis)

T. **Laparoscopy—**
Permits visualization of pelvis and intestines; obtains ovarian biopsy

U. **Mammography—**
Determines presence of benign or malignant breast disease and cysts and guides needle biopsy

V. **Myelography—**
Visualizes subarachnoid spaces; detects abnormalities of spinal cord and vertebrae

W. **Nuclear Medicine Scans—**
1. *Bone*—Detects focal defects in bone, infection, and fracture
2. *Brain*—Delineates subdural hematoma, arteriovenous malformation, thrombosis, abscess, neoplasms, glioma, or other metastatic tumors
3. *Gallium*—Determines presence of neoplasms, lymphoma, bronchogenic cancer, Hodgkin's disease, or inflammation

   4. *Liver and Spleen*—Detects lesions, cysts, hematomas, lacerations, and metastasis
   5. *Lung*—Examines pulmonary vascular circulation to locate pulmonary emboli
   6. *Multigated (Radionuclide) Angiogram*—Assesses indices of ventricular effectiveness, ejection fraction, and ventricular volume of heart
   7. *Renal*—Assesses kidney size, shape, location, and perfusion
   8. *Thallium*—Identifies myocardial fibrosis and ischemia; includes perfusion imaging, single photon emission computed tomography, Thallium 201
   9. *Thyroid*—Assess size, shape, and anatomic function of the thyroid
X. **Proctoscopy**—
   Examines anus, rectum, and sigmoid colon
Y. **Panendoscopy**—
   Provides visualization of larynx, bronchus, and nasopharynx for strictures, inflammation, or bleeding; performs biopsy for analysis
Z. **Magnetic Resonance Imaging**—
   Most common diagnostic tool used to evaluate suspected malignancies of the central nervous system because of its ability to perform multiplanar images and ease of instillation of contrast media
AA. **Positron Emission Tomography (PET)**—
   Uses nuclear medicine with precise localization to penetrate body's metabolism to measure blood flow/volume and protein metabolism. In oncology, metabolic changes precede anatomic changes; therefore PET is more accurate in detecting a variety of neoplasms. PET scanning is able to:
   1. Differentiate scar or radiation necrosis from active tumor
   2. Determine if a mass lesion is malignant or benign
   3. Characterize enlarged lymph nodes as malignant or benign
   4. Detect malignancy in normal-size lymph nodes or normal-appearing tissue
   5. Evaluate early tumor treatment response
BB. **Ultrasonography Doppler**—
   Uses sound waves to assess tissue function and blood flow velocity to determine if a lesion is cystic or solid. A cystic mass may feel tense with fluid.

Aspiration should reveal nonbloody fluid and result in complete resolution of the lesion. A biopsy is indicated if the fluid aspirated is bloody and the lesion does not resolve completely, or if the cyst recurs after repeated aspirations. Transrectal ultrasound is used in prostate cancer to determine if the disease is confined to the gland itself and to guide the needle biopsy process.

V. STAGING

Staging is the process of describing the extent or spread of the disease from the site of origin. This is essential to determine the choice of therapy and to assess prognosis. The cancer stage is based on the primary tumor's size and location in the body and whether it has spread to other areas of the body. The staging process used varies with the cancer disease site. Hematologic malignancies are not staged the same way as classifications for solid tumors. These malignant disorders are characterized by a proliferation of abnormal white blood cells, by an abnormality within the lymphoreticular system, or by both and therefore use a different system to accurately classify and stage the disease.

The basic staging system that is commonly used for many cancers is the TNM system. TNM is an expression of the anatomic extent of the disease and is based on the assessment of three components. The use of numbers in the subsets of TNM represents the progression or extent of the disease involvement.

- T   The extent of the primary tumor
- N   The absence or presence and extent of regional node involvement
- M   The absence or presence of distant metastasis

A. Primary Tumor—
- T_X Primary tumor cannot be assessed
- T_0 No evidence of primary tumor
- T_{is} Carcinoma in situ (e.g., intraductal, lobular)
- T_1 Tumor 2 cm or less in greatest dimension
- T_2 Tumor more than 2 cm but not more than 5 cm in greatest dimension
- T_3 Tumor more than 5 cm in greatest dimension
- T_4 Tumor of any size with direct extension to tissue (e.g., chest wall, skin)

B. Regional Lymph Nodes—
- N_X Regional lymph nodes cannot be assessed

N_0 No regional lymph node metastasis
N_1 Metastasis to movable lymph node(s)
N_2 Metastasis to lymph node(s), fixed to one another or to other structure
N_3 Metastasis to internal lymph node(s)

C. Distant Metastasis—
M_X Distant metastasis cannot be assessed
M_0 No distant metastasis
M_1 Distant metastasis (anatomic site organ identified)

D. Staging—
Staging is further classified by obtaining clinical disease information by the following methods:

1. *Clinical Classification (cTNM)*—cTNM is obtained from history and physical examination, imaging and endoscopy examinations, biopsy, or surgical exploration. The clinical stage is used as a guide for the selection of primary therapy.

2. *Pathologic Classification (pTNM)*—pTNM is obtained from the pathologic examination of the tissue removed during the surgical procedure. This information is added to the previous clinical classification and can be used as a guide for adjuvant therapy, for estimation of prognosis, and for reporting results.

3. *Retreatment Classification (rTNM)*—Retreatment classification occurs after a disease-free interval and now requires retreatment approaches. Information obtained assists in determining the stage of the recurrent tumor. A biopsy confirmation of this tissue is required.

4. *Autopsy Classification (aTNM)*—Information obtained at the time of patient death by an autopsy is used to determine the stage classification of the tumor.

VI. TISSUE ANALYSIS

Tissue analysis is used to determine tissue type and the degree of cell differentiation (grade) of the tumor. A *frozen section* is a small amount of tissue that is thinly sliced, quickly frozen, and then stained for *immediate examination.*

A. Immunoperoxidase Staining—
Identifies specific cell types using monoclonal or polyclonal antibodies against cellular antigens

B. **Polymerase Chain Reaction—**
   Identifies specific genetic changes or chromosomal abnormalities
C. **Receptor Status—**
   Includes those cells that have receptor assays in certain cancers (e.g., estrogen and progesterone in breast cancer; epidermal growth factor gene [HER/2*neu*] in breast, ovarian, lung, gastric, and oral cancers)

VII. TUMOR GRADE
The grade of a tumor is based on the degree of the differentiation of the cell(s). (For a complete listing of all tumor types refer to the American Joint Committee on Cancer (AJCC) *Cancer Staging Manual*)

A. **Pathologic Grade—**
   X   Grade cannot be assessed
   I   Well differentiated, mature cells
   II Moderately differentiated, cells have some immaturity
   III Poorly differentiated, immature cells; do not look like normal cells
   IV Undifferentiated cells very immature; difficult to determine tissue of origin

B. **Histologic Grade—**
   Histologic grade refers to the cellular arrangement or structure of the tumor.

C. **Nuclear Grade—**
   Nuclear grade refers to differentiation of the tumor cell nuclei, the shape and size of nuclei, and the number of mitoses.

Bibliography
Alexander J: Diagnosis and staging. In Otto SE, editor: *Oncology nursing*, ed 4, St. Louis, 2001, Mosby.
Carr MW, Grey ML: Magnetic resonance imaging, *Am J Nurs* 102(12):26, 2002.
Fleming I, Cooper JS, Henson DE, et al: *AJCC cancer staging manual*, ed 5, Philadelphia, 2002, Lippincott-Raven.
Goedegebuure PS, Eberlein TJ: Tumor biology and tumor markers. In Townsend CM Jr, Beauchamp RD, Evers BM, et al, editors: *Textbook of surgery, the biological basis of modern surgical practice*, ed 16, Philadelphia, 2001, WB Saunders.
Guyton AC, Hall T: *Textbook of medical physiology*, ed 9, Philadelphia, 1999, WB Saunders.

Henry JB, editor: *Clinical diagnosis and management by laboratory methods,* ed 20, Philadelphia, 2001, WB Saunders.

Lea DH, Williams JK: Genetic testing and screening, *Am J Nurs* 102(7):36, 2002.

Pagana KD, Pagana TJ: *Mosby's diagnostic and laboratory test reference,* St. Louis, 2002, Mosby.

Rosenberg SA: Principles of cancer management: surgical oncology. In DeVita VT Jr, Hellman S, Rosenberg SA, editors: *Cancer principles and practice of oncology,* ed 6, Philadelphia, 2001, JB Lippincott.

Sacher RA, McPherson RA, Campos JM: *Widmann's clinical interpretation of laboratory tests,* Philadelphia, 2000, FA Davis.

General Principles

6

Research and Cancer Clinical Trials

I. CLINICAL RESEARCH

The National Institutes of Health was founded in 1887 and supports research for the cause, diagnosis, prevention, and cure of human disease. By the 1930s, cancer was identified as a major health problem requiring a large-scale national plan of action. In 1937, Congress passed the *National Cancer Institute Act*, which appropriated funding to establish the National Cancer Institute (NCI), which remains the largest division of the 12 institutes that are part of the National Institutes of Health. Cancer clinical trials require the use of many resources to conduct the trials and follow all the research standards of investigation. The description of such settings and professional members who conduct this type of research is described later.

II. CLINICAL RESEARCH SETTINGS AND PROFESSIONALS

A. **Oncology Training Programs**—
   NCI-funded fellowship programs in medical oncology and radiotherapy
B. **Comprehensive Cancer Centers**—
   Centers that provide comprehensive cancer care and meet the eight criteria for basic research: mechanisms for technology transfer, clinical research, programs of high priority clinical trials, cancer prevention and control research, research training and continuing education programs, cancer information services, and community services and outreach activities
C. **Cooperative Research Groups**—
   Research groups that are funded by NCI, consisting of researchers who jointly develop and conduct cancer treatment clinical trials in a multi-institutional setting

D. **Community-Based Research Programs—**
   1. *Cooperative Group Outreach Programs*—Programs that consist of individual community oncologists, surgeons, or radiation therapists contracting with a member institution of a cooperative group to register patients on research protocols
   2. *Community Clinical Oncology Programs*—Groups of community-based physicians linked to cooperative groups and cancer centers that serve as their research base
   3. *Cancer Control*—Research implemented through the cooperative group members
   4. *Institutional Review Boards*—Composed of at least five individuals with professional competence, experience, and qualifications to review the protocols. This board should include both men and women and should represent a variety of backgrounds, races, and cultural considerations. At least one member of this board should be a nonmedical professional and one person with no direct affiliation with the institution performing the research. The protocol review process provides the investigator, the institution, and the patient the assurance that the research is medically and ethically sound.

III. DRUG DEVELOPMENT PROCESS

The NCI is the largest single sponsor of studies using antineoplastic agents followed by industry, such as pharmaceutical companies. This research process for drug development is extremely costly in terms of labor, time, and financial resources. It is not unusual for a drug to be in the developmental process for 8 to 10 years before it is commercially released to the national market.

A. **Drug Identification—**
   Using a scientific process for drug discovery in preclinical trials.
B. **Drug Screening—**
   Identified compounds are entered into the NCI Division of Cancer.
C. **Treatment Drug Testing Program—**
   These compounds undergo a screening process that uses both animal and human tumor systems.

D. **Formulation and Production—**
   Compounds that have successfully passed through the screening process are selected for identification, purification, and definition of a chemical structure for further studies.

E. **Toxicity Testing—**
   Preclinical testing for drug toxicity to predict the safest starting dose for clinical trials and to determine if and when organ system toxicity occurs.

F. **Investigational New Drug Application—**
   The research institution or company with a new drug submits an investigational new drug application to the Food and Drug Administration (FDA) to request permission to evaluate this new agent in human cancer.

G. **Faster Drug Approvals for Cancer Patients—**
   A process used to shorten the usual 30-month review of a new drug application. The Prescription Drug User Free Act of 1992 and FDA Modernization Act of 1997 were passed to make certain drugs available to patients such as docetaxel and irinotecan in 1996 and imatinib mesylate (Gleevec) in 2002.

H. **Physician Approval—**
   The FDA approval of physicians who wish to participate in the human clinical trials of investigational drugs, requiring these physicians to complete medical training and experience and assume responsibility for compliance with the protocol requirements for drug administration, data monitoring, and toxicity reporting.

IV. ETHICAL ISSUES AND REGULATIONS

The patient and cancer treatment selection process requires certain ethical and regulatory guidelines to ensure all patients participating in the research process will receive unbiased care.

A. **Autonomy—**
   The right of a person to make independent decisions about personal affairs (determine their own course or plan of action)

B. **Beneficence—**
   The duty to take positive steps to help others, prevent or remove harm, minimize risk, and maximize benefits to the participants

C. **Justice—**
   Fairness in distribution of research burdens and benefits

D. **Randomization—**
   To make the selection process random for scientific experimentation; usual process includes entering data into a computer system, with selection process made through the computer and thereafter patient identification occurring by assigned identification number.

E. **Stratification—**
   The process of developing different levels or groups to ensure an equal balance of choices (e.g., men/women; age groups 26–30/31–35).

F. **Blinding—**
   Restricting knowledge of the treatment from the study participants and the treating physician.

G. **Eligibility Criteria—**
   Criteria that are specific to the condition and the treatment being investigated such as disease, stage of disease process, age, or certain laboratory measurements (e.g., serum creatinine 0.7–1.4 mg/dl).

V. CANCER PROTOCOLS

A. **Description—**
   A protocol is a formal document written to clearly describe the proposed experiment. Protocols provide the rationale for the proposed study, the study objectives or questions to be answered, and a concise description of the treatment involved. The protocol is written by the principal investigator and must be approved by the study sponsor. This protocol can be amended as needed (e.g., change in drug dose related to a certain toxicity) by the study sponsor throughout the clinical trial. All professionals participating in the clinical trial will follow this protocol throughout the clinical trial process. The participant reads and signs (before initiation of protocol) an informed consent document (e.g., detailed description and purpose of the treatment and side effects), and a copy of this document is kept in the patient's medical record (see later for detailed description of informed consent).

B. **Elements—**
   1. Objective—Defines the intent of the study

2. *Background*—Describes previous studies and justification for current study
3. *Drug Information*—Describes animal toxicology studies, human toxicity previously observed, mechanisms of drug action, drug storage, preparation, administration, supplier
4. *Patient Eligibility*—Defines parameters of patient participation (disease confirmation, major organ function, performance status, and medical history)
5. *Treatment Plan*—Details initial and subsequent doses, administration guidelines and schedule, duration of treatment
6. *Study Parameters*—Schedule of required evaluations and treatment
7. *Criteria for Response*—Defines the disease response
   a. *Complete remission*—Absence of all clinical evidence of the tumor on physical examination and diagnostic studies. This response must be for at least 4 weeks.
   b. *Partial remission*—A decrease of 50% or greater in measurable tumor by physical examination and diagnostic studies
   c. *Stable disease*—Measurable disease that does not meet the definition for disease response or progression
   d. *Increasing disease*—A 25% increase in tumor size as measured by physical examination and diagnostic studies
8. *Discipline Review*—Verification of correct pathologic diagnosis and required therapy by a designated review panel (laboratory, pathology, radiology)
9. *Data Submission*—Defines required data forms and submission intervals
10. *Statistical Considerations*—Defines accrual goals, study design, statistical analysis
11. *Toxicity Criteria*—Grading of treatment-related toxicities according to standardized scale
12. *Informed Consent*—Sample form that must be modified to meet institutional guidelines; a person's agreement to allow something to happen such as participation in a clinical trial or undergoing a surgical procedure; the form includes the following basic steps:

a. Explanation of the procedure/treatment process
b. Purpose of the procedure/treatment process
c. Known risks and benefits of the procedure/treatment process
d. Alternatives and consequences of not accepting treatment
e. Right to refuse consent or withdraw consent at any time
f. Whom to contact about the research and patient's rights
g. Description of confidentiality; disclosure of possible FDA inspection
h. Instruction that participation is voluntary and results in no penalty or loss of benefits to which the subject is otherwise entitled
i. Adverse drug reaction definition and report responsibilities

VI. PHASES AND TYPES OF CLINICAL TRIALS

Clinical trials are research studies that follow certain guidelines to study the effects of drugs or treatments to determine the benefits in preventing, alleviating, or curing illness or injury. The four phases and types of clinical trials in human investigative research are outlined in the following sections.

A. **Phases of Clinical Trials—**
   1. *Phase I*—To determine the maximum tolerated dose in humans, to determine the most effective schedule of drug administration, and to identify and quantify drug toxicity effects in normal organ systems. A limited number (10 to 20) of patients are enrolled in these clinical trials. Comprehensive cancer centers most often are the clinical settings for phase I clinical trials.
   2. *Phase II*—To determine objective antitumor activity in a variety of cancers. Increased numbers (>20) of patients are enrolled in these clinical trials, and community clinical oncology programs are the usual settings for these clinical trials.
   3. *Phase III*—To establish the value of a new cancer treatment relative to the standard treatments by a randomized or comparative clinical study. Extensive numbers (>100) of patients are enrolled and longer time frames (3 to 5 years) are needed to completely evaluate the studies to determine drug(s),

dosage(s), drug combinations, and the best schedule for drug administration.

   4. *Phase IV*—To determine the optimal use of a treatment as a standard therapy.
B. **Types of Clinical Trials—**
   1. *Cancer Control/Prevention*—Trials that test new approaches such as medicine, vitamins, minerals, or other supplements that may decrease the risk for a certain type of cancer (subjects enrolled in these trials have never had cancer) or prevent a new cancer from occurring in subjects who have already had cancer such as the Breast Cancer Prevention Trial (STAR study) and the Prostate Cancer Prevention Trial (SELECT)
   2. *Cancer Treatment*—Trials that test new treatments, such as new drugs, new combinations of treatments, or new methods of treatment (e.g., gene therapy)
   3. *Cancer Screening*—Trials that test the best method to detect cancer, especially in the early stage of cancer development
   4. *Quality of Life*—Trials that explore different ways to improve comfort and quality of life for patients with cancer (e.g., pain, nausea/vomiting, fatigue)

VI. RESEARCH AND CANCER CLINICAL TRIALS RESOURCES

Following is a list of Internet websites that provide information regarding clinical trials, drugs, types, or clinical settings:

Cancer Research Institute:
www.cancerresearch.org/impower.html

Cancer Centers Branch:
www.cancer.gov/cancercenters

Clinical Trials Listings:
www.cancer.gov/clinicaltrials

Code of Federal Regulations and Federal Register:
www.access.gpo.gov/nara/cfr

Food and Drug Administration:
www.fda.gov

National Cancer Institute:
www.nci.nih.gov

National Institutes of Health:
www.nih.gov

World Medical Association
www.wma.net

Bibliography

Carroll-Johnson RM, Jassak PF, editors: Evidence-based oncology nursing practice: improving patient outcomes in the next millennium, *Oncol Nurs Forum 28(2):supplement to March, 2001.*

Chu E, Grever MR, Chabner BA: Cancer drug development. In DeVita VT Jr, Hellman S, Rosenberg SA, editors: *Cancer principles and practice of oncology*, ed 6, Philadelphia, 2001, JB Lippincott.

Cooley ME, Rutledge DN: Utilization and conduct of research. In Lin EM, editor: *Advanced practice in oncology nursing*, Philadelphia, 2001, WB Saunders.

Food and Drug Administration Modernization Act of 1997; list of documents issued by the Food and Drug Administration that apply to medical devices regulated by the Center for Biologic Evaluation and Research. Food and Drug Administration, HHS, *Fed Regist* 64(79):20312, 1999 (notice).

Frank-Stromberg M, Christensen, Elmhurst D: Nurse documentation: not done or worse, done the wrong way—Part I, *Oncol Nurs Forum* 28(4):697, 2001.

Goldspiel BL: Clinical cancer trials, *Highlights Oncol Pract* 18:1, 2000.

Gullatte MM, Otto SE: Cancer clinical trials. In Otto SE, editor: *Oncology nursing*, ed 4, St. Louis, 2001, Mosby.

Jennings-Dozier K, Mahon SM, editors: *Cancer prevention, detection, and control*, Pittsburgh, 2002, Oncology Nursing Press.

Johansen HK, Gotzsche PC: Improving the conduct and reporting of clinical trials, *JAMA* 283(21):2787, 2000.

Klimaszewski A, Aikin J, Bacon M, et al: *Manual for clinical trials nursing*, Pittsburgh, 2000, Oncology Nursing Press.

National Cancer Policy Board, Hewitt M, Somone J, editors: *Ensuring quality cancer care*. Washington, DC, 1999, National Academy Press.

National Cancer Institute: *From lab to patient care: the drug approval process*, Atlanta, 2000, National Cancer Institute.

Oncology Nursing Society: *Cancer chemotherapy guidelines and recommendations for practice*, Pittsburgh, 2001, Oncology Nursing Press.

Polit DF, Beck CT, Hungler BP: *Essentials of nursing research, methods, appraisal, and utilization,* ed 5, Philadelphia, 2001, Lippincott.

Trinkaus KM, Miller JP: Principles of clinical trials. In Govindan R, Arquette MA, editors: *The Washington manual of oncology,* Philadelphia, 2002, Lippincott Williams & Wilkins.

UNIT II

CANCER TYPES

Brain and Central Nervous System Cancers

I. INCIDENCE/MORTALITY

Cancers of the central nervous system (CNS) account for less than 1.4% of all malignancies, with an estimated 18,300 cases diagnosed in 2003. The peak incidence occurs from birth to 6 years and after age 45. CNS tumors are more common in the white population than in blacks, with men having a higher mortality rate than women. An estimated 13,100 deaths related to CNS cancer will occur in 2003.

II. ETIOLOGY/RISK FACTORS

Specific causes and risk factors for CNS cancer have not been identified. Chemical exposures that have been implicated include vinyl chloride, radiation, petrochemicals, inks, lubricating oils, solvents, and aspartame. Hereditary conditions such as retinoblastoma syndrome, von Hippel-Lindau syndrome, Li-Fraumeni syndrome, and Turçot syndrome have been linked to CNS tumor development.

III. PREVENTION, SCREENING, AND DETECTION

There are no known screening or prevention methods for CNS and brain cancers. The symptoms appear gradually and do not lend themselves to diagnostic pre-screening methods.

IV. CLASSIFICATION

Tumors of the CNS include both brain and spinal cord tumors. CNS tumors are classified as primary and metastatic in nature. Primary tumors may exist as intra-cerebral or extracerebral. Major *intracerebral* tumors include those within the brain, neuroglia, neurons, and cells of the blood vessels of the connective tissue. Extracerebral tumors originate outside of the brain and include meningiomas and acoustic nerve, pituitary, and pineal gland tumors.

Metastatic tumors may exist either inside or outside the brain, CNS, or elsewhere in the body (Table 7-1).

V. CLINICAL FEATURES
The clinical features manifested by CNS tumors vary (Figures 7-1 and 7-2). The most common symptom is headache and seizure activity. Headaches are commonly bifrontal and biooccipital and occur on awakening. Structural changes; memory defects; and speech, motor, and visual changes vary depending on tumor location and size. Accompanying symptoms may include weakness, loss of bowel and bladder function, brain tissue hemorrhages, or increased intracranial pressure.

VI. DIAGNOSIS AND STAGING
The diagnostic evaluation of cancer includes a thorough history and physical examination, noting onset and duration of symptoms as described earlier. Diagnostic examinations include computed tomography scans, magnetic resonance imaging, positron emission tomography scan, cerebral angiography studies, radionuclide angiograms, and tumor markers. A stereotatic needle biopsy is used to obtain tissue for the definitive diagnosis.

VII. METASTASIS
The spread of primary CNS tumors beyond the brain and spinal cord is rare. Seeding is the most common method of spread within the CNS and spinal cord. Medulloblastoma tumors have the greatest potential to develop metastatic lesions within the CNS.

VIII. SURVIVAL
The tumor's histology types, tumor grade, size and extent of tumor, patient's age, performance status, and residual tumor determine survival. The survival for patients with CNS tumors ranges from complete cure to rapid deterioration and death. For example, early stage grade I astrocytomas with complete surgical excision may have an 80% to 100% 10-year survival versus grade

Table 7-1 BRAIN AND SPINAL CORD TUMORS

Neoplasm	Percent of Tumors	Location	Characteristics	Cell of Origin
Gliomas				
Astrocytoma	20	Anywhere in brain or spinal cord	Grade I and II Slow growing, invasive	Supportive tissue, astrocytes, glial cells
Glioblastoma multiforme	30	Common in cerebral hemispheres	Grade III, IV Highly invasive and malignant	Thought to arise from mature astrocytes
Oligodendrocytoma	4	Common in frontal lobes deep in white matter; may arise in brain stem, cerebellum, and spinal cord	Avascular, tends to be encapsulated; more malignant form called oligodendroblastoma	Oligodendrites, glial cells
Ependymoma	5	Intramedullary; wall of ventricles; may arise in	Common in children, variable growth rates;	Ependymal cells

Continued

Cancer Types

Table 7-1 BRAIN AND SPINAL CORD TUMORS—cont'd

Neoplasm	Percent of Tumors	Location	Characteristics	Cell of Origin
Gliomas—cont'd		caudal tail of spinal cord	more malignant, invasive form called ependymoblastoma; may extend into ventricle or invade brain tissue	
Neurilemoma	4	Cranial nerves (most often vestibular division of cranial nerve VIII)	Slow growing	Schwann cells
Neurofibroma		Extramedullary: spinal cord	Slow growing	Neurilemma, Schwann cells
Pituitary tumors	8	Pituitary gland; may extend to or invade	Age linked, several types slow growing,	Pituitary cells, pituitary chromophobes,

		floor of third ventricle	macroadenomas and microadenomas may be secreting or nonsecreting	basophils, eosinophils
Pineal region tumors	1	Pineal region; pineal parenchyma, posterior or third ventricle	Several types (e.g., germinoma, pineocytoma, teratoma)	Several types with different cell origin
Blood vessel tumors				
Angioma	3	Predominantly in posterior cerebral hemispheres	Slow growing	Arising from congenitally malformed arteriovenous connections
Neuronal cell tumors				
Medulloblastoma	1	Posterior cerebellar vermis, root of fourth ventricle	Well demarcated, rapid growing, fills fourth ventricle	Embryonic cells

Continued

Cancer Types

Table 7-1 BRAIN AND SPINAL CORD TUMORS—cont'd

Neoplasm	Percent of Tumors	Location	Characteristics	Cell of Origin
Mesodermal tissue tumors				
Meningioma	20	Intradural, extramedullary; sylvian fissure region, superior parasagittal surface of frontal and parietal lobes, olfactory groove, wing of sphenoid bone, superior surface of cerebellum, cerebellopontine angle, spinal cord	Slow growing, circumscribed, encapsulated, sharply demarcated from normal tissues, compressive in nature	
Choroid plexus tumors				
Papilloma	1	Choroid plexus of ventricular system;	Usually benign; slow in expansion,	Epithelial cells

		lateral ventricle in children, fourth ventricle in adults	inducing hemorrhage and hydrocephalus; malignant tumor is rare	
Cranial nerve and spinal nerve root tumors				
Hemangioblastoma	2	Arises from blood vessels, predominant in cerebellum	Benign, slow growing	Embryonic vascular tissue
Lymphoma	1	Cerebral hemispheres	Metastasis common	B cells
Metastatic tumors	35 of all cancer patients	Cerebral cortex diencephalon	Malignant spread	From lung, breast, colon, kidney, thyroid, prostate

Modified from Monahan FD: Medical-surgical nursing: foundations of clinical practice, ed 2, Philadelphia, 1998, Saunders.

Cancer Types

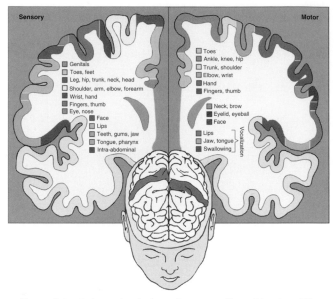

Figure 7-1 Brain and spinal cord tumors. (From Monahan FD: *Medical surgical nursing: foundations of clinical practice*, ed 2, Philadelphia, 1998, WB Saunders.)

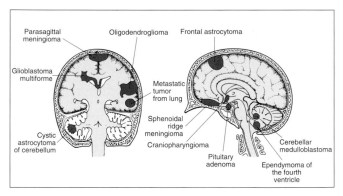

Figure 7-2 Common sites of intracranial tumors. (From McCance KL, Huether SE: *Pathophysiology: the biologic basis for disease in adults and children*, ed 3, St. Louis, 1998, Mosby.)

IV astrocytoma with aggressive treatment that has a mean survival of 12 to 14 months.

IX. TREATMENT MODALITIES

CNS tumors are treated with combination therapies such as surgery, radiation therapy, chemotherapy, and steroid therapy. Steroids (e.g., dexamethasone) are administered to produce an antiinflammatory response and to reduce the cerebral swelling. They may be administered before, during, or after surgery to reduce the immediate cerebral edema. Postoperative management includes the titration of such drugs and doses over a designated time period.

Surgery serves as a diagnostic (tissue sampling for histology) and treatment (craniotomy for debulking, dissection, tumor removal) modality for many of the CNS tumors. Stereotactic biopsies are used for the removal of smaller tumors and placement of radioactive substances to treat the nonresectable tumors.

Tumors that are inoperable or have only partial tumor resection may respond to radiation therapy. CNS tumors that are radiosensitive include medulloblastomas, high-grade astrocytoma, and metastatic brain tumors of breast, lung, myeloma, and sarcoma. Radiation treatments may be administered in a variety of doses and methods. The conventional dose therapy is usually given over a series of weeks, allowing healthy tissue to heal. Radiation therapy options include external beam therapy with or without hyperfractionation or particle-charged beams; use of radioactive sensitizers; or intensity modulator radiation therapy, which delivers a controlled intense beam to one target site with increased radiation to multiple sites in the tumor itself. Brachytherapy or interstitial therapy can be done through a computer-guided installation of radioactive seeds such as iodine-125 or iridium-192 into the tumor site.

Chemotherapy is used in combination with surgery or radiation for the treatment of gliomas and medulloblastomas. The most frequently used drugs are the nitrosoureas carmustine and lomustine. Additional agents used are cisplatin, cyclophosphamide, mechlorethamine, bleomycin, vincristine, etoposide, methotrexate, and procarbazine. Common routes include oral and intravenous administration. Additional methods include intraarterial administration into the carotid or vertebral artery. Another method is the use of Gliadel wafer to deliver carmustine directly into the resected cavity. The medication is slowly dispensed over a 3-week period. Administration of new medication temozolomide is used to treat refractory anoplastic astrocytomas.

Bibliography

Aft RL: Principles of surgical oncology. In Govindan R, Arquette MA, editors: *The Washington manual of oncology,* Philadelphia, 2002, Lippincott Williams & Wilkins.

American Cancer Society: *Cancer prevention and early detection, facts and figures 2003,* Atlanta, 2003, The Society.

American Cancer Society, *Cancer facts and figures 2003,* Atlanta, 2003, The Society.

Chu E, DeVita VT Jr: Principles of cancer management: chemotherapy. In DeVita VT Jr, Hellman S, Rosenberg SA, editors: *Cancer principles and practice of oncology,* ed 6, Philadelphia, 2001, JB Lippincott.

Cotran RS, Kumar V, Collins T: *Pathologic basis of disease,* ed 6, Philadelphia, 1999, WB Saunders.

Ferrell BR, Coyle N: An overview of palliative nursing care, *Am J Nurs* 102(5):26, 2002.

Fleming I, Cooper JS, Henson DE, et al: *AJCC cancer staging manual,* ed 5, Philadelphia, 2002, Lippincott-Raven.

Hawkins R: Mastering the intricate maze of metastasis, *Oncol Nurs Forum* 28(6):959, 2001.

Hellman S: Principles of cancer management: radiation therapy. In DeVita VT Jr, Hellman S, Rosenberg SA, editors: *Cancer principles and practice of oncology,* ed 6, Philadelphia, 2001, JB Lippincott.

Henry M: Descending into delirium, *Am J Nurs* 102(3):49, 2002.

Jemal A, Murray T, Samuels A, et al: Cancer statistics, 2003, *CA Cancer J Clin* 53(1):5, 2003.

Murphy ME: Cancers of the brain and central nervous system. In Otto SE, editor: *Oncology nursing,* ed 4, St. Louis, 2001, Mosby.

Paice JA: Managing psychological conditions in palliative care, *Am J Nurs* 102(11):36, 2002.

Quinn AM: CyberKnife: a robotic radiosurgery system, *Clin J Oncol Nurs* 6(3):149, 2002.

Redner A: Central nervous system malignancies. In Lanzkowsky P, editor: *Manual of pediatric hematology and oncology,* ed 3, San Diego, 2000, Academic Press.

Rivet D, Chicoine M, Simpson J, et al: Central nervous system tumors. In Govindan R, Arquette MA, editors: *The*

Washington manual of oncology, Philadelphia, 2002, Lippincott Williams & Wilkins.

Rosenberg SA: Principles of cancer management: surgical oncology. In DeVita VT Jr, Hellman S, Rosenberg SA, editors: *Cancer principles and practice of oncology*, ed 6, Philadelphia, 2001, JB Lippincott.

Smith RA, Cokkinides V, Eyre HJ: American Cancer Society guidelines for the early detection of cancer, 2003, *CA Cancer J Clin* 53(1):27, 2003.

Thompson JM, McFarland GK, Hirsch JE, et al: *Mosby's clinical nursing*, ed 5, St. Louis, 2002, Mosby.

Cancer Types

8

Breast Cancers

I. INCIDENCE

Approximately 211,300 new *invasive* cases of breast cancer will occur among women in the United States in 2003. Breast cancer rates among white women have slowly increased since the early 1980s. About 1300 new cases of breast cancer are expected in men in 2003. In addition to invasive breast cancer, 55,700 new cases of in situ breast cancer will occur among women in 2003. Approximately 88% of the in situ cases will be ductal carcinoma in situ (DCIS). The inherited susceptibility genes, *BRCA1* and *BRCA2*, account for about 5% of all breast cancer cases. The increase in the detection of DCIS and invasive breast cancer cases is related to the increased use of mammography screening.

II. MORTALITY

An estimated 40,200 deaths related to breast cancer (women, 39,800; men, 400) will occur in 2003. Breast cancer ranks first among cancers in incidence and second in cancer deaths for women in the United States.

III. ETIOLOGY/RISK FACTORS

The risk for breast cancer increases with age. The risk is greater for women who have a personal or family-history of breast cancer, biopsy-confirmed atypical hyperplasia, increased breast density, a prolonged menstrual history (early menarche and late menopause), obesity after menopause, or recent use of oral contraceptives or postmenopausal hormone replacement therapy and for women who have never had children or had their first child after age 30 or consume alcoholic beverages.

Factors known to decrease the risk for breast cancer include maintenance of a healthy body weight, vigorous physical activity, and selective estrogen receptor modulators such as tamoxifen or raloxifene.

IV. PREVENTION, SCREENING, AND DETECTION

The American Cancer Society maintains screening guidelines for asymptomatic women that incorporate the following three methods of early detection:

A. Breast Self-Examination—
Should be performed monthly by all women beginning at age 20.

B. Clinical Breast Examination—
By a health professional should be done every 3 years for women ages 20 to 39 and annually beginning at age 40.

C. Mammography—
(Routine screening mammography) should be performed every year beginning at age 40.

The Cancer Genetics Consortium has recommended that women who are known to carry a *BRCA1* or *BRAC2* mutation or who have a high likelihood of being a carrier should begin annual or semiannual clinical breast examination and annual mammography at age 25 to 35.

V. CLASSIFICATION

Breast cancer is most frequently staged according to the tumor, node, metastasis (TNM) classification system, which evaluates the tumor size, involvement of regional lymph nodes, and distant spread of the disease. The historical classification of the stage classifies it as local (no lymph nodes involved), regional (disease in lymph node), and distant (disease present).

VI. CLINICAL FEATURES

The earliest sign and symptom of breast cancer is a nodule or abnormality *noted in a mammogram* usually before it is felt or palpated by the woman while examining her breast. When this nodule or abnormality progresses in size to a *painless lump*, features such as thickening; swelling; tenderness; skin irritation or dimpling; and nipple pain, scaliness, ulceration, or retraction are noted. Breast pain is commonly caused by benign breast conditions and is not usually the initial symptom of breast cancer.

VII. DIAGNOSIS AND STAGING

The clinical diagnostic work-up for breast cancer includes a thorough history and physical examination;

bilateral mammography; complete blood count; liver function studies; and the evaluation of the bony structure, chest, liver, and brain, individualized by the patient's specific symptoms. Additional tests such as tumor markers are also performed.

Breast cancer is diagnosed with the cytologic cells or histologic tissue obtained by different biopsy methods. These methods include fine-needle aspiration (aspiration of material from the mass using a syringe and 21- to 23-gauge needle), core needle biopsy (core tissue from a dominant mass), needle localization biopsy (requires mammography guidance of wire or needle), stereotactic fine-needle aspiration (biopsy needle mechanically and precisely aligned by radiograph and computer), or ultrasound (guided biopsy to obtain adequate tissue specimen to ensure a definitive diagnosis).

VIII. METASTASIS
Breast cancer spreads by direct invasion of surrounding tissues, along the mammary ducts, or by way of lymphatic or blood vessels. The major site of regional spread is the axillary lymph nodes. These nodes are positive in approximately 50% of patients who have tumors that are 3 to 4 cm at diagnosis. Systemic or distant spread of the disease can occur in the bone, lung, pleura, liver, and adrenals. Less common sites are the brain, thyroid, leptomeninges, eye, pericardium, and ovary.

IX. SURVIVAL
The 5-year relative survival rate for localized breast cancer has increased from 72% in the 1940s to 96% in 2003. When the cancer has spread regionally, the 5-year survival rate is 78%, and for women with distant metastasis, the 5-year survival rate is 21%. Survival after a diagnosis of breast cancer continues to decline beyond 5 years, and survival at 10 years or more is also stage dependent, with the best survival rates observed in women diagnosed with early stage breast cancer.

X. TREATMENT MODALITIES
Treatment for all of the breast cancers are based on the tumor size, axillary lymph node status, estrogen and progesterone receptors, histologic and nuclear grade of the tumor, the DNA content of the cell (diploid-normal

DNA content and aneuploid-abnormal DNA), onco-genes (proto-oncogene her-2/*neu* or p53 gene), and lym-phatic and blood vessel invasion.

Often two or more treatment methods are used in combination for the treatment of breast cancer; for exam-ple, the treatment of DCIS includes local incision, radia-tion therapy, or tamoxifen. Surgical procedures used in breast cancer management include modified radical mastectomy, total mastectomy, lumpectomy, wide exci-sion, and quadrantectomy. Additional procedures include sentinel lymph node biopsy and breast reconstructive surgery. Significant advances in reconstruction tech-niques provide several options for breast reconstruction immediately after mastectomy.

Radiation therapy through external beam or brachy-therapy with a radiation boost to the original tumor site in conjunction with surgery, chemotherapy, or both is a treatment option. External beam radiotherapy, over 4 to 5 weeks, usually begins 2 to 4 weeks, and no later than 12 weeks, after surgery.

Systemic therapy involves the use of chemotherapy or endocrine manipulation to treat patients with axillary node involvement, poor prognosis, node-negative disease, advanced locoregional disease, or distant metastasis.

Multiple chemotherapy drug doses, combinations, or timing and scheduling of the chemotherapy administra-tion are available options. The current recommendations for adjuvant chemotherapy over 4 to 6 months include drug combinations of cyclophosphamide, methotrexate, doxorubicin, fluorouracil, paclitaxel, docetaxel, or the addition of trastuzumab for patients whose tumors overexpress the her-2/*neu* protein.

For women with locally advanced (>10 positive lymph nodes) or metastatic breast cancer, chemother-apy options may include high-dose chemotherapy with autologous peripheral blood stem cell transplantation. The recovery process is aided with the administration of growth factors (granulocyte, granulocyte-macrophage, epoetin alfa, or oprelvekin) to stimulate the recovery of white blood cells, red blood cells, and platelets.

Patients with tumors that are both estrogen and pro-gesterone receptor-positive respond to hormonal manip-ulation about 75% of the time, whereas only 10% of receptor-negative patients will respond. A variety of

Cancer Types

hormonal manipulations are available, but most types of hormonal therapy require several weeks to be effective. Hormonal drugs of choice include tamoxifen, anastrozole, letrozole, megestrol acetate, medroxyprogesterone acetate, and diethylstilbestrol (see Chapter 27, Hormonal Therapy).

Bibliography

American Cancer Society: *Cancer prevention and early detection, facts and figures 2003*, Atlanta, 2003, The Society.

American Cancer Society: *Cancer facts and figures 2003*, Atlanta, 2003, The Society.

Amgen, 2002, Aranesp (darbepoetin alfa) and Neulasta (pegfilgrastim), www.amgen.com

Bender CM, Kramer PA, Miaskowoski C: New direction in the management of cancer-related cognitive impairment, fatigue and pain, Raritan, NJ, 2002 Scientific Connexions. Ortho-Biotech Oncology.

Bland K, McCraw J, Copeland E: General principles of mastectomy: evaluation and therapeutic options. In Bland K, Copeland E, editors: *The breast: comprehensive management of benign and malignant diseases*, ed 2, Philadelphia, 1998, WB Saunders.

Bland K, Scott-Conner CE, Menck H, et al: Axillary dissection in breast-conserving surgery for stage I and II breast cancer: a National Cancer Data Base study of patterns of omission and implication for survival, *J Am Coll Surg* 188(6):586, 1999.

Brown HK, Healey JH: Metastatic cancer to the bone. In DeVita VT Jr, Hellman S, Rosenberg SA, editors: *Cancer principles and practice of oncology*, ed 6, Philadelphia, 2001, JB Lippincott.

Buchsel PC, Kapustay PM: *Stem cell transplantation: a clinical textbook*, Pittsburgh, 2000, Oncology Nursing Press.

Byers T, Nestle M, McTiernan A, et al: American Cancer Society Guidelines on nutrition and physical activity for cancer prevention: reducing the risks of cancer with healthy food choices and physical activity, *CA Cancer J Clin* 52(2):92, 2002.

Crane-Okada R: Breast cancers. In Otto SE, editor: *Oncology nursing*, ed 4, St. Louis, 2001, Mosby.

Erlichman C, Loprinzi CL: Hormonal therapies. In DeVita VT Jr, Hellman S, Rosenberg SA, editors: *Cancer principles and practice of oncology*, ed 6, Philadelphia, 2001, JB Lippincott.

Fleming I, Cooper JS, Henson DE, et al: *AJCC cancer staging manual*, ed 5, Philadelphia, 2002, Lippincott-Raven.

Jemal A, Murray T, Samuels A, et al: Cancer Statistics, 2003, *CA Cancer J Clin* 53(1):5, 2003.

Jennings-Dozier K, Mahon SM, editors: *Cancer prevention, detection, and control*, Pittsburgh, 2002, Oncology Nursing Press.

Lea DH, Williams JK: Genetic testing and screening, *Am J Nurs* 102(7):36, 2002.

Morrow M, Strom EA, Bassett LW: Standard for the management of ductal carcinoma in situ of the breast, *CA Cancer J Clin* 52(5):277, 2002.

Pasacreta JV, Jacobs L, Cataldo JK: Genetic testing for breast and ovarian cancer risk: the psychosocial issues, *Am J Nurs* 102(12):40, 2002.

Smith RA, Cokkinides V, Eyre HJ: American Cancer Society guidelines for the early detection of cancer, 2003, *CA Cancer J Clin* 53(1):27, 2003.

Winer EP, Morrow M, Osborne CK, et al: Malignant tumors of the breast. In DeVita VT Jr, Hellman S, Rosenberg SA, editors: *Cancer principles and practice of oncology*, ed 6, Philadelphia, 2001, JB Lippincott.

Zimmerman VL: BRCA gene mutations and cancer, *Am J Nurs* 102(8):28, 2002.

Cancer Types

9

Colorectal and Gastrointestinal Cancers

COLORECTAL

I. INCIDENCE/MORTALITY

In the United States, cancers of the colon and rectum combined (colorectal) are the third most common site of new cancer cases and cancer deaths in both men and women. There will be an estimated 147,500 new diagnosed cases and 57,100 deaths from this disease in 2003. Colorectal cancer (CRC) deaths decreased by 1.8% per year from 1992 to 1998. This has been attributed to improvements in nutrition, physical activity, and the timely use of existing CRC screening tests. Despite the effectiveness of several existing screening tests, the use of these tests for prevention remains extremely low.

II. ETIOLOGY/RISK FACTORS

An individual's lifetime risk for CRC in the United States is nearly 6%, with more than 90% of these cases occurring after age 50. Approximately 90% of CRC cases and deaths are thought to be *preventable*. The risk factors for CRC include obesity, alcohol and tobacco use, physical inactivity, and a diet high in fat or red meat. Additional risk factors include a strong family history of CRC or adenomatous polyps in a first-degree relative (parent or sibling younger than 60 years or in two first-degree relatives of any age); a personal history of CRC, polyps, or chronic inflammatory bowel disease; or a family history of hereditary CRC syndrome.

III. PREVENTION, SCREENING, AND DETECTION

The screening tests that could detect occult blood in the stool or identify adenomatous polyps (colonoscopy) can prevent the occurrence of CRC by allowing the detection and removal of these precancerous lesions before they undergo cellular malignant transformation.

A. The current recommendations for **prevention of CRC** include:
- Eat a variety of healthful foods, with an emphasis on plant sources.
- Adopt a physically active lifestyle.
- Maintain a healthful weight throughout life.
- Avoid or limit consumption of alcoholic beverages.

B. **Current CRC screening and surveillance** for early detection of colorectal adenomas and cancer include beginning at age 50 years (Table 9-1). In addition, both men and women should follow at least one of the following five options:
1. *Fecal occult blood test*—yearly test for men and women, plus flexible sigmoidoscopy every 5 years
2. *Flexible sigmoidoscopy*—every 5 years
3. *Colonoscopy*—every 10 years
4. *Double-contrast barium enema*—every 5 years
5. *Digital rectal examination*—every year. During the digital rectal examination, the clinician inserts a gloved finger into the rectum to feel for anything that is irregular or abnormal. This test can detect cancers of the rectum but *not* the colon.

IV. CLASSIFICATION

The site of presentation is primarily the sigmoidorectal area. The majority (40% to 50%) of lesions occur in the rectum, and 20% to 35% occur in the descending and sigmoid colon. Only 8% occur in the transverse colon and 16% in the cecum and ascending colon. A small percentage (4% to 8%) occurs as a second primary site. The

Table 9-1 AMERICAN CANCER SOCIETY GUIDELINES ON SCREENING AND SURVEILLANCE FOR THE EARLY DETECTION OF COLORECTAL ADENOMAS AND CANCER—WOMEN AND MEN AT INCREASED RISK OR AT HIGH RISK

Risk Category	Age to Begin	Recommendation	Comment
Increased Risk			
People with a single, small (<1 cm) adenoma	3–6 years after the initial polypectomy	Colonoscopy*	If the exam is normal, the patient can thereafter be screened as per average-risk guidelines.
People with a large (1 cm +) adenoma, multiple adenomas, or adenomas with high-grade dysplasia or villous change	Within 3 years after the initial polypectomy	Colonoscopy*	If normal, repeat examination in 3 years; If normal then, the patient can thereafter be screened as per average-risk guidelines.
Personal history of curative-intent resection of colorectal cancer	Within 1 year after cancer resection	Colonoscopy*	If normal, repeat examination in 3 years; If normal then, repeat examination every 5 years.

Either colorectal cancer or adenomatous polyps, in any first-degree relative before age 60, or in two or more first-degree relatives at any age (if not a hereditary syndrome)	Age 40, or 10 years before the youngest case in the immediate family	Colonoscopy*	Every 5–10 years. Colorectal cancer in relatives more distant than first-degree does not increase risk substantially above the average-risk group.
High Risk			
Family history of familial adenomatous polyposis (FAP)	Puberty	Early surveillance with endoscopy, and counseling to consider genetic testing	If the genetic test is positive, colectomy is indicated. These patients are best referred to a center with experience in the management of FAP.
Family history of hereditary non-polyposis colon cancer (HNPCC)	Age 21	Colonoscopy and counseling to consider genetic testing	If the genetic test is positive or if the patient has not had genetic testing, every 1–2 years until age 40, then annually. These patients are best

Continued

Cancer Types

Table 9-1 AMERICAN CANCER SOCIETY GUIDELINES ON SCREENING AND SURVEILLANCE FOR THE EARLY DETECTION OF COLORECTAL ADENOMAS AND CANCER—WOMEN AND MEN AT INCREASED RISK OR AT HIGH RISK—cont'd

Risk Category	Age to Begin	Recommendation	Comment
High Risk—cont'd			referred to a center with experience in the management of HNPCC.
Inflammatory bowel disease Chronic ulcerative colitis Crohn's disease	Cancer risk begins to be significant 8 years after the onset of pancolitis, or 12–15 years after the onset of left-sided colitis.	Colonoscopy with biopsies for dysplasia	Every 1–2 years. These patients are best referred to a center with experience in the surveillance and management of inflammatory bowel disease.

Source: Smith RA, Cokkinides V, Eyre HJ: American Cancer Society guidelines for the early detection of cancer, 2003, *CA Cancer J Clin,* 53(1):27–43, 2003.

*If colonoscopy is unavailable, not feasible, or not desired by the patient, double contrast barium enema (DCBE) alone or the combination of flexible sigmoidoscopy and double contrast barium enema are acceptable alternatives. Adding flexible sigmoidoscopy to DCBE may provide a more comprehensive diagnostic evaluation than DCBE alone in finding significant lesions. A supplementary DCBE may be needed if a colonoscopic exam fails to reach the cecum, and a supplementary colonoscopy may be needed if a DCBE identifies a possible lesion, or does not adequately visualize the entire colorectum.

tumor, node, metastasis classification system is used to determine disease stage.

V. CLINICAL FEATURES
Most of the CRCs begin as a polyp, a small noncancerous growth in the lining of the colon. Over time, the polyp changes in size and shape and becomes malignant. As they grow in size, polyps can bleed or obstruct the colon, and symptoms such as rectal bleeding or blood in stool, change in stool shape or color, cramping pain in the lower abdomen, or abdominal discomfort with an urge to have a bowel movement may occur. Other symptoms include fatigue, unexplained anemia, anorexia, and weight loss.

VI. DIAGNOSIS AND STAGING
A thorough history and physical examination including inspection, palpation, and auscultation of the abdomen is necessary for diagnosis. Multiple laboratory tests (complete blood count, liver function studies, and carcinoembryonic antigens [CEA]) and diagnostic examinations (barium enema, colonoscopy, chest radiograph, with scans of liver and bone) are performed to determine extent of disease. The diagnosis is confirmed by a tissue biopsy from the suspected site.

VII. METASTASIS
Most CRCs spread by direct extension and penetration into the layers of the bowel. Local invasion occurs to surrounding organs. The lymph node involvement and invasion into the vascular bed allow for disseminated disease. These nodal chains follow the pathway of the superior and mesenteric arteries, thus spreading to the liver. Approximately 25% of patients with CRC have liver metastasis at the time of initial disease presentation. Additional sites of metastasis include the brain, bone, adrenal glands, and lung.

VIII. SURVIVAL
The survival rate for patients with CRC is greatest when the disease is diagnosed early. The 1- and 5-year survival rates for patients with CRC are 81% and 61%, respectively. If the disease is detected *early*, however, the 5-year survival is approximately 90%. *Only* 37% of all CRCs are

Cancer Types

found at this early stage. When the disease has spread to adjacent organs or lymph nodes, the 5-year survival rate decreases to 64%, and the 5-year survival is only 8% when the disease is metastasized to distant areas.

IX. TREATMENT MODALITIES

If the colon cancer is detected at an early stage, a polypectomy or a local excision of disease tissue with a small margin of nondisease tissue is removed. Segmental colon resections with a temporary or permanent colostomy are performed when larger sections of the bowel are involved or there is lymph node involvement. The three major surgical procedures performed are colon resection with reanastomosis, colostomy (temporary or permanent), and abdominal perineal resection. A wide excision of the tumor with a distal margin of approximately 5 cm is recommended for curative surgery.

Radiation therapy is used primarily to treat rectal cancer; it is used less often in treatment for colon cancer. The goal of radiation therapy is to prevent metastatic disease caused by the spread of cancer cells that may be missed in the surgical procedures. Radiation therapy can also be administered before surgery to shrink the tumor, allowing the surgeon a better opportunity for surgical resection. Intraoperative radiation therapy in conjunction with surgery is an option dependent on tumor location and extent of disease.

Adjuvant chemotherapy has become a mainstay in the treatment of CRC. The various forms of drug combinations include fluorouracil (5-FU), leucovorin, levamisole, and the newer agent irinotecan. Chemotherapy is administered through an intravenous route; however, when CRC disease extends to the liver, drugs such as floxuridine, or combinations of floxuridine with mitomycin C or 5-FU, are administered intraarterially through an implantable infusion pump.

ESOPHAGUS

I. INCIDENCE/MORTALITY

Cancer of the esophagus is a fairly uncommon cancer in the United States, but the incidence varies greatly throughout the world. In the United States, there will be an estimated 13,900 new cases diagnosed in 2003, and 13,000 of these patients will die from this disease.

II. ETIOLOGY/RISK FACTORS
The cause of esophageal cancer is not well known. Some identified risk factors are associated with chronic irritation of the esophagus. In the United States, alcohol ingestion and smoking are the most prominent factors. Other factors include a previous history of squamous cell carcinoma of the esophagus, oropharyngeal leukoplakia, tylosis palmaris, head and neck cancer, caustic injury, prior irradiation, and a variety of nutritional deficiencies.

III. PREVENTION, SCREENING, AND DETECTION
Prevention of this disease focuses on counseling regarding alcohol and tobacco use and instructing patients with risk factors to report any problems with dysphagia or pain on swallowing. Dietary instructions regarding ensuring fresh citrus fruits, vegetables high in carotenoids, milk, and enriched flour as a source of riboflavin should be explained to the patient. Individuals at high risk for this cancer should undergo periodic endoscopy examination with biopsies every 2 to 3 years as directed by their physician.

IV. CLASSIFICATION
Adenocarcinoma and squamous cell carcinoma are the most common types of esophageal cancer in the United States. Other less common esophageal tumors include mucoepidermoid carcinoma, small-cell carcinoma, sarcoma, adenoid cystic carcinoma, and lymphoma.

V. CLINICAL FEATURES
Dysphagia, weight loss, and pain when swallowing are the most common symptoms of esophageal cancer. A weight loss greater than 10% total body weight may occur before the patient seeks medical attention. Because of this delay, most patients present with advanced disease.

VI. DIAGNOSIS AND STAGING
Endoscopy examinations usually follow the barium swallow and are required to confirm the presence of a tumor.

Biopsies and brushings can be obtained through the endoscope to confirm the histology of the lesion. Ultrasonography may be used to identify invasion of the tumor into the tissue layers to aid in staging of the disease.

VII. METASTASIS/SURVIVAL
Esophageal cancer can spread to almost any part of the body. Primary sites of metastasis include the lymph nodes, lung, liver, adrenals, bronchus, and bone. The presence of metastatic disease is indicative of a poor prognosis. Survival with proven metastasis is less than 7 months.

VIII. TREATMENT MODALITIES
The most effective approach to the treatment of esophageal cancer is a combined modality therapy. Surgery offers the best chance for a cure. Resection, removal, or both of the affected tissue with surgical bypass or anastomosis and esophagectomy with reconstruction are options depending on the location of the tumor. The latter procedure continues to be associated with high mortality and morbidity rates.

Radiation therapy is seldom used as a primary therapy because studies have demonstrated chemotherapy plus radiation therapy is far superior. Preoperative chemoradiation has been found to provide improved disease-free survival and a higher frequency of curative resections. Cisplatin-based combination chemotherapy (5-FU and cisplatin or paclitaxel, 5-FU, and cisplatin) is frequently used. A number of studies are under way to explore the benefit of concurrent neoadjuvant chemotherapy and radiation therapy.

GALLBLADDER

I. INCIDENCE/MORTALITY
Gallbladder cancer is an uncommon cancer with an estimated 6800 new cases diagnosed and approximately 3500 related adult deaths in the United States in 2003.

II. ETIOLOGY/RISK FACTORS
This disease is more common in women than men (3:1 ratio). The median age of presentation is 73 years. There is a correlation between gallbladder cancer and

cholelithiasis or calcified gallbladders and typhoid carriers.

III. PREVENTION, SCREENING, AND DETECTION

No prevention/screening/detection (PSD) methods are available for the screening or early detection of cancer of the gallbladder.

IV. CLASSIFICATION/METASTASIS

The most common tumor type is adenocarcinoma, accounting for 85% of cases, with the remaining 15% being squamous cell or mixed tumors. This disease most often spreads through the lymphatic or hematogenous routes into the adjacent tissues (biliary tract, liver, pancreas, and omentum).

V. CLINICAL FEATURES/SURVIVAL

In the early stages of gallbladder cancer the patient is often asymptomatic. However, once the symptoms are present the disease is in an advanced state. The most common symptoms are nonspecific and include pain in the right upper quadrant of the abdomen (75% to 95%), nausea and vomiting (40% to 64%), weight loss (37% to 77%), and jaundice (45%). The overall 5-year survival rate is less than 15%.

VI. DIAGNOSIS AND STAGING/TREATMENT MODALITIES

The diagnostic evaluation includes ultrasound and computed tomography (CT) scans with a fine-needle aspiration biopsy for tissue sampling to confirm the diagnosis. Additional CT scans of the chest and abdomen with laboratory tests are performed to detect extent of the disease. The treatment of choice is surgical resection; however, only 40% of the patients are found to have resectable disease at the time of diagnosis. A small number of patients may be diagnosed during a cholecystectomy for chronic cholecystitis, when the surgery alone is adequate. Those patients with more extensive disease require more radical procedures. Because there is little evidence that radiation therapy improves survival, this modality is used more often for palliation of biliary tract obstruction.

Cancer Types

The role of chemotherapy has been well defined, but it is usually offered to patients with metastatic disease or unresectable disease. Drugs commonly used include a combination of 5-FU, doxorubicin, and mitomycin. Although patients who receive chemotherapy have slightly improved survival rates, more than 90% of patients with unresectable disease die within 1 year.

GASTRIC

I. INCIDENCE/MORTALITY
In the United States, an estimated 22,400 new cases of gastric cancer will be diagnosed in 2003, and a total of 12,100 deaths will be attributed to this disease.

II. ETIOLOGY/RISK FACTORS
Several nutritional (low-fat foods, salted meat or fish, high nitrate consumption), environmental (poor food preparation, lack of refrigeration, poor drinking water), and medical factors (prior gastric surgery, *Helicobacter pylori* infection, gastric atrophy) have been associated with the development of gastric cancer.

III. PREVENTION, SCREENING, AND DETECTION
The key to prevention of cancer of the stomach lies in dietary intake. People of geographic areas and socioeconomic groups associated with the lowest incidence consume a diet different from those in the highest incidence groups. Nutrition counseling for the prevention of gastric cancers should emphasize the importance of eating a balanced diet high in fruits and vegetables with moderate amounts of animal protein. Salted, pickled, and smoked foods should be consumed sparingly.

IV. CLASSIFICATION
Adenocarcinomas represent almost 95% of gastric malignancies; lymphomas, carcinoid, leiomyosarcoma, and squamous cell carcinoma comprise the remaining 5%. Several classification systems are used for gastric cancers and the most widely accepted system identifies the two main groups of gastric cancers: diffuse gastric

cancer (33%) and intestinal gastric cancer (53%); the remaining 14% are unclassified.

V. CLINICAL FEATURES/METASTASIS

Symptoms of gastric cancer are usually nonspecific and may have been present for several months. They include indigestion and epigastric discomfort (67%), nausea and vomiting (40%), hematemesis (15%), and anorexia (25%). The majority of patients present with locally advanced disease or metastatic disease. In addition to local extension to nearby organs and tissue, gastric cancer metastasizes most frequently to liver, lungs, peritoneum, and bone marrow.

VI. DIAGNOSIS AND STAGING

The two most useful diagnostic procedures for gastric cancer are the esophagogastroduodenoscopy and the double-contrast upper gastrointestinal series. Additional examinations include CT scan of chest, abdomen, and pelvis to evaluate tumor extent, nodal involvement, and distant metastasis. Endoscopic ultrasonography is highly accurate in staging the depth of invasion of the primary tumor and in assessing local lymph involvement.

VII. SURVIVAL

The overall survival for patients with gastric cancer depends on the extent of the disease and on the treatment. Most cases are diagnosed at an advanced stage, and even after surgery disease is known to reoccur in 80% of patients. The 5-year survival rate in the United States ranges from 5% to 15%.

VIII. TREATMENT MODALITIES

The primary treatment for gastric cancer is surgical resection. Irrespective of the specific surgical procedure (resection or partial gastrectomy with en bloc dissection of lymphatic tissue) used for treatment of gastric cancer, the effectiveness of surgical resection is poor. When survival of node-positive patients is examined after gastric resection, the overall survival rate is only 30% in the United States.

A variety of combination chemotherapy regimens have been widely used in the palliative management

Cancer Types

of patients with gastric cancer. None of these regimens results in the cure of metastatic adenocarcinoma of the stomach; however, some regimens produce complete response rates as high as 15%, although these complete responses are not durable. Drugs used frequently in these combination therapies include 5-FU, doxorubicin, mitomycin, and leucovorin. Combined modalities including surgery, radiation therapy, and chemotherapy are undergoing clinical trials. Newer approaches to gastric cancer management, including antiangiogenesis strategies, with either monoclonal antibodies or small molecule inhibitors of epidermal growth factor receptor activity may be of benefit to patients with gastric cancer.

HEPATOCELLULAR (LIVER)

I. INCIDENCE/MORTALITY
Hepatocellular cancer (HCC) is one of the most common cancers. In general, the incidence of HCC is greater in men, increases with age, and reaches its peak between the fifth and seventh decade of life. Geographic regions such as Asia and sub-Saharan Africa have the highest incidence rates. In the United States this malignancy is less common, with an estimated 17,300 new cases diagnosed and an estimated 14,400 deaths in 2003.

II. ETIOLOGY/RISK FACTORS
HCC arises from long-standing cirrhosis from hepatitis B virus (HBV) and hepatitis C virus (HCV) infections. Epidemiologic factors vary with different geographic regions such as those in China, Taiwan, and sub-Saharan Africa where HBV is prevalent. An excessive alcohol intake over a prolonged time or ingesting food products such as aflatoxin B1 (a product of the *Aspergillus* fungus found in stored grains in hot humid environments such as Africa and China) places the individual at an increased risk. Additional underlying factors include autoimmune chronic active hepatitis, primary biliary cirrhosis, hemochromatosis, and deletions of *p16* and *p53* mutations, which have a role in hepatocarcinogenesis in HCV and aflatoxin-related HCC.

III. PREVENTION, SCREENING, AND DETECTION

Prevention of virus-related HCC is dependent on minimizing HBV and HCV exposures. Universal vaccination against HBV has helped somewhat, but there are no prophylactic measures that exist for HCV. All blood donors are routinely screened for both HBV and HCV, thereby eliminating posttransfusion hepatitis. Changes in lifestyle behaviors such as safe sexual practices and eliminating intravenous drug abuse could reduce the number of HBV infections.

IV. CLASSIFICATION/METASTASIS

Hepatocellular carcinoma accounts for more than 90% of the adult primary cancers of the liver. Three classifications have been identified: nodular, diffuse, and massive. The massive type forms a large discrete mass involving most or all of one lobe. The diffuse type is associated with cirrhosis. Diffuse and massive types account for more than 90% of all liver cancer cases. The usual sites for HCC metastasis are the regional nodes, lung, bone, adrenal gland, and brain.

V. CLINICAL FEATURES/SURVIVAL

The majority of patients have nonspecific symptoms such as weakness, anorexia, malaise, weight loss, upper abdominal pain, or abdominal fullness. Hematemesis may occur because of esophageal varices. Jaundice occurs because of biliary duct obstruction. An early diagnosis of HCC is uncommon and most patients present with advanced disease. Those patients who have stage III or IV at the time of diagnosis have a median survival of 4 months or less. Patients with regional lymph node involvement have a median survival of 7 months.

VI. DIAGNOSIS AND STAGING

The diagnostic work-up with staging uses spiral CT scans and CT scan angiography, ultrasonography, magnetic resonance imaging, with multiple laboratory studies, tumor markers, and chemistries to determine extent of the disease. Serum α-fetoprotein (AFP) levels greater than 4000 ng/ml in hepatitis B or C antigen-positive patients and greater than 400 ng/ml in the surface antigen-negative patients are indicative of an HCC

Cancer Types

diagnosis. A liver biopsy, preferably a core biopsy, is required for the definitive diagnosis of HCC. The tumor, node, metastasis staging system is used to classify the extent of the disease.

VII. TREATMENT MODALITIES

Surgical resection, total hepatectomy, and orthotopic (graft of organ) liver transplantation are the only potentially curative treatments for HCC, with *disease only in the liver*. Because of high cancer recurrence rates and limited donor organs, these procedures are controversial. Hepatic resections are based on anatomic segments of the liver—the type, size, number, and location of excisions required to ensure disease-free margins. Cryosurgery is a procedure used to treat multiple or bilobar unresectable primary and metastatic liver tumors.

Percutaneous ethanol injection involves the direct injection of 95% ethanol into a tumor using ultrasound guidance. This is used for patients with 2 or 3 lesions less than 4 cm each who are ineligible for a resection. The treatments are repeated 1 to 2 times a week for a total of 6 to 8 treatments, and they provide disease palliation.

Regional chemotherapy infusion through the intraarterial route can be administered through temporary catheter placement into the axillary or femoral artery, then threaded into the hepatic artery of the liver. Drugs can also be administered through an implantable pump, which offers the advantages of allowing the patient to remain ambulatory and reducing catheter-related complications. The agents most frequently used for intraarterial chemotherapy are floxuridine and 5-FU. Other drugs used in combination with floxuridine and 5-FU include cisplatin, doxorubicin, mitomycin C, leucovorin, vinblastine, vincristine, and IL-2.

PANCREAS

I. INCIDENCE/MORTALITY

An estimated 30,700 new cases in pancreatic cancer with approximately 30,000 related deaths are expected to occur in 2003. The death rates from pancreatic cancer among men has declined slightly, whereas those in women have slightly increased.

II. ETIOLOGY/RISK FACTORS

Cigarette and cigar smoking increases the risk for pancreatic cancer. Incidence rates are more than twice as high for smokers than for nonsmokers. Additive risks include obesity, physical inactivity, chronic pancreatitis, diabetes, and cirrhosis. Pancreatic cancer rates are greater in countries whose populations eat a diet high in fat.

III. PREVENTION, SCREENING, AND DETECTION

PSD for pancreatic cancer is not applicable because there are no identified tests that show evidence of the disease at an early stage. Currently, only a biopsy yields a certain diagnosis. Because of the "silent" clinical course of the disease, the need for biopsy may only become obvious with advanced disease.

IV. CLASSIFICATION/METASTASIS

Ninety-five percent of cancers involving the pancreas arise from the exocrine gland ductal system. Ductal adenocarcinoma accounts for 85% of all pancreatic cancers. Two thirds of these carcinomas occur in the pancreas head, with the remaining in the body and tail of the pancreas. This cancer most likely is metastasized at time of diagnosis, occurring through the regional nodes, to the liver and peritoneum. Distant metastatic sites include lung, adrenal glands, and ovary.

V. CLINICAL FEATURES/SURVIVAL

Cancer of the pancreas usually develops *without early* symptoms. If the tumor develops in an area of the pancreas near the common bile duct, its blockage may lead to jaundice, which sometimes allows the tumor to be diagnosed at an early stage. Many patients report pain that is dull, constant, and aching or radiating to the middle or upper back. Anorexia and weight loss are often reported at the time of diagnosis. Because of the clinical presentation of the disease, survival rates for pancreatic cancer are poor. For all stages combined, the 1-year relative survival rate is only 21% and the 5-year rate is about 5%.

VI. DIAGNOSIS AND STAGING

The diagnostic work-up includes CT scans with contrast media, magnetic resonance imaging and angiography

Cancer Types

studies, and endoscopic retrograde cholangiopancreatography accompanied by a fine-needle aspiration biopsy to confirm the tissue diagnosis.

VII. TREATMENT MODALITIES

Surgery, radiation therapy, and chemotherapy are treatment options that can extend the survival or relieve the symptoms in many patients but seldom offer a disease cure. Only 10% to 20% of patients with pancreatic cancer can be considered candidates for curative resection. These patients will undergo a pancreaticoduodenectomy (Whipple procedure) that includes the removal of the distal stomach, gallbladder, common bile duct, head of the pancreas, the duodenum, and the upper jejunum. The second surgical procedure is a total pancreatectomy that is an extension of the pancreaticoduodenectomy and in addition involves the removal of the body and tail of the pancreas, the spleen, and a more extensive lymphadenectomy. Controversy continues regarding the advantages and disadvantages of each of these extensive procedures.

The current practice of giving chemotherapy before as well as after surgery is being investigated. The chemotherapy drugs most commonly administered for pancreatic cancer include many gemcitabine-containing combinations. At least 53 different studies of these regimens have been explored in phase I, II, and III trials during the past 2 years. Some of these gemcitabine-containing combinations include: gemcitabine + 5-FU with or without leucovorin; gemcitabine + 5-FU + paclitaxel; gemcitabine + cisplatin; gemcitabine + capecitabine; and gemcitabine + 5-FU + leucovorin + oxaliplatin. Additional investigational agents include monoclonal antibodies, epidermal growth factors, the topoisomerase I inhibitors, and the cyclooxygenase-2 inhibitor celecoxib.

Radiation therapy plus chemotherapy (radiation with gemcitabine; or radiation with paclitaxel, mitomycin C, and cisplatin, alone or in combination with 5-FU) is currently in clinical trials. Survival thus far has been reported with ranges of 7.7 to 40 months with a median survival of 12 months.

SMALL INTESTINE

I. INCIDENCE/MORTALITY
Cancers of the small intestines are rare. An estimated 5300 new cases will be diagnosed with an estimated 1100 related deaths in 2003.

II. ETIOLOGY/RISK FACTORS
Risk factors that have been associated with small-bowel cancers include adenomatous polyposis, Crohn's disease, celiac disease, urinary-ileo anastomosis, ileostomy, nodular lymphoid hyperplasia, and immunodeficiency.

III. PREVENTION, SCREENING, AND DETECTION
No PSD methods are available for the screening or early detection of cancer in the small intestine.

IV. CLASSIFICATION/METASTASIS
The four primary types of tumors found in the small intestines are: adenocarcinoma (42%), carcinoid (29%), lymphoma (18%), and leiomyosarcoma (11%). These tumors often spread to the liver before the diagnosis is made; the patient initially presents with symptoms of a carcinoid syndrome (flushing of head and neck and watery secretory diarrhea).

V. CLINICAL FEATURES/SURVIVAL
The symptoms of cancer of the small intestine are vague and not localizing, occurring late in the disease course. Because of these vague symptoms and the rarity of the malignancy, there is usually a delay of months before a diagnosis is made. Patients have advanced disease symptoms including pain (35% to 86%), perforation (10%), bleeding (20% to 54%), and weight loss (32% to 67%). The 5-year survival rate varies widely from 0% to 60% because of the lymph node metastasis.

VI. DIAGNOSIS AND STAGING/TREATMENT MODALITIES
The diagnostic evaluation includes multiple gastrointestinal scopes that have the capability of tissue sampling to

Cancer Types

confirm the diagnosis. Additional examinations include ultrasound examinations and CT scans of the chest and abdomen with laboratory tests, which are performed to detect extent of the disease. The treatment depends on the histologic type of the tumor and location. The most common approach to curative treatment is surgery, with tumor removal, resection, or debulking of the tumor. Procedures may include segmental resections or primary anastomosis of the bowel, or both. Adjuvant chemotherapy follows the surgical procedure and radiation therapy is considered to be high risk and is not often used.

Bibliography

Aft RL: Principles of surgical oncology. In Govindan R, Arquette MA, editors: *The Washington manual of oncology,* Philadelphia, 2002, Lippincott Williams & Wilkins.

American Cancer Society: *Cancer prevention and early detection, facts and figures 2003,* Atlanta, 2003, The Society.

American Cancer Society: *Cancer Facts and Figures 2003,* Atlanta, 2003, The Society.

Beyers T, Nestle M, McTiernan A, et al: American Cancer Society Guidelines on nutrition and physical activity for cancer prevention: reducing the risks of cancer with healthy food choices and physical activity, *CA Cancer J Clin* 52(2):92, 2002.

Cotran RS, Kumar V, Collins T: *Pathologic basis of disease,* ed 6, Philadelphia, 1999, WB Saunders.

Daniel BT: Gastrointestinal cancers. In Otto SE, editor: *Oncology nursing,* ed 4, St. Louis, 2001, Mosby.

Desjardins LA: Hepatocellular carcinoma, *Clin J Oncol Nurs* 6(2):107, 2002.

Ferrell BR, Coyle N: An overview of palliative nursing care, *Am J Nurs* 102(5):26, 2002.

Fleming I, Cooper JS, Henson DE, et al: *AJCC cancer staging manual,* ed 5, Philadelphia, 2002, Lippincott Williams & Wilkins.

Jemal A, Murry T, Samuels A, et al: Cancer statistics, 2003, *CA Cancer J Clin* 53(1):5–26, 2003.

Jennings-Dozier K, Mahon SM, editors: *Cancer prevention, detection, and control,* Pittsburgh, 2002, Oncology Nursing Press.

Kemeny N, Fata F: Hepatic-arterial chemotherapy, *Lancet Oncol* 2(7):418, 2001.

Levin B, Brooks D, Smith RA, et al: Emerging technologies screening for colorectal cancer: CT colonoscopy, immunochemical fecal occult blood tests, and stool screening using molecular markers, *CA Cancer J Clin* 53(1):44–55, 2003.

Macdonald JS: Gastric cancer, *Clinical Oncology Updates* 4(3):1, 2001.

Murphy ME: Colorectal cancers. In Otto SE, editor: *Oncology Nursing*, ed 4, St. Louis, 2001, Mosby.

O'Brien B: Advances in the treatment of colorectal cancer, *Oncol Nurs* 9(2):1, 2002.

Rosenberg SA: Principles of cancer management: surgical oncology. In DeVita VT Jr, Hellman S, Rosenberg SA, editors: *Cancer principles and practice of oncology*, ed 6, Philadelphia, 2001, JB Lippincott.

Smith RA, Cokkinides V, Eyre HJ: American Cancer Society Guidelines for the early detection of cancer, 2003, *CA Cancer J Clin* 53(1):27–43, 2003.

Thompson JM, McFarland GK, Hirsch JE, et al: *Mosby's clinical nursing*, ed 5, St. Louis, 2002, Mosby, 2002.

Von Hoff DD, Mahadevan D, Bearss DJ: New developments in the treatment of patients with pancreatic cancer, *Clinical Oncology Updates* 4(4):1, 2001.

Cancer Types

10 Genitourinary Cancers

BLADDER

I. INCIDENCE
An estimated 57,400 new cases of cancer of the bladder will occur in 2003. From 1992 through 1998, bladder cancer incidence rates declined slightly in both men and women. Overall, bladder cancer incidence in 2003 is about four times greater in men (42,200) than in women (15,200), and about two times higher in whites than in blacks.

II. MORTALITY
An estimated 12,500 deaths related to bladder cancer will occur in 2003. Between the early 1970s and the late 1980s, mortality rates for bladder cancer decreased significantly in both whites and blacks; during the 1990s, mortality rates continued to decline among blacks, but remained constant among whites.

III. ETIOLOGY/RISK FACTORS
Smoking is the greatest risk factor for bladder cancer; the risk for smokers is twice as great as that for nonsmokers. Numerous studies have identified a variety of agents associated with the development of bladder cancer such as aromatic amine compounds used in textile, rubber, paint, cable, and printing industries. Additional occupational exposure risk is experienced by aluminum workers, motor vehicle operators, dry cleaners, chemical workers, pesticide applicators, miners, chimney sweeps, and cooks.

IV. PREVENTION, SCREENING, AND DETECTION
There are no prevention, screening, and detection (PSD) methods currently used for bladder cancer.

V. CLASSIFICATION
The World Health Organization and the International Society of Urologic Pathology recommends use of the term *transitional cell* to be replaced with *urothelial cell or urothelium*, and further recommends the term *superficial* be abandoned. Urothelial carcinoma accounts for 90% of all the bladder cancer cases, 5% of squamous cell carcinomas, and less than 1% of adenocarcinoma. The two staging systems currently in use are the Jewett-Strong system and the American Joint Committee on Cancer.

VI. CLINICAL FEATURES
The most common clinical feature of bladder cancer is blood in the urine, usually associated with increased frequency of urination. Secondary symptoms include urgency, dysuria, bladder irritability, and the patient having more than one episode of intermittent bleeding over a 6-month period before seeking a clinical examination. Back pain, rectal pain, or suprapubic pain may suggest metastatic disease.

VII. DIAGNOSIS AND STAGING
Multiple radiography studies such as intravenous pyelogram or excretory urogram, cystoscopy with random biopsies, urine cytology studies, computed tomography (CT) scans, DNA flow cytometry (identifies the DNA content within the urine), ultrasound, ureteroscopy, and magnetic resonance imaging (MRI) are used in the diagnostic work-up.

VIII. METASTASIS
Metastatic disease occurs through the tumor invasion outside the bladder walls into the adjacent pelvic structure.

IX. SURVIVAL
When diagnosed at a localized stage, the 5-year relative survival rate for patients with bladder cancer is 94%; approximately 74% of these cancers are detected at an early stage. For regional and distant stages, the 5-year relative survival rates are 48% and 6%, respectively.

X. TREATMENT MODALITIES

Surgery, alone or in combination with other treatments, is used for more than 90% of bladder cancer cases. The standard treatment for tumors invading the muscle is surgical removal of the bladder by radical cystectomy. Women undergo both cystectomy and hysterectomy. For men, the procedure involves a cystoprostatectomy. Urinary diversions are created in the form of ileal conduits or by direction urine flow into an internal urinary reservoir with drainage into the abdominal wall or to the urethra.

Superficial, localized cancers may be treated by administration of immunotherapy or chemotherapy drugs (directly into the bladder, i.e., intravesical therapy). Examples of agents in current use include thiotepa, mitomycin C, epirubicin, doxorubicin, and mitoxantrone. Chemotherapy alone or with radiation therapy *before cystectomy* has improved some of the invasive treatment results. Laser treatment and photodynamic therapy may be used for patients with recurrent localized disease.

PENILE

I. INCIDENCE/MORTALITY

Approximately 1400 new cases of penile cancer will occur in 2003 with 200 deaths related to this cancer.

II. ETIOLOGY/RISK FACTORS

Penile cancer is usually associated with an older age, with most cases occurring in men in the sixth or seventh decade of life. The cause is unknown, but nearly 100% of the cases are in men who are uncircumcised. The human papillomavirus (HPV), specifically HPV type 16, is linked to the disease.

III. PREVENTION, SCREENING, AND DETECTION

There are no PSD methods used for penile cancer.

IV. CLASSIFICATION

Several staging systems are in use including the tumor, node, metastasis (TNM) system and the Jackson system that categorizes the disease by the following:

A. **Stage I—**
   Tumors limited to glans, prepuce, or both
B. **Stage II—**
   Tumors invading the shaft
C. **Stage III—**
   Tumors with operable metastatic nodes
D. **Stage IV—**
   Tumors invading adjacent structures or with inoperable nodes or distant metastasis

Lesions may be further classified as precancerous, carcinoma in situ, Kaposi's sarcoma, or squamous cell that accounts for 95% of all penile cancers.

V. CLINICAL FEATURES
Common clinical presentation includes an ulcerated nodule or a nonhealing ulcer on the penis. Swelling or discharge from the prepuce may also precede the diagnosis.

VI. DIAGNOSIS AND STAGING
Diagnostic evaluation includes urethroscopy and cavenosography with contrast media. Ultrasound examinations and MRI scans are used to identify the adjacent structures. Additional investigative examinations include CT scanning, fine-needle aspiration, and bipedal lymphangiography.

VII. METASTASIS
The metastatic process generally occurs throughout the lymphatic channels by lymphatic embolization. The depth of tumor invasion and tumor grade is directly related to nodal metastases.

VIII. SURVIVAL
Long-term survival is directly related to the nodal status. Five-year survival rates approach 85% with negative nodes, compared with 56% with unilateral nodal metastasis only.

IX. TREATMENT MODALITIES
Surgery, alone or in combination with other treatments, is used for the majority of invasive penile cancer cases. Radical inguinal or ileoguinal lymphadenectomy may be included in the surgical procedure.

Cancer Types

Laser surgery is routinely performed for superficial lesions, precancerous lesions, and in situ lesions. Radiotherapy offers a conservative approach for early stage (T1N1) tumors less than 4 cm in diameter. Both external beam therapy and brachytherapy are used. A circumcision is performed before brachytherapy.

PROSTATE

I. INCIDENCE
Approximately 220,900 new prostate cancer cases will occur in 2003. Prostate cancer incidence rates remain significantly greater for the black male than for the white male. Since the onset of using the prostate-specific antigen (PSA) blood test, incidence rates have declined and leveled off especially in the elderly.

II. MORTALITY
An estimated 28,900 deaths will occur in 2003 as the result of prostate cancer. Although the mortality rates have declined among white and black men, rates in *black men remain more than twice as high* as rates in white men.

III. ETIOLOGY/RISK FACTORS
The incidence of prostate cancer increases with age; with more than 70% of the cases diagnosed in men older than 65 years. Blacks have the *highest* prostate cancer incidence rates in the world. Recent genetic studies suggest that significant familial predisposition may be responsible for 5% to 10% of the cases, and international studies suggest dietary fat may also be a risk factor.

IV. PREVENTION, SCREENING, AND DETECTION
The PSA test with the digital rectal examination should be performed beginning at age 50 years to men who have a life expectancy of at least 10 years. Black men and men who have a first-degree relative diagnosed with prostate cancer at a young age should begin this testing process at age 45. Currently, there are two prostate cancer prevention trials sponsored by the National Cancer Institute. One trial is a double-blind, placebo-controlled trial, with men randomized to receive finasteride 5 mg/d or a placebo for 7 years. The second trial began in 2001, with an expected enrollment of 32,000 men over a 5-year

period. This trial will have four study groups: (1) 200 µg selenium daily plus vitamin E-appearing placebo; (2) 400 mg vitamin E daily plus a selenium-appearing placebo; (3) both the selenium and vitamin doses, and (4) both placebos.

V. CLASSIFICATION
Ninety-five percent of prostate cancers are *adenocarcinomas.* Ductal carcinomas, transitional and squamous cell carcinomas, endometrioid carcinomas, and sarcomas account for the remaining 5%.

VI. CLINICAL FEATURES
The most common presenting symptoms include weak or interrupted urine flow, inability to urinate, difficulty starting or stopping the urine flow, and nocturia. Symptoms associated with advanced disease may include pain or burning on urination, hematuria, continual pain in lower back, pelvis, or upper thighs, or weight loss.

VII. DIAGNOSIS AND STAGING
The diagnostic work-up includes the physical examination, PSA test, transrectal ultrasound, MRI, and spiral or helical CT scanning. Bone scans are recommended for patients with PSA levels more than 20 ng/ml. Biopsy is performed using an 18-gauge, spring-loaded needle to obtain multiple specimens.

VIII. METASTASIS
Prostate cancer spreads by direct extension to the seminal vesicles and contiguous structures, bladder, membranous urethra, and pelvic sidewall.

IX. SURVIVAL
Eighty-three percent of all prostate cancers are discovered in the locoregional stages. The 5-year survival rates for patients whose tumors are diagnosed at these stages are 100%. The overall survival for all stages combined is 96%. The relative 10-year survival is 75%, and the 15-year survival is 54%.

X. TREATMENT MODALITIES
Depending on the patient's age, stage of the cancer, and other medical conditions, surgery, radiation therapy, or

both is usually selected. Hormonal therapy and chemotherapy options are considered for metastatic disease. Treatment options are summarized as follows:

A. Stage I Disease—
Careful observation without further treatment for most patients, and more definitive therapy for younger men in good health

B. Stage II Disease—
Radical prostatectomy, external beam or interstitial implant radiotherapy, and watchful waiting

C. Stage III Disease—
External beam radiotherapy with or without hormonal manipulation, hormonal manipulation alone, radical prostatectomy in limited cases; watchful waiting is an additional option for older men or those men who are asymptomatic with coexisting medical conditions

D. Stage IV Disease—
Hormonal therapy, orchiectomy, external beam radiotherapy, palliative pain management with radioisotopes or external beam radiation therapy, watchful waiting, chemotherapy for hormone refractory disease

RENAL

I. INCIDENCE
Approximately 31,900 new renal cancer cases will occur in 2003. The ratio of men (19,500 cases) to women (12,400) with renal cancer is 1.5:1.0. Renal cell cancer represents about 3% of adult malignancies, and most cases occur in persons aged 50 to 60 years.

II. MORTALITY
In 2003, approximately 11,900 adults will die from renal cancer, with 7400 deaths in men and 4500 in women.

III. ETIOLOGY/RISK FACTORS
The etiologic factors are unknown, but renal cancer has been associated with abnormalities with deviations involving chromosome 3, *p53*, and the von Hippel-Lindau disease (*VHL*) gene. Environmental, genetic, cellular, and hormonal factors have been examined including obesity, dietary fat intake, tobacco use, phenacetin, and occupational exposure to asbestos and petroleum.

IV. PREVENTION, SCREENING, AND DETECTION
There are no known PSD methods used to detect renal cell carcinoma.

V. CLASSIFICATION
More than 95% of parenchymal tumors are adenocarcinomas and are referred to as *hypernephroma, renal cell carcinoma, clear cell cancer*, or *Grawitz tumor.* Squamous cell carcinoma and nephroblastoma are also identified in the adult. The American Joint Committee on Cancer TNM system is used in renal cancer. The staging system for renal cell cancer is based on the degree of tumor spread beyond the kidney. Blood vessel involvement may not always be a *poor* prognostic indicator.

VI. CLINICAL FEATURES
The classic triad of hematuria, palpable flank mass, and costovertebral pain is associated with advanced tumors and occurs in only 10% to 20% of patients. Early stage renal cell cancer is *usually silent* and is coincidentally detected when the patient is undergoing diagnostic examinations such as cardiac angiography or gallbladder ultrasound. Approximately 88% of patients with renal cell carcinoma have a hypochromic anemia as a result of hemolysis or hematuria.

VII. DIAGNOSIS AND STAGING
Multiple diagnostic examinations—CT, MRI, ultrasound, arteriography, and excretory urography—are used.

VIII. METASTASIS
The most common sites for nonlymphatic metastases are: lung: 75%; bone: 20%; liver: 18%; and soft tissues: 36%. Renal cell carcinoma can metastasize to unusual sites such as the testes and skin.

IX. SURVIVAL
The survival of renal cell carcinoma is equated with an early diagnosis of the disease. Patients experiencing relapsing, recurring, or progressive disease regardless of the cell type have *poor* survival rates. Local recurrence occurs infrequently, and treatment failure is related to metastasis through nodal or hematogenous spread.

X. TREATMENT MODALITIES

A surgical procedure such as radical nephrectomy is used most often and has proven to be an effective treatment modality for localized renal carcinoma. Following radical nephrectomy, 20% to 30% of patients with localized tumors will experience disease relapse. Median time to relapse is 2 to 3 years. Renal cell carcinoma is refractory to chemotherapy. Current clinical trials investigating circadian-based floxuridine (FUDR) have failed to show patient improvement. Continued clinical investigation exists with the use of cytokine therapy (IL-2) and exploring gene therapy for renal cell tumors.

TESTICULAR

I. INCIDENCE/MORTALITY

Approximately 7600 new cancer cases will occur in 2003, and approximately 400 deaths will occur from testicular cancer. This is the *most common solid tumor* in men aged 15 to 35 years and is the *second most common solid tumor* in men aged 35 to 39 years.

II. ETIOLOGY/RISK FACTORS

The cause of testicular cancer is unknown, but it has an increased incidence in men with atrophic testis or a cryptorchid (undescended) testis. A family history of testicular cancer is associated with risk 3 to 12 times greater than the average, a history of a prior germ cell testicular tumor is associated with 23 to 27 times greater risk, and certain intersex syndromes are associated with greater than 100 times the average risk. Organ transplant patients experience a 20 to 50 times greater risk for testicular cancer than the general male population.

III. PREVENTION, SCREENING, AND DETECTION

Early detection of testicular cancer is best accomplished through monthly testicular self-examination (TSE). TSE is facilitated by heat of a warm bath or shower, examining each testicle with both hands. The index finger and middle fingers are placed on one side on the testicle with the thumbs on the other side, and a gentle rolling motion should be used to allow a complete palpation of each testicle. The ACS recommends TSE beginning at puberty for all men.

IV. CLASSIFICATION

Testicular tumor categories include germ cell tumors (seminomas, embryonic cancers, teratomas, choriocarcinomas, and yolk sac tumors), sex cord-stromal/gonadal stromal tumors, mixed germ and stromal cell tumors, adnexal and paratesticular tumors, and other malignancies such as mesothelioma and lymphoma. In addition, the testes may be the site of metastatic disease from other cancer types. Approximately 95% of all testicular tumors are germ cell and more than 90% of this tumor type is cured.

V. CLINICAL FEATURES

The classic presentation of a testicular tumor is a small-sized painless mass ranging from several millimeters to centimeters.

VI. DIAGNOSIS AND CLINICAL STAGING

Diagnostic work-up includes history and physical examination, urinalysis and culture/sensitivity, α-fetoprotein (AFP) and human chorionic gonadotropin (HCG) levels, chemistry profile, and chest radiograph. A radical inguinal orchiectomy usually follows, after the patient has been informed about options regarding storing sperm in a sperm bank. Both the clinical examination and the radical orchiectomy are required for clinical staging. Staging is accomplished using the TNM system.

VII. METASTASIS

Testicular cancer metastasizes to the brain, lung, and bone.

VIII. SURVIVAL

The cure rate for stage I nonseminoma approaches 95%. Stage II nonseminoma has rates greater than 95%, and the cure rate for stage III nonseminoma is about 70%. Relapse-free survival is nearly 100%. Approximately 90% of patients with seminoma advanced disease will achieve a cure with platinum-based chemotherapy regimens.

IX. TREATMENT MODALITIES

Testicular cancer treatment is based on the major categories of seminoma therapy and nonseminoma therapy

Cancer Types

with fertility planning included for both groups. Removal of the affected testicle (radical inguinal orchiectomy) is the initial treatment for all stages of seminomas. Most often this procedure is performed on an outpatient basis. After the orchiectomy, stage I seminomas are treated with radiation therapy to the retroperitoneal nodes and ipsilateral lymph nodes. Combination chemotherapy with cisplatin, etoposide, and bleomycin is effective in treating bulky type tumors. Approximately 90% of these patients achieve a cure even when advanced disease is present.

Nonseminoma therapy for stage I disease approaches 95% cure rate after a radical inguinal orchiectomy with or without retroperitoneal lymph node dissection. If retroperitoneal lymph node dissection reveals no nodal involvement, no adjuvant chemotherapy is administered; however, if nodes are positive, adjuvant chemotherapy is indicated. Combination chemotherapy drugs include etoposide and cisplatin or bleomycin, cisplatin, and etoposide. Patients with brain metastases are treated with chemotherapy and simultaneous whole brain irradiation and consideration of surgical excision. Those patients who do not have a complete response to the initial chemotherapy or who have a relapse are treated with salvage therapy regimens containing cisplatin, ifosfamide, and vinblastine.

Bibliography

American Cancer Society: *Cancer facts and figures 2003,* Atlanta, 2003, The Society.

American Cancer Society: *Cancer prevention and early detection, facts and figures 2003,* Atlanta, 2003, The Society.

Bosl GJ, Bajorin DF, Sheinfeld J, et al: Cancer of the testes. In DeVita VT Jr, Hellman S, Rosenberg S, editors: *Cancer: principles and practice of oncology,* ed 5, Philadelphia, 1997, Lippincott-Raven.

Bradley JD, Perez CA: Fundamentals of patient management in radiation oncology. In Govindan R, Arquette MA, editors: *The Washington manual of oncology,* Philadelphia, 2002, Lippincott Williams & Wilkins.

Brown HK, Healey JH: Metastatic cancer to the bone. In DeVita VT Jr, Hellman S, Rosenberg SA, editors: *Cancer principles and practice of oncology,* ed 6, Philadelphia, 2001, JB Lippincott.

Erlichman C, Loprinzi CL: Hormonal therapies. In DeVita VT Jr, Hellman S, Rosenberg SA, editors: *Cancer principles and practice of oncology,* ed 6, Philadelphia, 2001, JB Lippincott.

Fleming I, Cooper JS, Henson DE, et al: *AJCC cancer staging manual*, ed 5, Philadelphia, 2002, Lippincott Williams & Wilkins.

Held-Warmkessel J: What your patient needs to know about prostate cancer, *Nursing* 32(12):36, 2002.

Hellerstedt BA, Pienta KJ: The current status of hormonal therapy for prostate cancer, *CA Cancer J Clin* 52(3):154, 2002.

Hellman S: Principles of cancer management: radiation therapy. In DeVita VT Jr, Hellman S, Rosenberg SA, editors: *Cancer principles and practice of oncology*, ed 6, Philadelphia, 2001, JB Lippincott.

Jemal A, Murray T, Samuels A, et al: Cancer statistics, 2003, *CA Cancer J Clin* 53(1):5, 2003.

Maher KE: Male genitourinary cancers. In Dow KH, Bucholtz JD, Iwamoto R, et al, editors: *Nursing care in radiation oncology*, ed 2, Philadelphia, 1997, WB Saunders.

O'Rouke ME: Genitourinary cancers. In Otto SE, editor: *Oncology nursing*, ed 4, St. Louis, 2001, Mosby.

Rosenberg SA: Principles of cancer management: surgical oncology. In DeVita VT Jr, Hellman S, Rosenberg SA, editors: *Cancer principles and practice of oncology*, ed 6, Philadelphia, 2001, JB Lippincott.

Smith RA, Cokkinides V, Eyre HJ: American Cancer Society guidelines for the early detection of cancer, 2003, *CA Cancer J Clin* 53(1):27, 2003.

Weinrich SP, Weinrich MC, Priest J, et al: Self-reported reasons men decide not to participate in free prostate cancer screening, *Oncol Nurs Forum* 30(1):10, 2003.

Cancer Types

Gynecologic Cancers

CERVIX

I. INCIDENCE
An estimated 12,200 cases of invasive cervical cancer are expected to occur in 2003. Incidence rates have decreased steadily over the past several decades including incidence rates for black women (11.3/100,000) and white women (7.0/100,000) from 1994 through 1998.

II. MORTALITY
An estimated 4100 deaths related to cervical cancer will occur in 2003. Since 1982, cervical cancer mortality rates have declined by an average of 1.6% per year.

III. ETIOLOGY/RISK FACTORS
Cervical cancer risk is closely linked to sexual behavior and to sexually transmitted infections with certain types of human papillomavirus. Women who have sex at an early age, many sexual partners, or have partners who have had many sexual partners are at greater risk for cervical cancer. Tobacco use such as cigarette smoking is also associated with cervical cancer.

IV. PREVENTION, SCREENING, AND DETECTION
Prevention is the key by limiting the number of sexual partners and using barrier contraceptives such as condoms or diaphragms. The Pap test should be performed annually with a bimanual pelvic examination in women

who are, or have been, sexually active or who have reached the age of 18. After three or more consecutive annual examinations with normal findings, the Pap test may be performed less frequently at the discretion of the physician.

V. CLASSIFICATION

Squamous cell carcinomas account for 80% of cervical cancers; of the remaining 20%, 11% to 16% are adenocarcinomas or adenosquamous carcinomas. The latter two diagnoses occur more often in women younger than 35 years. When adenomatous features are present, a poorer prognosis is associated with the disease.

VI. CLINICAL FEATURES

The most common presenting signs and symptoms of cervical cancer are abnormal vaginal bleeding (decrease in the interval between periods, or an increase in the amount or length of menstrual flow), spotting, and abnormal vaginal discharge. Episodes of "contact bleeding" after intercourse or douching may also be reported.

VII. DIAGNOSIS AND STAGING

The diagnosis and staging process for cervical cancer include the clinical examination (inspection, palpation, colposcopy), radiographic examinations (chest, kidneys, sigmoid colon and rectum, skeleton, intravenous pyelogram [IVP]), barium enema, cystoscopy, or proctoscopy, with a pathologic evaluation of biopsy and curettage materials used to determine the disease extent and ultimately plan treatment. The tumor, node, metastasis (TNM) system is used to stage cervical cancer.

VIII. METASTASIS

Cervical cancers are slow growing tumors that invade by direct extension into the adjacent tissue of the uterus, vagina, rectum, bladder, and parametrial tissues. Lymphatic invasion also occurs in regional and distant lymphatic channels.

IX. SURVIVAL

The survival rate for patients with preinvasive lesions is almost 100%. Eighty-nine percent of patients with cervical cancer survive 1 year after diagnosis and 70% survive 5 years. When detected at an early stage, invasive cervical cancer is one of the most successfully treatable cancers with a 5-year survival rate of 92% for localized cancers. Approximately 56% of invasive cervical cancers are among white women, and 44% of cancers among black women are diagnosed at a localized stage.

X. TREATMENT MODALITIES

Preinvasive cervical lesions or changes in the cervix may be treated by cryotherapy, electrocautery, cold-knife conization, laser ablation, or local surgery. Invasive cervical cancers are treated by surgery (radical hysterectomy with bilateral pelvic lymphadenectomy) or radiation therapy (external beam and internal or interstitial beam, or both), and chemotherapy may be used in some cases. Pelvic exenteration is considered a curative treatment for women with recurrent disease if no evidence of extrapelvic disease, tumor fixed to the pelvic wall, or ureteral obstruction from the tumor is present before surgery. This procedure consists of removal of the uterus, cervix, vagina, rectum, bladder, urethra, and lateral supporting tissues and has significant morbidity.

OVARY

I. INCIDENCE/MORTALITY

The 25,400 new cases of ovarian cancer will account for approximately 30% of all the gynecologic cancers diagnosed in 2003. Ovarian cancer will cause 14,300 deaths and will account for 35% of all the death related to gynecologic cancer and 6% of all cancer deaths among women in 2003.

II. ETIOLOGY/RISK FACTORS

The etiologic factors of ovarian cancer are unknown; however, age, genetics, history of other cancers, and abnormal menstrual history have been associated with an increased incidence of the disease. A familial or personal history of other cancers, including breast, colon, and uterine cancers, increase the risk for ovarian cancer.

III. PREVENTION, SCREENING, AND DETECTION

No known cost-effective tests or tumor markers are recommended for early detection of ovarian cancer. Certain hereditary syndromes have been described and include hereditary breast/ovarian cancer syndromes associated with changes at chromosome 17q (BRAC1) and chromosome 13q (BRAC2) (see Chapter 2). These familial cancers typically appear at a younger age than sporadic ovarian cancer. Options regarding prevention of ovarian cancer in women at high risk may include prophylactic oophorectomy, tubal ligation, or both. Additional factors that offer some degree of protection include oral contraceptives, pregnancy, breast-feeding, and following a low-fat, high-fiber diet.

IV. CLASSIFICATION

Ovarian cancers are classified as epithelial, sex cord-stromal (5%) or germ cell (5%) tumors. Epithelial tumors found in women 40 to 65 years of age account for 90% of all ovarian malignancies.

V. CLINICAL FEATURES

Vague gastrointestinal symptoms such as dyspepsia, indigestion, anorexia, and early satiety may be some of the initial symptoms of ovarian cancer. Increased pressure of the tumor on the rectum and bladder may result in symptoms of urinary frequency, constipation, or pelvic discomfort. Progressive disease is noted by an increase in the abdominal girth, pain, shortness of breath, or intestinal or ureteral obstruction.

VI. DIAGNOSIS AND STAGING

Tissue sampling and inspection of the abdominal cavity at the time of exploratory laparotomy achieve diagnosis and staging goals for women with ovarian cancer. A careful and methodical approach is used to remove (debulk) as much of the tumor burden as possible at this time.

VII. METASTASIS

Ovarian cancer spreads by direct extension to adjacent pelvic organs such as opposite ovary, uterus, fallopian tubes, bladder, rectum, and peritoneum and by seeding of the peritoneal cavity and lymphatic and vascular channels.

Cancer Types

VIII. SURVIVAL
Prognostic outcomes for ovarian cancer that are associated with poorer survival include age (older patients), grade (poorly differentiated lesions), histology type (clear cell and mucinous types), stage (more extensive disease), and volume of disease (stage III with a larger volume of residual cells). Five-year survival rates according to the stage are 95% for early stage disease and disease treated aggressively, 81% for regional disease, and 29% for distant disease. The overall survival rate for all stages combined is 52%.

IX. TREATMENT MODALITIES
The treatment of ovarian cancer is based on the surgical staging of the disease, malignant potential of the tumor, and the bulk of the remaining disease. Surgery (surgical removal of uterus, cervix, fallopian, and ovaries) with the debulking of any remaining disease is performed with resection of the bladder, colon, or omentum if indicated. Radiation therapy is delivered through instillation of radioactive isotopes in the peritoneal cavity and has been used in women with early stage disease. Chemotherapy drugs including cisplatin-based therapy at conventional doses without paclitaxel; paclitaxel plus cisplatin at conventional doses; or other drugs such as gemcitabine, topotecan, or trastuzumab are used in many chemotherapy regimens. High-dose chemotherapy with autologous stem cell transplantation is used in varied treatment regimens.

UTERUS

I. INCIDENCE
An estimated 40,100 cases of cancer of the uterine corpus (endometrium or lining of the uterus) will occur in 2003. Incidence rates are greater among white women (22.9/100,000) than among black women (15.7/100,000).

II. MORTALITY
Approximately 6800 deaths related to uterine cancer will occur in 2003, with mortality rates of 5.7/100,000

in black women compared with 3.1/100,000 in white women.

III. ETIOLOGY/RISK FACTORS

High cumulative exposure to estrogen is the major risk factor for the most common type of cancer of the uterine corpus. Estrogen-related exposure including estrogen replacement therapy or hormone replacement therapy (HRT), tamoxifen, early menarche, never having children, and a history of failure to ovulate have all been shown to increase the risk for endometrial cancer. Progesterone plus HRT is believed to largely offset the increased risk related to HRT using *only* estrogen. Additional risk factors include infertility, diabetes, gallbladder disease, hypertension, and obesity. Pregnancy and the use of contraceptives appear to provide protection against endometrial cancer. Hereditary nonpolyposis colon cancer, a genetic syndrome, also has been associated with endometrial and ovarian cancer.

IV. PREVENTION, SCREENING, AND DETECTION

Primary prevention is targeted toward women at high risk. Maintenance of ideal body weight is recommended to avoid obesity and to decrease the risk for hypertension and diabetes. No reliable, valid, or cost-effective tests are recommended for periodic screening of asymptomatic women for endometrial cancer. An annual history to review risk factors with a physical examination to evaluate the size, consistency, and shape of the uterus is recommended. An endometrial biopsy is obtained for histologic confirmation of the disease.

V. CLASSIFICATION

The primary types of endometrial cancer are adenocarcinoma, sarcoma, mucinous carcinoma, serous carcinoma, clear cell carcinoma, and epidermoid carcinoma.

VI. CLINICAL FEATURES

Usual reporting signs and symptoms include abnormal uterine bleeding or spotting. This abnormal bleeding is usually prolonged, excessive, irregular premenopausal or postmenopausal bleeding. Women with advanced disease may have pain, intestinal obstruction, ascites, jaundice, respiratory distress, or hemorrhage.

VII. DIAGNOSIS AND STAGING

The diagnostic evaluation includes physical examination, vaginal probe ultrasonography, color flow–Doppler studies, and tissue sampling with laboratory and radiographic studies to determine the histologic type, degree of differentiation, and extent of disease. Cervical biopsies and endocervical curettage are collected to minimize the risk for contamination of the cervical specimen with the endometrial tissue. Additional studies include complete blood count, cancer antigen 125 levels, blood, renal and chemistries, chest x-ray, magnetic resonance imaging (MRI), and computed tomography (CT) scans. If involvement of the bladder or rectum is suspected, an IVP, barium enema, cystoscopy, and proctosigmoidoscopy may also be performed. The TNM staging system is used for endometrial cancer.

VIII. METASTASIS

Most endometrial cancers originate in the fundus of the uterus and spread by direct extension to the entire endometrium through the layers of the uterine wall or through the endocervical canal to the cervix.

IX. SURVIVAL

The 1-year relative survival rate for endometrial cancer is 93%. The 5-year relative survival is 96% for local disease, 63% for regional disease, and 26% if the disease is diagnosed at a distant stage.

X. TREATMENT MODALITIES

Endometrial cancers are usually treated with surgery, radiation therapy, hormonal therapy, or chemotherapy depending on the disease stage. Surgical removal (total abdominal hysterectomy and bilateral salpingo-oophorectomy) is the most common primary treatment for women with early stage disease. Radiation therapy may consist of intracavity brachytherapy, vaginal cuff irradiation, and external beam. Hormonal manipulation therapy is used either as adjuvant or as treatment for recurrent disease. Chemotherapy is reserved for women who have estrogen- and progesterone-negative tumors, who have not responded to hormone therapy, or who have disseminated disease. Agents typically used include cisplatin, docetaxel, doxorubicin, vincristine, carboplatin, hexamethylmelamine, and ifosfamide.

VAGINA

I. INCIDENCE/MORTALITY
Approximately 2000 new vaginal cancer cases with approximately 800 deaths related to vaginal cancer will occur in 2003.

II. ETIOLOGY/RISK FACTORS
The cause of vaginal cancer is unknown; however, prior radiation to a field including the vagina, diethylstilbestrol (DES) exposure in utero, and increasing age place women at greater risk for the disease.

III. PREVENTION, SCREENING, AND DETECTION
No recommendations exist for the prevention and screening of women for vaginal cancer. An annual physical examination including inspection and palpation of the vaginal tissues, cervical cytology, and bimanual pelvic examination should be done routinely for women who are sexually active or are 18 years or older.

IV. CLASSIFICATION
Most carcinomas of the vagina are squamous cell cancers (93% to 97%). Other cell types include clear cell carcinoma associated with exposure to DES in utero, malignant melanoma, and sarcoma.

V. CLINICAL FEATURES
Most patients have postcoital, perimenopausal, or postmenopausal *painless bleeding*.

VI. DIAGNOSIS AND STAGING
Definitive diagnosis of preinvasive and invasive carcinoma of the vagina is made by tissue biopsy of a gross or colposcopic detected lesion. Staging is done clinically based on inspection, palpation, and bimanual examination. Radiographic studies, a biochemical profile, chest

Cancer Types

x-ray, IVP, barium enema, cystoscopy, proctoscopy, MRI, and CT scans are used in the diagnostic work-up. The TNM system is used to stage vaginal cancer.

VII. METASTASIS

Squamous cell carcinoma of the vagina spreads primarily by direct extension to adjacent tissues, including the urethra, bladder, rectum, parametria, and pelvic sidewall.

VIII. SURVIVAL

Survival at 5 years after diagnosis of primary vaginal cancer is as follows: 65% to 85% for stage I, 50% to 66% for stage II, 15% to 39% for stage III, and 0% to 25% for stage IV. Overall survival for all stages combined range from 42% to 56%.

IX. TREATMENT MODALITIES

Surgery is recommended as treatment for women with stage I and II disease. This treatment may consist of radical hysterectomy, vaginectomy with formation of split thickness of skin graft neovagina, and lymphoidectomy. Radiation therapy alone or in combination with surgery is recommended for women with stage II and higher carcinoma of the vagina. Chemotherapy has not shown a benefit for women with vaginal cancer.

VULVA

I. INCIDENCE/MORTALITY

Approximately 4000 new vulvar cancer cases and approximately 800 deaths related to vulvar cancer will occur in 2003.

II. ETIOLOGY/RISK FACTORS

The etiologic factors of vulvar cancer are unknown; however, factors associated with an increased disease incidence include concurrent diseases such as hypertension, diabetes, cardiovascular disease, obesity, cervical cancer, early menopause, nulliparity, and chronic vulvar irritation.

III. PREVENTION, SCREENING, AND DETECTION
Nonspecific measures are recommended for the prevention of vulvar cancer.

IV. CLASSIFICATION
Invasive cancers of the vulva are classified as squamous cell, basal cell, adenocarcinoma, and malignant melanoma. Ninety percent of all cancers of the vulva are squamous cell carcinomas.

V. CLINICAL FEATURES
Most women with vulvar cancer are asymptomatic; therefore a thorough history and physical examination with inspection and palpation of vulvar tissue for abnormalities are necessary.

VI. DIAGNOSIS AND STAGING
Diagnostic and staging examinations consist of cystoscopy, proctoscopy, barium enema, IVP, lymphangiography, CT scans, MRI, and a wedge biopsy for clinically staging vulvar cancer. The TNM classification system is used for staging.

VII. METASTASIS
Direct extension occurs in adjacent structures including the vagina, perineum, clitoris, and anus. Lymphatic embolization to regional nodes may occur early in the disease.

VIII. SURVIVAL
Five-year survival for patients with vulvar cancer treated with a curative intent are as follows: 92% for stage I, 80% for stage II, 53% for stage III, and 15% for stage IV. Overall patient survival for stages I to IV is 71%. The overall 5-year survival of patients with positive lymph nodes is 50%, and the overall survival rate for patients treated with palliation is 47%.

IX. TREATMENT MODALITIES
The treatment of vulvar cancer is based on the size and extent of the lesion, depth of stromal invasion, and evidence of metastatic disease.

Cancer Types

For women with preinvasive disease (vulvar intraepithelial neoplasm or carcinoma in situ) in a limited area, a conservative approach with topical fluorouracil, cryotherapy, laser therapy, wide local excision, or simple vulvectomy can be used. When more extensive disease (>2 cm in diameter and >5 mm invasion) is present, a radical vulvectomy with complete, bilateral groin dissection is performed. Chemotherapy has been used (fluorouracil, cisplatin, methotrexate, cyclophosphamide, bleomycin, and mitomycin C) through single-agent administration or combination therapy. Radiation therapy has been used before and after surgery in conjunction with surgery for women with locally advanced disease.

FALLOPIAN TUBE

I. INCIDENCE/MORTALITY
Cancer of the fallopian tube accounts for only 0.1% of all cancers of the female reproductive tract with approximately 300 cases reported annually.

II. ETIOLOGY/RISK FACTORS
The etiologic factors of cancer of the fallopian tubes are unknown, but chronic inflammation of the tubes may contribute to the disease. This cancer usually occurs in the fifth or sixth decade of life, with ages ranging from 14 years to 88 years and a mean age of 57 years.

III. PREVENTION, SCREENING, AND DETECTION
No known recommendations are made specifically for the prevention of and screening for cancer of the fallopian tubes.

IV. CLASSIFICATION
Adenocarcinoma is the most common histologic type of cancer of the fallopian tube. Sarcomas, mixed mesodermal tumors, lymphomas, hydatidiform moles, and choriocarcinoma have been reported.

V. CLINICAL FEATURES
Postmenopausal women may present with symptoms of vaginal bleeding; intermittent, colicky, dull, aching

pain; and profuse watery serosanguineous vaginal discharge.

VI. DIAGNOSIS AND STAGING
Diagnosis of fallopian cancer is made at the time of surgery for the definitive treatment of a pelvic mass.

VII. METASTASIS
Carcinoma of the fallopian tube metastasizes primarily by direct extension to adjacent tissues and organs, seeding of the abdominal cavity, and lymphatic spread to locoregional nodes.

VIII. SURVIVAL
The survival rates for patients with fallopian tube cancer are similar to that of patients with ovarian cancer. The survival rate for all stages combined has been reported to be 40%, but it is as high as 88% in patients with stage I disease.

IX. TREATMENT MODALITIES
Surgery is the cornerstone of the initial treatment and usually follows the practice for epithelial ovarian cancer. Usually a total abdominal hysterectomy–bilateral salpingo-oophorectomy and omentectomy are performed followed by removing as much tumor as possible with collection of ascitic or peritoneal fluid, sampling of pelvic and para-aortic lymph nodes, and a careful examination of the extent of the disease. Interperitoneal radioactive isotopes or systemic single-agent or combination chemotherapy with cyclophosphamide, doxorubicin, progestins, cisplatin, or chlorambucil is recommended.

GESTATIONAL TROPHOBLASTIC DISEASE

I. INCIDENCE/MORTALITY
Gestational trophoblastic disease (GTD) consists of several disorders that arise from placental trophoblastic tissue after abnormal fertilization. These include hydatidiform mole, choriocarcinoma, chorioadenoma, and placental site trophoblastic tumor. It accounts

for only 1% of all cancers of the female reproductive system.

II. ETIOLOGY/RISK FACTORS

As previously stated, GTD includes a variety of tumors that originate in the trophoblastic layer of the chorionic villi during pregnancy. A woman who has had a hydatidiform mole has an approximately 1000-fold greater chance for choriocarcinoma development than a woman who has a live birth.

III. PREVENTION, SCREENING, AND DETECTION

No recommendations for prevention or screening of asymptomatic women for GTD are available. The detection of GTD is based on a careful review of findings on the history, clinical examination, and laboratory studies. Disparities such as uterine size inconsistent with estimated gestational age and abnormal human chorionic gonadotropin (HCG) levels are the keys to early detection.

IV. CLASSIFICATION

GTD classified morphologically as hydatidiform moles, invasive moles, or choriocarcinoma has a greater incidence of metastasis to surrounding tissues and thus has a poor prognosis.

V. CLINICAL FEATURES

The most common symptom of GTD is vaginal bleeding, particularly during the first trimester. A history of hyperemesis, enlargement of the uterus in excess of estimated length of gestation, an abnormal ultrasound appearance of the intrauterine contents, abnormal fetal heart sounds, and fetal parts that cannot be palpated are also signs of GTD.

VI. DIAGNOSIS AND STAGING

Diagnosis of GTD is confirmed by tissue examination from expulsion of grapelike villi, vaginal bleeding, or evacuation of tissues from the uterus.

Staging of GTD is classified by two major categories:

I   Nonmetastatic disease: no evidence of disease outside the uterus

II   Metastatic disease: any disease outside of uterus

VII. METASTASIS

Metastasis from GTD occurs primarily by local extension to surrounding tissues of the pelvis or through hematogenous spread. The most common sites of distant metastases include lungs, brain, and liver.

VIII. SURVIVAL

Survival for GTD is reported based on the percentage of patients who achieve remission with treatment. For patients with nonmetastatic disease, remission (HCG levels within normal range for 3 consecutive weeks) rates with single-agent chemotherapy range from 90% to 100%. Remission rates for patients with metastatic disease to lungs or vagina who received combination chemotherapy and radiation therapy are 74%.

IX. TREATMENT MODALITIES

Hysterectomy as primary therapy for hydatidiform mole is acceptable for women who have completed childbearing. Patients with nonmetastatic disease and low-risk metastatic disease are treated with single-agent chemotherapy using methotrexate or actinomycin D. Radiation therapy has a role in the treatment of women with metastatic disease. The cure rate of GTD exceeds 90%. Measurement of HCG values provides a reliable means to determine the response to therapy and to detect recurrent disease in cases of molar pregnancy and gestational trophoblastic neoplasia.

Patients should be monitored with serum HCG monthly for at least 1 year. Contraception is needed for a minimum of 6 months, but 12 months is preferred. If pregnancy should develop, an early ultrasound should be performed to document an intrauterine pregnancy.

Bibliography

American Cancer Society: *Cancer facts and figures 2003*, Atlanta, 2003, The Society.

American Cancer Society: *Cancer prevention and early detection, facts and figures 2003*, Atlanta, 2003, The Society.

Boyle D: Psychosocial issues. In Lin EM, editor: *Advanced practice in oncology nursing*, Philadelphia, 2001, WB Saunders.

Chu E, DeVita VT Jr: Principles of cancer management: chemotherapy. In DeVita VT Jr, Hellman S, Rosenberg SA, editors:

Cancer Types

Cancer principles and practice of oncology, ed 6, Philadelphia, 2001, JB Lippincott.

Cooper DL, Seropian S: Autologous stem cell transplantation. In DeVita VT Jr, Hellman S, Rosenberg SA, editors: *Cancer principles and practice of oncology,* ed 6, Philadelphia, 2001, JB Lippincott.

Fleming I, Cooper JS, Henson DE: *AJCC cancer staging manual,* ed 5, Philadelphia, 2002, Lippincott Williams & Wilkins.

Goedegebuure PS, Eberlein TJ: Tumor biology and tumor markers. In Townsend CM Jr, Beauchamp RD, Evers BM, et al, editors: *Textbook of surgery, the biological basis of modern surgical practice,* ed 16, Philadelphia, 2001, WB Saunders.

Giarelli E: Ethical issues in genetic testing, *J Infus Nurs* 24(5):310, 2001.

Hoskins WM: Surveying the field of gynecologic oncology, *Oncology Spectrum* 2(5):312, 2001.

Jemal A, Murray T, Samuels A, et al: Cancer statistics, 2003, *CA Cancer J Clin* 53(1):5, 2003.

Jennings-Dozier K, Mahon SM, editors: *Cancer prevention, detection, and control,* Pittsburgh, 2002, Oncology Nursing Press.

Lea DH, Williams JK: Genetic testing and screening, *Am J Nurs* 102(7):36, 2002.

McGuire WP: Treatment of advanced epithelial ovarian cancer, *Clinical Oncology Updates* 5(1):1, 2002.

Otto SE, editor: *Oncology nursing,* ed 4, St. Louis, 2001, Mosby.

Pasacreta JV, Jacobs L, Cataldo JK: Genetic testing for breast and ovarian cancer risk: the psychosocial issues, *Am J Nurs* 102(12):40, 2002.

Rosenberg SA: Principles of cancer management: surgical oncology. In DeVita VT Jr, Hellman S, Rosenberg SA, editors: *Cancer principles and practice of oncology,* ed 6, Philadelphia, 2001, JB Lippincott.

Smith RA, Cokkinides V, Eyre HJ: American Cancer Society Guidelines for the early detection of cancer, 2003, *CA Cancer J Clin* 53(1):27, 2003.

Zimmerman VL: BRCA gene mutations and cancer, *Am J Nurs* 102(8):28, 2002.

12 Head and Neck Cancers

I. INCIDENCE
Head and neck (H&N) cancers will account for an estimated total of 27,700 new cancer cases in 2003. This number includes tongue (7100), mouth (9200), pharynx (8300), and other parts of the oral cavity (3100). The incidence rates are more than *twice* as high in *men* as in women and are greatest in men who are older than 40 years.

II. MORTALITY
As estimated total of 7200 deaths related to H&N cancer will occur in 2003, with a distribution among the following regions: tongue (1700), mouth (1900), pharynx (2000), and other sites (1600). The mortality rates for H&N cancer have been decreasing by about 1.3% per year.

III. ETIOLOGY/RISK FACTORS
Cigarette, cigar, or pipe smoking; use of smokeless tobacco; and excessive alcohol intake are the major risk factors associated with H&N cancer. Environmental and occupational exposures to ultraviolet rays of sun, asbestos, radiation, certain chemicals, coke ovens, or wood or nickel refining also increase the risk for H&N cancer.

IV. PREVENTION, SCREENING, AND DETECTION
Dentists and primary care clinicians most often detect abnormalities in the oral cavity such as a red or white lesion on the tongue, gums, or floor of the mouth. When lesions are detected early and prompt intervention is provided, this early stage cancer can be cured. All

individuals should participate in biannual dental examinations and annual health examinations.

V. CLINICAL FEATURES

A sore that bleeds easily and does not heal, a lump or thickening, or a red or white lesion on the tongue or in the mouth are among the most common symptoms. Additional patient-reported complaints include difficulty in chewing, swallowing, or moving the tongue around in the mouth; persistent headaches; bloody drainage from nose; hoarseness; and pain in ear or neck areas.

VI. CLASSIFICATION/DIAGNOSIS AND STAGING

The optimal treatment and patient survival require accurate identification of the primary tumor, locoregional disease spread, and distant metastasis. A thorough examination of the head and neck region with the use of a mirror or fiberoptic nasopharyngolaryngoscope is essential. In addition, radiologic examinations, magnetic resonance imaging, computed tomography scans, direct triple endoscopy examinations, bronchoscopy, and multiple biopsies are performed to attain the definitive diagnosis.

The TNM staging system is used to classify the disease for the following differential anatomic sites: nasopharynx, oropharynx, hypopharynx, nasal cavity, oral cavity, and larynx. Squamous cell carcinoma (95%) is the most common histologic cell type for H&N cancer. Prior to any definitive treatment, consultative assessments are completed for dental, pulmonary, nutritional, psychosocial, communication, and cognitive motor skills, and an evaluation of rehabilitation needs is assessed.

VII. METASTASIS

Most H&N cancers spread by direct extension and penetration into the tissue layers. Local invasion occurs to adjacent structures in the head and neck region. Lymph node involvement and invasion into the vascular bed allow for disseminated disease. Primary metastatic sites include brain, lung, and bone.

VIII. SURVIVAL

For all stages combined, about 81% of oral cavity and pharynx cancer patients survive 1 year after the diagnosis. The 5- and 10-year relative survival rates are 56% and 41%, respectively.

IX. TREATMENT MODALITIES

Combined multimodality therapy (surgery, radiation therapy, and chemotherapy) is the common approach for the treatment of H&N cancers. If the disease is detected at an early stage, surgery, radiation, or both therapies are usually selected. When lymph nodes are involved, disease extension into adjacent tissue, distant disease, or both is present; all three therapies are used in combination. For example, chemotherapy, radiation therapy, or both may be given before surgery to shrink the tumor mass, thus allowing a more optimal surgical resection of the involved tissue. Chemotherapy, radiation therapy, or both are then administered after surgery to prevent metastatic disease caused by the spread of cancer cells that may be missed in the surgical procedures.

The specific surgical procedure(s) may include removal, resection, nodal dissection, or procedures such as laryngectomy, tracheostomy, and radical neck dissection, with sequential grafts and flaps used in the reconstructive process. Each surgical procedure is based on the anatomic disease site, extent of disease, and functional outcome for the patient.

Chemotherapy scheduling and timing such as neoadjuvant, concurrent (postoperative with surgery), sandwich (used after surgery or before radiotherapy), and maintenance (used after surgery and radiotherapy) have demonstrated effectiveness in patient survival outcomes. Drugs selected for these regimens include doxorubicin, methotrexate, bleomycin, cyclophosphamide, cisplatin, carboplatin, fluorouracil, vinblastine, and vincristine. Newer drugs such as paclitaxel, ifosfamide, gemcitabine, topotecan, amonafide, and uracil have been added to the many drug combinations to improve the patient's response to therapy.

Bibliography

Aft RL: Principles of surgical oncology. In Govindan R, Arquette MA, editors: *The Washington manual of oncology*, Philadelphia, 2002, Lippincott Williams & Wilkins.

American Cancer Society, *Cancer prevention and early detection, facts and figures 2003*, Atlanta, 2003, The Society.

American Cancer Society, *Cancer facts and figures 2003*, Atlanta, 2003, The Society.

Arquette MA: Head and neck cancer. In Govindan R, Arquette MA, editors: *The Washington manual of oncology*, Philadelphia, 2002, Lippincott Williams & Wilkins.

Beyers T, Nestle M, McTiernan A, et al: American Cancer Society Guidelines on nutrition and physical activity for cancer prevention: reducing the risks of cancer with healthy food choices and physical activity, *CA Cancer J Clin* 52(2):92, 2002.

Bradley JD, Perez CA: Fundamentals of patient management in radiation oncology. In Govindan R, Arquette MA, editors: *The Washington manual of oncology*, Philadelphia, 2002, Lippincott Williams & Wilkins.

Camp-Sorrell D: Surviving the cancer, surviving the treatment: acute cardiac and pulmonary toxicity, *Oncol Nurs Forum* 26(6):983, 1999.

Chu E, DeVita VT Jr: Principles of cancer management: chemotherapy, In DeVita VT Jr, Hellman S, Rosenberg SA, editors: *Cancer principles and practice of oncology*, ed 6, Philadelphia, 2001, JB Lippincott.

Cotran RS, Kumar V, Collins T: *Pathologic basis of disease*, ed 6, Philadelphia, 1999, WB Saunders.

Fleming I, Cooper JS, Henson DE, et al: *AJCC cancer staging manual*, ed 5, Philadelphia, 2002, Lippincott Williams & Wilkins.

Haggood AS: Head and neck cancers. In Otto SE, editor: *Oncology nursing*, ed 2, St. Louis, 2001, Mosby.

Hawkins R: Mastering the intricate maze of metastasis, *Oncol Nurs Forum* 28(6):959, 2001.

Hellman S: Principles of cancer management: Radiation therapy. In DeVita VT Jr, Hellman S, Rosenberg SA, editors: *Cancer principles and practice of oncology*, ed 6, Philadelphia, 2001, JB Lippincott.

Hodgson BB, Kizior RJ: *Saunders nursing drug handbook 2003*, Philadelphia, 2003, WB Saunders.

Holland JF, editor: *Cancer medicine*, ed 5, Philadelphia, American Cancer Society, Hamilton, Ontario, 2000, BC Decker.

Jemal A, Murray T, Samuels A, et al: Cancer Statistics, 2003, *CA Cancer J Clin* 53(1):5, 2003.

McCaffery M, Pasero C: *Pain: clinical manual*, ed 2, St. Louis, 1999, Mosby.

Oncology Nursing Society: *Cancer chemotherapy guidelines and recommendations for practice*, Pittsburgh, 2001, Oncology Nursing Press.

Smith RA, Cokkinides V, Eyre HJ: American Cancer Society Guidelines for the early detection of cancer, 2003, *CA Cancer J Clin* 53(1):27, 2003.

Thompson JM, McFarland GK, Hirsch JE, et al: *Mosby's clinical nursing*, ed 5, St. Louis, 2002, Mosby.

Human Immunodeficiency Virus and Related Cancers

I. INCIDENCE

In the early 1980s an illness later defined as acquired immunodeficiency syndrome (AIDS) was reported by the California health care providers to the Centers for Disease Control and Prevention (CDC). Currently, human immunodeficiency virus (HIV)/AIDS remains a significant global health problem. More than 40 million people worldwide are infected with the HIV virus that causes AIDS. Almost half of the new adult infections are among those 15 to 24 years old. Twelve million teenagers and young adults are living with HIV, with more than 6000 becoming infected each day. In addition, 14 million children living today have lost one or both parents to AIDS-related deaths. In the United States, approximately 40,000 new HIV cases occur annually.

II. MORTALITY

In 2000, HIV disease accounted for 10,074 deaths in men 20 to 59 years old, 3365 deaths occurred in women 20 to 59 years old, and 60 deaths occurred in children 1 to 14 years old. In the United States, the HIV death rate began to decline in the 1990s with the availability of antiretroviral therapy; HIV/AIDS-related deaths decreased from 49,895 in 1996 to 17,171 in 1998.

III. ETIOLOGY/RISK FACTORS

The routes for transmission of HIV include intimate sexual contact, parenteral exposure to blood, exposure to blood-containing body fluids and blood products, and mother-to-child contact during the perinatal period.

Although HIV has been identified in a variety of body fluids, those consistently shown to be infectious are blood, semen, and vaginal secretions. Transmission has also been associated with breast milk. HIV is directly transmitted from person to person through sexual contact; through direct inoculation with contaminated blood products, needles, or syringes; and from an infected mother to her newborn.

IV. PREVENTION, SCREENING, AND DETECTION
To decrease infection rates, the CDC has begun a new strategy called SAFE (Serostatus Approach to Fighting the HIV Epidemic). This program intends to decrease new cases of HIV infection in the United States by 50% by the end of 2005. The major program components include the following:

- Increasing efforts to assist all infected people in learning their HIV-positive status (a campaign called "Know Now" will make testing more widely available)
- Helping people infected with HIV adopt and maintain safe behaviors and have better access to treatment
- Promoting adherence to prescribed HIV antiretroviral therapy
- Improving prevention programs for people who are at high risk for HIV infection

V. CLASSIFICATION/CLINICAL FEATURES
At the initial infectious event, many people are unaware they carry the virus that causes AIDS. Although a viral-type syndrome resembling influenza or mononucleosis may develop in some people within a few days or weeks of the infection, most individuals are unaware and do not relate it to the initial infection. The acute infection period is followed by a long period (5 to 10 years) of asymptomatic HIV infection.

As HIV progresses and depletes the body of sufficient numbers of T4 helper cells, subtle symptoms of immunodeficiency may emerge. Persistent generalized lymphadenopathy or minor dermatologic manifestations begin to develop. It is during this time that a slow, persistent destruction of the immune system occurs with a gradual decline in the number of CD4 cells. With a continued destruction of the immune system, opportunistic infections and malignancies begin to develop and cause clinical symptoms. The clinical findings that often signal the rapid progression to end-stage HIV/AIDS disease include unexplained severe weight loss greater than 10% of usual body weight, persistent fever, diarrhea, and night sweats longer than 2 weeks in duration.

VI. DIAGNOSIS AND STAGING/METASTASIS

The single most important advance in HIV care is viral load testing that allows the clinician to more accurately stage the patient with HIV disease based on the measurable status of the immune system. Viral load studies measure the level of plasma HIV-1 RNA, which is proportional to the rate of viral replication and CD4 lymphocyte destruction. Viral load testing is the single most important predictor of HIV progression. For example, the report reads as CD4 count less than 350 to 500 cells/mm^3 or viral load greater than 20,000 copies/ml with recommendations to treat with combination antiretrovirals.

HIV is a chronic, progressive disease characterized in four distinct categories as listed in the CDC classification system for HIV infections in adults as follows:

A. **Stage I—**
Acute infection: occurs at initial HIV infection may last days to weeks

B. **Stage II—**
Asymptomatic infection: occurs after stage I and may last for several years

C. **Stage III—**
Persistent generalized lymphadenopathy: characterized by palpable lymph nodes persisting for more than 3 months

D. **Stage IV—**
Presence of other diseases (neurologic), opportunistic infections, secondary cancers (Kaposi's sarcoma, non-Hodgkin's lymphoma, primary lymphoma of brain)

HIV disease is a chronic, systemic infection. The infection itself primarily infects a specific group of lymphocytes (the CD4 lymphocytes) but also has the potential for direct infection of the monocytes and macrophages and possibly muscle and nerve cells. Many patients also experience HIV infection directly affecting the CNS and illness affecting the skin, mucous membranes, and respiratory and gastrointestinal tracts. The disease progresses as described earlier in the staging categories until the patient's immune system is no longer functional and succumbs to the stage IV–related complications.

VII. SURVIVAL

Highly active antiretroviral therapy, better prophylaxis, and effective treatment of opportunistic infections contribute to the survival of patients with AIDS. With HIV infection, cancer risk increases gradually, and with prolonged survival in patients with AIDS, the probability exists for more neoplasms to develop in these patients.

VIII. TREATMENT MODALITIES

Several treatment options are available to slow the disease progression of the illness, but currently no cure exists for HIV disease. Drug therapy for HIV/AIDS has progressed rapidly since the 1980s when the focus of treatment was for *Pneumocystis carinii* pneumonia and other opportunistic infections. Current therapy targets HIV with multiple antiretroviral drugs aimed at interrupting the viral replication. The following antiretroviral drugs work inside the infected CD4+ cells by inhibiting the action of enzymes necessary for HIV replication.

- Nonnucleoside reverse transcriptase inhibitors attach to the reverse transcriptase enzyme, preventing the enzyme from converting HIV RNA to DNA.
- Nucleoside reverse transcriptase inhibitors (NRTIs) become a part of HIV DNA and derail the building process. The damaged viral DNA is unable to take control of the cell's DNA.
- Protease inhibitors work at a later stage in the replication process, preventing the protease enzyme from cutting HIV viral proteins into the virions that infect new CD4+ cells. The new copies of HIV will be defective and unable to infect other CD4+ cells. Combining drugs from these categories allows them to block the HIV at several points in the replication process, thus slowing its spread in the body.

Additional therapies include biotherapy agents such as growth factors for treatment of anemia and leukopenia. Multiple other drugs such as antiemetics, antifungals, antimicrobials, and analgesics are used to manage the varied complications or symptoms that accompany the declining immune system or the treatment drug side effects (see Chapter 25).

IX. HIV-RELATED CANCERS

People with AIDS are at an increased risk for Kaposi's sarcoma, non-Hodgkin's lymphoma, and Hodgkin's disease. These cancers also have been associated with specific human viruses, for example, human herpes virus infections. Additional cancers that occur in the AIDS population include primary central nervous system lymphoma and cervical and anal carcinoma. The diagnostic evaluation and specific treatment for these HIV-related cancers receive similar interventions to those discussed in other chapters throughout this book. Unfortunately, patients with HIV/AIDS have a moderate to severe immunosuppression that may limit certain drugs or dosing principles specifically impacting the bone marrow.

Bibliography

American Cancer Society: *Cancer prevention and early detection, facts and figures 2003*, Atlanta, 2003, The Society.

American Cancer Society: *Cancer facts and figures 2003*, Atlanta, 2003, The Society.

Brogdon C: Human immunodeficiency virus (HIV). In Otto SE, editor: *Oncology nursing*, ed 4, St. Louis, 2001, Mosby.

Coyne PJ, Lyne ME, Watson AC: Symptom management in people with AIDS, *Am J Nurs* 102(9):48, 2002.

Greenwald SL, Goodman M, Frogge M, et al: *Cancer nursing: principles and practice*, ed 5, Boston, 2000, Jones and Bartlett.

Jemal A, Murray T, Samuels A, et al: Cancer statistics, 2003, *CA Cancer J Clin* 53(1):5, 2003.

Paice JA: Managing psychological conditions in palliative care, *Am J Nurs* 102(11):36, 2002.

Jones SG: Taking HAART, how to support patients with HIV/AIDS, *Nursing* 31(12):36, 2001.

Pagana KD, Pagana TJ: *Mosby's diagnostic and laboratory test reference*, St. Louis, 2002, Mosby.

Tan B, Ratner L: AIDS-associated malignancies. In Govindan R, Arquette MA, editors: *The Washington manual of oncology*, Philadelphia, 2002, Lippincott Williams & Wilkins.

Thompson JM, McFarland GK, Hirsch JE, et al: *Mosby's clinical nursing*, ed 5, St. Louis, 2002, Mosby.

Cancer Types

14
Leukemia

I. INCIDENCE

Approximately 30,600 new cases of leukemia are expected to occur in 2003, with those numbers evenly divided between acute and chronic leukemia cases. Leukemia is diagnosed 10 times more frequently in adults than in children. Acute lymphocytic leukemia accounts for approximately 2200 cases in children. In the adult, the most common types are acute myeloid leukemia (10,500 cases) and chronic lymphocytic leukemia (7300 cases). Acute myeloid leukemia has increased in adults by 1.8% from 1992 to 1998, with most of this increase in the elderly; this escalation may also be related to cigarette smoking.

II. MORTALITY

An estimated 21,900 deaths from leukemia are expected in 2003.

III. ETIOLOGY/RISK FACTORS

Leukemia affects both sexes and all ages. Specific causes are unknown. The incidence of leukemia is greater among patients with Down syndrome or genetic alterations. Excessive exposure to ionizing radiation, certain chemicals such as benzene, and cigarette smoke also increase the risk for leukemia. It can also occur as a side effect related to cancer treatment. Certain leukemias and lymphomas are caused by a retrovirus, human T-cell leukemia/lymphoma virus-1.

IV. PREVENTION, SCREENING, AND DETECTION
The prevention and detection of leukemia are not applicable because there are no identified preventable risks, and early detection is hampered by the vagueness of the common symptoms. Leukemia can be difficult to diagnose in the early stages; therefore patients are encouraged to seek prompt medical attention for persistent, common clinical features.

V. CLASSIFICATION
Leukemia is a malignant hematologic disorder characterized by a proliferation of abnormal white blood cells (WBCs) that infiltrate the bone marrow, peripheral blood, and other organs and may present as an acute or chronic disease process. Leukemias are classified by their stem cell of origin—erythroid, megakaroid, myeloid, or lymphoid committed cells. Multiple classification systems exist to classify the different types of leukemia.

A. French-American British (FAB) Classification—

   1. Acute Lymphocytic Leukemia (ALL)—Classification for ALL is as follows:
   - L1 (80% of childhood leukemias and 30% of leukemias in adults)
   - L2 (adult form of lymphocytic leukemia)
   - L3 (rare leukemia that is present in 2% to 7% of patients with leukemia and resembles Burkitt's lymphoma)

   ALL is characterized by presence of fever, presence of infection, adenopathy present in 80% of cases, headaches, and *blast cells* (very immature WBC) at a rate of less than 50,000 mm^3 in 60% of cases. Further definitive classifications include the following:
   - WBC count >10,000 mm^3 in 50% to 60% of cases
   - WBC count <100,000 mm^3 in 30% to 40% of cases
   - WBC count >100,000 mm^3 in 10% of cases
   - Platelet count <50,000 mm^3 in 60% of cases
   - Bone marrow: hypercellular, blasts 30% or greater, and a decreased red blood cell count
   - Cerebrospinal fluid: cytology infiltration with leukemic cells at diagnosis—children 5% and adults <10%

2. *Acute Myeloid Leukemia (AML)*—Classification of AML is as follows:
   - M0: 7%
   - M1 myeloblastic (without myeloid maturation): 20%
   - M2 myeloblastic (with myeloid maturation): 30%
   - M3 promyelocytic: 10%
   - M3-variant (M3V)
   - M4 myelomonocytic: 15% to 20%
   - M4E: 5% to 10%
   - M5 monocytic: subtype A, 5%; subtype B, 5%
   - M6 erythroleukemia: <5%
   - M7 megakaryocytic: <5%

AML is characterized by presence of serious infections (30%), significant bleeding (30%), intracutaneous bleeding (75%), elevated uric and lactate dehydrogenase, and the following:
   - WBC count decreased, <10,000 initially, then WBC count increases (30%)
   - WBC count normal, 5000 to 10,000 mm^3, then WBC count increases (30%)
   - WBC count >50,000 mm^3 (25%)
   - Platelet count <20,000 mm^3 (common)
   - Bone marrow: hypercellular, blasts 30% or greater and an increased erythroid element
   - Cerebrospinal fluid: cytology infiltration with leukemic cells at diagnosis less than 5%; greater risk for occurrence in M1 and M2

B. **Rai and Binet Staging Systems**—
   1. *Chronic Lymphocytic Leukemia (CLL)*—Classification for CLL is as follows:
      a. *Rai*
         - Stage 0: Low risk—lymphocytes in blood and marrow only
         - Stage I: Intermediate risk—lymphocytosis + lymphadenectomy + splenomegaly ± hepatomegaly
         - Stage II
         - Stage III: High risk—lymphocytosis + anemia, thrombocytopenia, or both
         - Stage IV
      b. *Binet*
         - A: <3 node-bearing areas

- B: ≥3 node-bearing areas
- C: Anemia, thrombocytopenia, or both

CLL is characterized by chronic, subtle onset of elevated peripheral WBC (WBC counts >100,000 mm^3); nearly 50% of bone marrow is infiltrated before the peripheral blood counts are compromised.

C. Philadelphia Chromosome—

1. ***Chronic Myelogenous Leukemia (CML)*—**In CML, chromosome 22 is missing part of its long arm, which is translocated to the long arm of chromosome 9. A new hybrid BCR-ABL oncogene is formed. Most patients with CML express a 210-kD BCR-ABL protein.

   CML is characterized by the following:

   a. *Chronic phase:* WBC often >100,000 mm^3, blasts <5%, hypercellular bone marrow, mature and immature granulocytes, and mild anemia

   b. *Accelerated phase:* WBC often >100,000 mm^3, basophils >15%, blasts >15%, thrombocytopenia <100,000 platelets, hemoglobin <7.0 g/dl with presence of >10% blasts in the bone marrow; and symptoms (fever, night sweats, weight loss, splenomegaly, and bone pain)

   c. *Blast phase:* WBC >100,000 mm^3, blasts >30%, plus same characteristics as accelerated phase; bone marrow: blasts in clumps and >30%, and leukemic infiltrates lymph nodes palpable

D. Myelodysplastic Syndrome (MDS)—

Subtypes of MDS are classified by bone marrow aspirates, achieved by examining the peripheral blood blasts (Pbb) and the bone marrow blasts (Bmb). MDS is characterized by Pbb and Bmb as follows:

1. ***Refractory anemia (RA):*** Pbb <1%, Bmb <5%
2. ***RA with ringed sideroblasts (RARS):*** Pbb <1%, Bmb <5%, >15% ring sideroblasts
3. ***RA, erythroblastic (RAEB):*** Pbb ≤5%, Bmb 5% to 20%
4. ***RA with excess blasts in transition (RAEBt):*** Pbb ≥5%, + Auer rods, Bmb 21% to 30%
5. ***Chronic myelomonocytic leukemia:*** Pbb <5%, monocytes >1000 mm^3, Bmb ≤20%

Severe pancytopenia, respiratory or gram-negative infections, bleeding as the result of thrombocytopenia, and splenomegaly (10% of cases) are the usual presenting signs and symptoms with the definitive criteria listed earlier and are present in the majority of MDS cases.

E. **Hairy Cell Leukemia (HCL)—**

HCL is identified by a certain "hairy cell" in the blood, bone marrow, and reticuloendothelial organs. Patients are diagnosed based on the presence of cytopenia, hairy cells in the peripheral blood, splenomegaly, and bone marrow aspiration and biopsy.

VI. CLINICAL FEATURES

The common clinical signs and symptoms reported for leukemia include fatigue, pallor, weight loss, repeated infections that do not respond to treatment, petechiae, bruising easily, or nosebleeds. Depending on the extent of the disease's acceleration, the patient may report dyspnea, tachycardia, and fever. Chronic leukemia usually has a slow subtle onset and can progress with minimal or no symptoms.

VII. DIAGNOSIS AND STAGING

The diagnostic process includes a thorough history and physical examination with evaluation of the clinical features. Multiple laboratory and diagnostic studies are performed. Placement of a durable vascular access is done on confirmation of the diagnosis to obtain the daily and ongoing laboratory samplings required for the diagnostic work-up and for monitoring the response to therapy. Bone marrow aspiration with biopsy is essential to finalize the diagnosis and provide specimens for histochemical staining, immunophenotyping, and cytogenetics. Laboratory blood tests include blood chemistries, complete blood count, coagulation studies, uric acid, pregnancy test, and urinalysis. Additional diagnostic examinations include chest x-ray, multiple-gated acquisition scan, lumbar puncture for cerebrospinal fluid analysis, and oxygen saturation; specific culture and sensitivity studies may be ordered for the febrile patient.

VIII. METASTASIS

Leukemia cells infiltrate to multiple sites including the spleen, liver, retina, testes, cerebrospinal fluid, or into the bone marrow.

IX. SURVIVAL
The 1-year relative survival rate for patients with leukemia is 64%. Survival rates decrease somewhat 5 years (46% 5-year survival) after the diagnosis, which is attributed to the poor survival associated with certain types of leukemia such as acute myeloid leukemia. Conversely, the 5-year survival rate for adult patients with ALL is 63% for adults and 85% for children.

X. TREATMENT MODALITIES
The treatment for leukemia varies with the *type* (acute or chronic); the *classification* with *subset* (e.g., FAB M4), such as lymphocytic, myeloid, hairy cell, and MDS; *cytogenetics*; specific *disease prognostic factors*; patient age; *bone marrow aspiration studies;* presence of leukemia cells in organs or tissue; and previous therapies for cancer treatment. The overall goal is cure, disease remission, or supportive care. Some form of chemotherapy or combinations with radiation therapy and peripheral blood stem cell transplantation (PBSCT) are used for all of the types of leukemia disease. Chemotherapy is administered through various drugs or drug combinations with varying dosages (standard to high dose), routes (intravenous, oral, or intrathecal), regimens (e.g., every 12 hours for 7 days), and periods of time (days, weeks, months). The courses of chemotherapy are as follows:

A. **Induction Therapy—**
   The primary goal for induction therapy is to induce a complete disease remission with drugs such as vincristine, prednisone, doxorubicin, daunorubicin, idarubicin, L-asparaginase, cyclophosphamide, methotrexate, cytarabine, ifosfamide, or gemtuzumab ozogamicin.

B. **Central Nervous System Treatment—**
   Intrathecal chemotherapy with methotrexate or cytarabine with or without high-dose systemic chemotherapy is used to treat the leukemia cells in the central nervous system. Cranial irradiation may be used in certain conditions.

C. **Consolidation—**
   Consolidation therapy drug regimens are almost as intense as the induction course, and the drugs are given over a period of months after the attainment of

Cancer Types

a complete remission; drugs such as cytarabine are used for consolidation.

D. **Intensification—**

An intensified schedule of drugs given is similar to those used during the induction course. The most frequently used agent is high-dose cytarabine alone or in combination with other drugs.

E. **Maintenance Therapy—**

Maintenance therapy is usually a lower dose treatment administered continuously for 2 to 3 years; the drugs/doses and schedule based on the type and classification of the leukemia. Drugs such as 6-mercaptopurine and 6-thioguanine are administered orally for ALL, leustatin is given for hairy-cell leukemia, hydroxyurea or chlorambucil is administered to treat chronic lymphocytic leukemia, and imatinib is used in the treatment of chronic myeloid leukemia.

F. **Ablative Therapy—**

Multiple drugs (carmustine, busulfan, etoposide, cyclophosphamide, and thiotepa) are administered at a high dose to prepare the patient for PBSCT. The goal is to destroy all leukemia cells in the marrow, create space in the bone marrow, and suppress the immune system in preparation for stem cell transplantation.

G. **Autologous/Allogeneic–PBSCT (A-PBSCT)—**

A-PBSCT after high-dose chemotherapy and radiation therapy is the only potentially curative treatment for some leukemia diseases such as CML. The best results occur when the transplant is performed early while the patient's disease is in complete remission.

H. **Scheduled Evaluations—**

After each course of therapy (e.g., induction) and before the patient is scheduled for the next course (e.g., consolidation), evaluative bone marrow aspiration studies are performed to determine the patient's response to that specific course. The goal is to have less than 5% blast cells (immature WBCs, leukemia cells) in the patient's bone marrow before proceeding to the next scheduled therapy course.

Bibliography

Almadrones L, Armstrong T, Gilbert M, et al: *Chemotherapy-induced neurotoxicity: Current trends in management, a multi-*

disciplinary approach, Philadelphia, 2002, Phillips Group Oncology Communications.

American Association of Blood Banks: *Technical manual,* ed 14, Bethesda, MD, 2001, American Association of Blood Banks.

American Cancer Society: *Cancer prevention and early detection, facts and figures 2003,* Atlanta, 2003, The Society.

American Cancer Society: *Cancer facts and figures 2003,* Atlanta, 2003, The Society.

Camp-Sorrell D: Surviving the cancer, surviving the treatment: acute cardiac and pulmonary toxicity, *Oncol Nurs Forum* 26(6):983, 1999.

Childs RW: Allogeneic stem cell transplantation. In DeVita VT Jr, Hellman S, Rosenberg SA, editors: *Cancer principles and practice of oncology,* ed 6, Philadelphia, 2001, JB Lippincott.

Chu E, DeVita VT Jr: Principles of cancer management: chemotherapy. In DeVita VT Jr, Hellman S, Rosenberg SA, editors: *Cancer principles and practice of oncology,* ed 6, Philadelphia, 2001, JB Lippincott.

Griffin JD: Hematopoietic growth factors. In DeVita VT Jr, Hellman S, Rosenberg SA, editors: *Cancer principles and practice of oncology,* ed 6, Philadelphia, 2001, JB Lippincott.

Jemal A, Murray T, Samuels A, et al: Cancer statistics, 2003, *CA Cancer J Clin* 53(1):5, 2003.

Moran AB, Camp-Sorrell D: Maintenance of venous access devices in patients with neutropenia, *Clin J Oncol Nurs* 6(3):126, 2002.

Osoki RE: Leukemia. In Otto SE, editor: *Oncology nursing,* ed 4, St. Louis, 2001, Mosby.

Schenberg DA, Maslak P, Weiss M: Acute leukemias. In DeVita VT Jr, Hellman S, Rosenberg SA, editors: *Cancer principles and practice of oncology,* ed 6, Philadelphia, 2001, JB Lippincott.

Segal BH, Walsh TJ, Holland SM: Infections in the cancer patient. In DeVita VT Jr, Hellman S, Rosenberg SA, editors: *Cancer principles and practice of oncology,* ed 6, Philadelphia, 2001, JB Lippincott.

Smith RA, Cokkinides V, Eyre HJ: American Cancer Society guidelines for the early detection of cancer, 2003, *CA Cancer J Clin* 53(1):27, 2003.

Cancer Types

15
Lung Cancers

I. INCIDENCE
Approximately 171,900 new cases of lung cancer will occur in 2003, accounting for about 13% of all cancer diagnoses. The incidence rate decreased in men from 86.5/100,000 in 1984 to 69.8/100,000 in 1998. The incidence rate for women was 43.4/100,000 in 1998.

II. MORTALITY
An estimated 157,200 deaths related to lung cancer will occur in 2003, accounting for 31% of male cancer deaths and 25% of female cancer deaths. Decreasing lung cancer incidence and mortality rates are most likely the result of decreased smoking rates over the past 30 years. In 2003, lung cancer deaths in *men* will be greater than the total cancer deaths for prostate, colorectal, pancreas, and non–Hodgkin's lymphoma; in *women,* deaths related to lung cancer will be greater than breast and colorectal cancer deaths combined.

III. ETIOLOGY/RISK FACTORS
Tobacco use is by far the most important risk factor in the development of lung cancer. Other risks include exposure to certain industrial substances such as arsenic; some organic chemicals; occupational or environmental exposures to radon and asbestos; radiation exposure from occupational, medical, and environmental sources; air pollution; tuberculosis; and for nonsmokers, environmental tobacco smoke.

IV. PREVENTION, SCREENING, AND DETECTION
Early detection currently has not been shown to improve survival. Chest x-ray, sputum cell cytology studies, and fiberoptic examination of the bronchial passages have

shown only limited effectiveness in early lung cancer detection. More recent tests such as low-dose helical computed tomography (CT) scan and molecular markers in sputum are currently being investigated in screening and detection clinical trials. The new CT helical scan can image the entire lung in 20 to 30 seconds and can produce three-dimensional images. These studies will explore the most clinically effective, cost-effective, and efficient method for detecting early-stage lung cancer.

Prevention strategies for smoking cessation include screening individuals for tobacco use through selective questions (asked by the healthcare professional) such as "Do you smoke?" and "Do you want to quit?" Patients willing to quit require assistance such as the following interventions:

- **Ask**—Identify the tobacco users
- **Advise**—Strongly urge/suggest tobacco users to quit
- **Assess**—Determine the smoker's willingness to quit
- **Assist**—Help the person to quit by developing a plan to quit, providing counseling, or recommending pharmacotherapy
- **Arrange**—Arrange a follow-up meeting to assess plan and strategies for quitting

V. CLASSIFICATION

The World Health Organization has identified numerous categories of lung cancers or lesions, but the majority (90%) consists of one of five types: small-cell anaplastic, squamous cell carcinoma, adenocarcinoma, large-cell anaplastic carcinoma, and mixed cell types. The two major categories are small cell and non-small cell.

A. Small-Cell Lung Cancer (SCLC)—
Biologically and clinically different from all other types (arising from the basal cell lining of the bronchial mucosa called a *Kulchitsky-type cell*), SCLC often presents at diagnosis in the central part of the chest with metastasis, has a large growth fraction and aggressive nature, and is most sensitive of all the lung cancers to both single agent and combination chemotherapy and radiation therapy. SCLC sometimes is referred to as *oat cell carcinoma* because of its small, round, spindle shape and microscopic resemblance to oats. SCLC accounts for about 20% to 25% of all lung cancers.

Cancer Types

B. **Non–Small-Cell Lung Cancer (NSCLC)—**
   The categories of NSCLC include the following:
   1. *Squamous cell carcinoma* arises in the central portion of the chest, may present as a Pancoast's tumor (high in the lung apex, causing a classic shoulder pain that radiates down the ulnar nerve), often is associated with a sudden onset of hypercalcemia resulting from the production of a parathyroid hormone-like substance, and is not associated with bone metastasis.
   2. *Adenocarcinoma* is recognized microscopically by its glandular appearance and mucin production, and patients with adenocarcinoma often have or will have metastasis to brain, liver, adrenal, or bone.
   3. *Large-cell anaplastic syndrome* appears microscopically as large cells lacking any distinguishing features with clinical features similar to those with adenocarcinoma.
   4. *Mixed cell types* have the same stem cell origin with different histologic cell types.
   All of the NSCLC categories account for 75% to 80% of all lung cancer.

VI. CLINICAL FEATURES
The most common presenting signs and symptoms include a persistent cough, sputum streaked with blood, chest pain, dyspnea, stridor, fatigue, weight loss, and recurrent pneumonia or bronchitis unresponsive to antimicrobials.

VII. DIAGNOSIS AND STAGING
Multiple diagnostic examinations are used for SCLC and NSCLC work-up, including chest x-ray, CT scans (bone, abdomen, liver), pulmonary function studies, magnetic resonance imaging, complete blood count, fiberoptic bronchoscopy with biopsy or washings, mediastinoscopy with biopsy, thoracentesis for cytology, and biopsy of other nodes at accessible metastatic sites (bone). The tumor, node, metastasis system is used for the classification of the different stages.

VIII. METASTASIS
Both SCLC and NSCLC metastasize to the other lung and pleura, brain, bone, liver, and lymph nodes. Cancers of the lung find many other sanctuaries, including bone

marrow, pericardium and heart, kidney, and adrenal gland.

IX. SURVIVAL

The 1-year relative survival rate for all lung cancers has increased from 34% in 1975 to 41% in 1997. The 5-year relative survival rate for all stages combined is only 15%. The survival rate is 48% for patients when the disease is detected early, but only 15% of lung cancer cases are diagnosed at this early stage. Non–small-cell cancer 5-year survival rates by *clinical stage* are as follows:

Stage IA	68%
Stage IB	38%
Stage IIA	34%
Stage IIB	24%
Stage IIIA	13%
Stage IIIB	5%
Stage IV	1%

X. TREATMENT MODALITIES

The treatment options for lung cancers are determined by the type (small cell vs. non-small cell) and stage (early vs. late stage) of the cancer and include surgery, radiation therapy, and chemotherapy.

A. NSCLC—

Surgery is the treatment of choice for stages I and II, which represent 25% of all lung cancers; surgery is the primary hope for cure. Additional surgical options for NSCLC include pneumonectomy and laser therapy procedures. Radiation therapy treatments for NSCLC include hyperfractionation-external beam, high-dose rate brachytherapy with placement of catheters close to the tumor, or both. High-dose rate iridium is introduced into the catheter using a computerized remote control. Chemotherapy agents such as cisplatin, carboplatin, gemcitabine, vinorelbine, paclitaxel, etoposide, ifosfamide, irinotecan, and docetaxel have been used as single agents or in multiple drug and drug dose combinations and have led to improvement in patient outcomes.

B. SCLC—

Concurrent radiation therapy (external beam and prophylactic cranial irradiation) with chemotherapy or alternating chemotherapy with radiotherapy have been shown to be the best treatment options. Chemotherapy single agent selection or combination regimens include cyclophosphamide, ifosfamide, epirubicin, doxorubicin, etoposide, carboplatin, cisplatin, topotecan, vincristine, and methotrexate.

Bibliography

American Cancer Society, *Cancer prevention and early detection, facts and figures 2003*, Atlanta, 2003, The Society.

American Cancer Society, *Cancer facts and figures 2003*, Atlanta, 2003, The Society.

Camp-Sorrell D: Surviving the cancer, surviving the treatment: acute cardiac and pulmonary toxicity, *Oncol Nurs Forum* 26(6):983, 1999.

Ferrell BR, Coyle N: An overview of palliative nursing care, *Am J Nurs* 102(5):26, 2002.

Fish-Steagall A: Multidisciplinary care in the management of non-small cell lung cancer, Princeton, NJ, 2000, Bristol-Myers Squibb Oncology.

Fleming I, Cooper JS, Henson DE, et al: *AJCC cancer staging manual*, ed 5, Philadelphia, 2002, Lippincott Williams & Wilkins.

Giarelli E: To screen or not to screen: using spiral computerized tomography in early detection of lung cancer, *Clin J Oncol Nurs* 6(4):1, 2002.

Ginsberg RJ, Vokes EE, Rosenzweig K: Non-small-cell lung cancer. In DeVita VT Jr, Hellman S, Rosenberg SA, editors: *Cancer principles and practice of oncology*, ed 6, Philadelphia, 2001, JB Lippincott.

Hawkins R: Mastering the intricate maze of metastasis, *Oncol Nurs Forum* 28(6):959, 2001.

Hellman S: Principles of cancer management: radiation therapy. In DeVita VT Jr, Hellman S, Rosenberg SA, editors: *Cancer principles and practice of oncology*, ed 6, Philadelphia, 2001, JB Lippincott.

Jemal A, Murrary T, Samuels A, et al: Cancer statistics, 2003, *CA Cancer J Clin* 53(1):5, 2003.

Joyce M, Houlihan N: Current strategies in the diagnosis and treatment of lung cancer, *Oncol Nurs* 8(1):1, 2001.

Murrin J, Glatstein E, Pass HI: Small-cell lung cancer. In DeVita VT Jr, Hellman S, Rosenberg SA, editors: *Cancer principles and practice of oncology*, ed 6, Philadelphia, 2001, JB Lippincott.

Nail LM: I'm coping as fast as I can: psychological adjustment to cancer & cancer treatment, *Oncol Nurs Forum* 28(6):967, 2001.

Otto SE, editor: *Oncology nursing*, ed 4, St. Louis, 2001, Mosby.

Paice JA: Managing psychological conditions in palliative care, *Am J Nurs* 102(11):36, 2002.

Rosenberg SA: Principles of cancer management: surgical oncology. In DeVita VT Jr, Hellman S, Rosenberg SA, editors: *Cancer principles and practice of oncology,* ed 6, Philadelphia, 2001, JB Lippincott.

Smith RA, Cokkinides V, Eyre HJ: American Cancer Society guidelines for the early detection of cancer, 2003, *CA Cancer J Clin* 53(1):27, 2003.

Wickham R: Dyspnea: recognizing and managing an invisible problem, *Oncol Nurs Forum* 29(6):925, 2002.

Cancer Types

Malignant Lymphoma

I. INCIDENCE

An estimated 61,000 new cases of malignant lymphoma will occur in 2003, including 7600 cases of Hodgkin's disease (HD) and 53,400 cases of non–Hodgkin's lymphoma (NHL). Since the early 1970s the incidence rates for NHL have nearly doubled, whereas the overall incidence rates of HD have declined.

II. MORTALITY

An estimated 24,700 malignant lymphoma–related deaths will occur in 2003, with 23,400 resulting from NHL and 1300 from HD.

III. ETIOLOGY/RISK FACTORS

The risk factors for NHL and HD are unknown but are related to exposure to certain infectious agents, occupational exposure to herbicides or chemicals, and having a reduced immune function. Persons with organ transplants are at higher risk because of the altered immune function. Human immunodeficiency virus and human T-cell leukemia/lymphoma virus-1 are associated with an increased risk for NHL.

IV. PREVENTION, SCREENING, AND DETECTION

Prevention, screening, and detection of HD and NHL is not applicable because there are no identified preventable risks, and early detection is hampered by the vagueness of the common symptoms. Patients are encouraged to seek medical attention for persistent, common, clinical features.

V. CLASSIFICATION

A. Hodgkin's Disease—

HD is classified according to the Cotswald's Staging Classification as follows:

1. *Stage I*—Involvement of a single node region or structure
2. *Stage II*—Involvement of two or more lymph node regions on the same side of the diaphragm; number of anatomic sites identified by suffix (e.g., II)
3. *Stage III*—Involvement of lymph node regions or structures on both sides of the diaphragm with or without other nodal presentation (splenic hilar, celiac, portal, paraaortic, iliac, or mesenteric)
4. *Stage IV*—Involvement of extranodal site(s); includes categories of no symptoms; B symptoms include fever, drenching sweats, weight loss; bulky disease; involvement of nodes contiguous or proximal to known nodal site

B. Non–Hodgkin's Lymphoma—

NHL is classified by the World Health Organization Classification of Neoplastic Disease of Hematopoietic and Lymphoid Tissue with the Revised European American Lymphoma classification system that recognizes the three major categories of lymphoid malignancies: B cell, T/natural killer, and HD. B-cell NHL accounts for the majority of NHL malignancies and is further classified by the following:

1. *Indolent B-Cell Lymphomas*
2. *Aggressive B-Cell Lymphomas*
3. *Very aggressive B-Cell Lymphomas*

VI. CLINICAL FEATURES

Enlarged lymph nodes, severe itching, night sweats, fatigue, weight loss, and alcohol-induced pain are the most common presenting signs and symptoms. Fever and night sweats episodes can last for several days or weeks.

VII. DIAGNOSIS AND STAGING

The diagnostic work-up varies according to HD or NHL and may include the following: history and physical examination focusing on presence of B symptoms and duration and rate of lymph node involvement; multiple laboratory studies; chest, gallium, bone, and positron emission tomography scans; magnetic

Cancer Types

resonance imaging; cytology of pleural effusion; bone marrow aspiration and biopsy; and excisional biopsy of certain lymph nodes.

VIII. METASTASIS

HD spreads contiguously from one lymph node chain to an adjacent nodal chain, until eventually the malignant cells invade the blood vessels and spread to other organs. Involvement of the retroperitoneal nodes, lungs, liver, spleen, and bone marrow occurs after HD has generalized. The metastatic process for NHL varies with lymphoma type (follicular: bone marrow involvement; diffuse: disseminates quickly and involves areas such as the central nervous system, bone, and gastrointestinal tract).

IX. SURVIVAL

Survival rates for malignant lymphoma vary significantly by the cell type and disease stage. The 1-year survival rates for HD and NHL are 95% and 77%, respectively. The 5-year survival rate for HD is 84%, the 10-year survival rate is 75%, and the 15-year survival rate is 68%. The 5-, 10-, and 15-year survival rates for NHL are 55%, 40%, and 38%, respectively.

X. TREATMENT MODALITIES

A. Hodgkin's Disease—
   Chemotherapy alone or with radiotherapy is used for most patients with HD. In the early stage, localized lymph node disease is treated with radiotherapy. Patients with disease in later stages are treated with chemotherapy or with chemotherapy/radiation therapy combinations and high-dose chemotherapy with autologous peripheral blood stem cell transplantation (PBSCT). Selected chemotherapy regimens in the treatment of HD may include mechlorethamine, vincristine, procarbazine, and prednisone (MOPP); cytarabine, bleomycin, vinblastine, and dacarbazine (ABVD); chlorambucil, vinblastine, procarbazine, and prednisone (Ch1VPP); and doxorubicin, vinblastine, mechlorethamine, vincristine, bleomycin, etoposide, and prednisone (Stanford V).

B. Non-Hodgkin's Lymphoma—
   The treatment approaches to NHL are based on the specific histology of the neoplasm, stage of disease,

and the prognosis and physiologic status of the patient. Similar therapies such as radiation therapy, with chemotherapy combinations or high-dose chemotherapy with autologous and allogeneic PBSCT are used in multiple treatment regimens. Similar chemotherapy drugs and drug combinations to those used in HD management are used in the treatment of NHL. New treatment programs using highly specific monoclonal antibodies (rituximab), those with radioisotopes attached (tositumomab or ibritumomab with yttrium-90), or both, directed at lymphoma cells, are being tested in selected patients. High-dose chemotherapy with autologous or allogeneic PBSCT may be used in combination with the monoclonal antibodies.

Passive immunotherapy with active vaccination protocols is being investigated for NHL. Studies are being evaluated to improve the number of patients who can mount an immune response and also to improve the quality of the immune response. Multiple products are being investigated such as use of dendrite cells, protein-based vaccines, use of alternative adjuvants to improve the response such as sargramostim, and use of a CD40-activated lymphoma to stimulate T cells for adoptive transfer.

Cancer Types

Bibliography

American Cancer Society: *Cancer prevention and early detection, facts and figures 2003,* Atlanta, 2003, The Society.

American Cancer Society: *Cancer facts and figures 2003,* Atlanta, 2003, The Society.

Armitage JO, Mauch PM, Harris NL, et al: Non-Hodgkin's lymphoma. In DeVita VT Jr, Hellman S, Rosenberg SA, editors: *Cancer principles and practice of oncology,* ed 6, Philadelphia, 2001, JB Lippincott.

Bradley JD, Perez CA: Fundamentals of patient management in radiation oncology. In Govindan R, Arquette MA, editors: The Washington manual of oncology, Philadelphia, 2002, Lippincott Williams & Wilkins.

Buchsel PC, Kapustay PM: *Stem cell transplantation: a clinical textbook,* Pittsburgh, 2000, Oncology Nursing Press.

Childs RW: Allogeneic stem cell transplantation. In DeVita VT Jr, Hellman S, Rosenberg SA, editors: *Cancer principles and practice of oncology,* ed 6, Philadelphia, 2001, JB Lippincott.

Chu E, DeVita VT Jr: Principles of cancer management: chemotherapy. In DeVita VT Jr, Hellman S, Rosenberg SA, editors: *Cancer principles and practice of oncology,* ed 6, Philadelphia, 2001, JB Lippincott.

Daniel BT: Malignant lymphoma. In Otto SE, editor: *Oncology Nursing,* ed 4, St. Louis, 2001, Mosby.

Diehl V, Mauch PM, Harris NL: Hodgkin's disease. In DeVita VT Jr, Hellman S, Rosenberg SA, editors: *Cancer principles and practice of oncology,* ed 6, Philadelphia, 2001, JB Lippincott.

Fleming I, Cooper JS, Henson DE, et al: *AJCC cancer staging manual,* ed 5, Philadelphia, 2002, Lippincott Williams & Wilkins.

Hellman S: Principles of cancer management: radiation therapy. In DeVita VT Jr, Hellman S, Rosenberg SA, editors: *Cancer principles and practice of oncology,* ed 6, Philadelphia, 2001, JB Lippincott.

Hendrix CS, de Leon C, Dillman RO: Radioimmunotherapy for non-Hodgkin's lymphoma with yttrium 90 ibritumomab tiuxetan, *Clin J Oncol Nurs* 6(3):144, 2002.

Jemal A, Murray T, Samuels A, et al: Cancer Statistics, 2003, *CA Cancer J Clin* 53(1):5, 2003.

Smith RA, Cokkinides V, Eyre HJ: American Cancer Society guidelines for the early detection of cancer, 2003, *CA Cancer J Clin* 53(1):27, 2003.

Thomas M, Doss D: Thalidomide nursing roundtable update, American Academy of CME and OmegaMed, 2002, Skillman, NJ.

Tuma RS: Update on radioimmunotherapy in NHL, *Oncology Times,* January 25, 2003, special edition.

Vose JM: Immunotherapy for non-Hodgkin's lymphoma, *Clin Oncol Updates* 6(4):1, 2002.

17 Multiple Myeloma

I. INCIDENCE/MORTALITY

Multiple myeloma (MM) is a rare malignancy of plasma cells that accounts for only 1.1% of all hematologic malignancies diagnosed in the United States. It is diagnosed equally among men and women but occurs 14 times more frequently in blacks than in whites. The median patient age is 65 years. An estimated 14,600 new cases of MM will occur in 2003, with an estimated 10,900 related deaths.

II. ETIOLOGY/RISK FACTORS

The cause of MM is not understood, but research models have identified factors such as chromosomal abnormalities, host-genetic factors, chronic antigenic stimulation, viruses, and growth factors as possible contributors to the development of plasma cell dyscrasias. Additional host factors such as age, race, and occupational exposure to petroleum products, rubber, farming-related chemicals, asbestos, and radiation may contribute to the increased risk for the disease.

III. PREVENTION, SCREENING, AND DETECTION

No recommendations exist for the prevention or screening of asymptomatic individuals for MM.

IV. CLINICAL FEATURES

Although some individuals may be asymptomatic, at examination most patients report a history of weakness, anorexia, weight loss, and fatigue. The symptoms of more advanced disease include bone pain (back region); anemia; recurrent infections; changes in urinary patterns; and cognitive, sensory, or motor changes.

V. CLASSIFICATION/DIAGNOSIS AND STAGING

The diagnosis is based on the findings of the history and physical examinations and findings obtained from laboratory and radiograph studies. Serum and urine electrophoretic and immunologic studies reveal elevations in IgG, IgA, and light chain levels. Additional laboratory tests include blood chemistries and Bence-Jones urine protein levels. Radiographic studies include skeletal survey (skull, pelvis, femurs, and humeri), bone scans, or magnetic resonance imaging to detect presence of osteoporosis, osteolytic lesions, or pathologic fractures. Finally, a bone marrow aspiration with biopsy is performed to determine bone marrow percentage involvement with plasma cells. For a diagnosis of MM to be made one or more of the following criteria must exist:

- Plasma cell infiltration of the bone marrow of at least 10%
- A monoclonal spike on serum or urine electrophoresis
- Radiograph confirmation of osteoporosis and osteolytic lesions
- Soft tissue plasma cell tumors
- No universal staging system for MM currently exists.

VI. METASTASIS

The metastatic process occurs through the hematogenous route with spread to bone marrow and with renal and respiratory involvement.

VII. SURVIVAL

The majority of MM cases are not curable. The course of the disease progression is determined by the organ involvement at the time of diagnosis and the response to active treatment. Asymptomatic patients may live with the disease for months to years without active treatment. A pattern of response tends to occur with those receiving chemotherapy alone or with autologous or allogeneic peripheral blood stem cell transplantation (PBSCT). Survival can range from a few months to years. In 2002, survival rates include 33% at 5 years and 28% at 7 years; for stage I disease, the 5-year survival rate for patients receiving autologous or allogeneic PBSCT was 53%.

VIII. TREATMENT MODALITIES

Chemotherapy alone or in combination with radiation therapy, biologic response modifiers, or PBSCT is used most often for treatment of MM. Radiation therapy is used to treat patients with chemotherapy-resistant disease, to relieve bone pain, and to treat spinal cord compression. Biologic response modifier therapy is used to treat the chemotherapy-related side effects of anemia, thrombocytopenia, and neutropenia.

Clinicians have used combinations of prednisone, high-dose melphalan, vincristine, carmustine, cyclophosphamide, and doxorubicin. Systemic combination chemotherapy has demonstrated a survival ranging from 18 months to 36 months, with a greater than median survival of 24 months. The drug thalidomide is currently being used in multiple clinical trials as a single agent or in combination with prednisone.

Additional therapies include PBSCT for selected patients with MM depending on age (younger than 70 years), stage of disease, and favorable response to the initial chemotherapy. Donor leukocyte/lymphocyte infusion is an additive infusion to accompany allogeneic PBSCT. Donor lymphocytes from the original donor marrow are obtained by leukapheresis in one to three sessions. The purpose of the donor leukocyte/lymphocyte infusion is to induce a state of host-versus-graft tolerance, thereby giving donor derived T-lymphocytes the opportunity to recognize and eradicate host-derived tumor cells such as anti–graft-versus-host disease, thus providing the patient with a chance for a better survival outcome.

Bibliography

American Cancer Society: *Cancer facts and figures 2003,* Atlanta, 2003, The Society.

Buchsel PC, Kapustay PM: *Stem cell transplantation: a clinical textbook,* Pittsburgh, 2000, Oncology Nursing Press.

Desikan R, Barlogie B, Sawyer J, et al: Results of high-dose therapy for 1000 patients with multiple myeloma: durable complete remissions and superior survival in the absence of chromosome 13 abnormalities, *Blood* 95(12):4008, 2000.

Diel IJ, Solomayer EF, Bastert G: Bisphosphonates and the prevention of metastasis: first evidence from preclinical and clinical studies, *Cancer* 88(12 suppl):3080, 2000.

Fleming I, Cooper JS, Henson DE, et al: *AJCC cancer staging manual*, ed 5, Philadelphia, 2002, Lippincott Williams & Wilkins.

Gado K, Domjan G, Hegyesi H, et al: Role of interleukin-6 in the pathogenesis of multiple myeloma, *Cell Biol Int* 24(4):195, 2000.

Gahrton G, Bjorkstrand B: Progression hematopoietic stem cell transplantation for multiple myeloma. *J Intern Med* 248(3): 185, 2000.

Gillespie TW: Effects of cancer-related anemia on clinical and quality-of-life outcomes, *Clin J Oncol Nurs* 6(4):206, 2002.

Jemal A, Murray T, Samuels A, et al: Cancer statistics, 2003, *CA Cancer J Clin* 53:5, 2003.

Kanis JA, McCloskey EV: Bisphonates in multiple myeloma, *Cancer* 88 (suppl 12):3022, 2000.

Leger CS: Autologous blood and marrow transplantation in patients 60 years and older, *Biol Blood Marrow Transplant* 6(2A):204, 2000.

Lokhorst HM, Schattenberg A, Cornelissen JJ, et al: Donor leukocyte infections are effective in relapsed multiple myeloma after allogeneic bone marrow transplantation, *Blood* 90(10):4206, 1997.

Lokhorst HM, Schattenberg A, Cornelissen JJ, et al: Donor lymphocyte infusion for relapsed multiple myeloma after all-BMT: predictive factors for response and long-term outcome, *J Clin Oncol* 18(16):3031, 2000.

Poole P, Greer E: Immune suppression in transplantation, *Crit Care Nurs Clin North Am* 12(3):315, 2000.

Smith RA, Cokkinides V, Eyre HJ: American Cancer Society guidelines for the early detection of cancer, 2003, *CA Cancer J Clin* 53(1):27, 2003.

Stiff P: Mucositis associated with stem cell transplantation: current status and innovative approaches for management, *Bone Marrow Transplant* 27 (suppl 2) S3-S11, 2001.

Zaidl AA, Vesole DH: Multiple myeloma, an old disease with new hope for the future, *CA Cancer J Clin* 51:273, 2001.

18 Skin Cancers

I. INCIDENCE

More than 1 million cases of highly curable basal cell cancer (BCC) and squamous cell cancer (SCC) occur annually. The most serious form of skin cancer is melanoma, with an expected 54,200 new cases to be diagnosed in 2003. Melanoma is most common among whites, who have incidence rates 10 times greater than blacks. Since 1981, the rate of increase for melanoma is about 3% per year.

II. MORTALITY

As estimated 9800 deaths related to skin cancer will occur in 2003, with 7600 resulting from malignant melanoma and 2200 from other skin cancers. Recent melanoma mortality rates have shown slight increases for white men but has stabilized for white women.

III. ETIOLOGY/RISK FACTORS

The significant risk factors for skin cancer include *excessive exposure* to ultraviolet radiation; fair complexion; occupational exposure to coal tar, pitch, creosote, arsenic compounds, or radium; positive family history; and multiple or atypical nevi (moles).

IV. PREVENTION, SCREENING, AND DETECTION

Prevention is accomplished by avoidance of exposure to the sun during the midday hours (10 AM to 4 PM). When outdoors, wear protective clothing such as a long-sleeve shirt; a hat that shades the face, neck, and ears; and sunglasses to protect the eyes. Use a sunscreen with a solar protection factor (SPF) of 15 or greater. Children should follow the same prevention guidelines as adults. When children experience severe sunburn at an early age they have an increased risk for melanoma in later life.

Recognizing and reporting changes in skin growths are the best detection methods for skin cancers. All adults should practice monthly skin self-examinations. A physician should promptly evaluate any suspicious lesion. BCC and SCC often appear as a pale, waxlike, pearly nodule or as a red, scaly, sharply outlined patch. Any sudden or progressive changes should be investigated.

Melanomas often start as a small molelike growth that increases in size, changes color, or both. The ABCD rule outlines the warning signals of melanoma as follows:

A. Asymmetry—
   One half of the mole does not match the other half
B. Border Irregularity—
   The border edges are ragged, notched, or blurred
C. Color—
   The pigmentation is not uniform with varying degrees of tan, brown, or black
D. Diameter—
   The diameter of the mole is greater than 6 mm (tip of pencil eraser)

V. CLASSIFICATION

Skin cancers are classified according to specific tissue type and histology, such as:

A. Basal Cell Cancer—
   BCC is classified as nodular, superficial, pigmented, morpheaform (sclerotic), and keratosic.
B. Squamous Cell Cancer—
   SCC is classified by the presenting symptoms, tissue source, and histologic differences: ischemic ulceration, Bowen's disease, actinic cheilitis, and verrucous.
C. Malignant Melanoma—
   Malignant melanoma is classified by four different types: superficial spreading, nodular, lentigo maligna, and acral lentiginous.

VI. CLINICAL FEATURES

Clinical features of skin cancer include any change on the skin, especially in the size or color of a mole or other dark pigmented growth or spot; scaliness, oozing, bleeding, or a change in the appearance of a bump or nodule; the spread of pigmentation beyond the border; or a change in sensations, itchiness, tenderness, or pain. In addition, any skin lesion that does not heal should be investigated by a clinician.

VII. DIAGNOSIS AND STAGING
The initial clinical staging for melanoma includes a medical history and physical examination including careful skin examination; complete blood count; chemistries; lactate dehydrogenase; chest x-ray; computed tomography scan of chest, pelvis, or abdomen; bone scan; computed tomography scan/magnetic resonance imaging of the brain; or a positron emission tomography scan. An excisional biopsy, punch biopsy, or both are performed to have an adequate tissue specimen for pathologic examination to determine the clinical diagnosis and identifying features of the various tissue classifications. The BCC and SCC diagnostic work-up includes all of these tests with the *exception* of computed tomography or positron emission tomography scans, magnetic resonance imaging, and bone scans.

VIII. METASTASIS
Metastatic disease rarely occurs with BCC and incidence ranges from 0.3% to 3.7%, with related death resulting in 75% of patients with SCC. Melanoma has a radial and vertical growth pattern and can metastasize to skin (intracutaneous or subcutaneous metastasis) or spread to any organ or remote viscera such as bone, brain, lung, and liver.

IX. SURVIVAL
Basal cell and squamous cell cancers are highly curable if detected and treated early. When melanoma is detected at its earliest stage and treated properly, it is also highly curable. The 5-year survival rate for patients with melanoma is 89%. The 5-year survival rates for localized, regional, and distant stage disease are 96%, 61%, 12%, respectively. Approximately 82% of melanoma cancers are diagnosed at a localized stage.

X. TREATMENT MODALITIES
The treatment for BCC and SCC includes surgery (electrodessication, cryosurgery, and laser therapy) in 90% of cases. Radiation therapy is also used in BCC and SCC treatment.

For malignant melanoma, the primary tumor must be adequately excised with a wide disease-free margin of tissue and biopsy or removal of the surrounding lymph nodes. A sentinel lymph node biopsy performed at the time of the wide local excision has revolutionized the surgical staging and treatment of melanoma. Through lymphatic mapping and limited sampling of one or two nodes, sentinel lymph node biopsy allows determination of regional lymph node involvement without the need for an extensive procedure. Only patients with positive sentinel lymph nodes will then undergo complete lymph node dissection. Melanoma disease that has spread beyond the lymph nodes is usually treated with radiation therapy, immunotherapy, or chemotherapy in conjunction with the surgical procedure.

Immunotherapy agents such as interferon-α-2b and IL-2 have been used as single agents or in combination with chemotherapy and have led to improved patient outcomes with prolonged relapse-free and overall survival. Chemotherapy drugs selected for the treatment of melanoma include dacarbazine, vincristine, vinblastine, cisplatin, carboplatin, and carmustine. Dacarbazine has demonstrated far superior results versus the others drugs listed.

Finally, a treatment shown to be of benefit for melanoma is hyperthermic regional perfusion. This technique, also called *limb perfusion*, is effective in treating melanoma of the limbs. It is the perfusion of chemotherapy (cisplatin, dacarbazine, or melphalen) directly into the extremity. The limb is then perfused for 1 hour with a high concentration of drug at 39° C to 41° C (102.2° F to 105.8° F) with a perfusion pump and extracorporeal circulator. The hyperthermia enhances the cytotoxic effect so that the total dose of the drug may be reduced, while delivering a high drug concentration to area of disease recurrences with minimal side effects.

Bibliography

American Cancer Society: *Cancer prevention and early detection, facts and figures 2003,* Atlanta, 2003, The Society.

American Cancer Society: *Cancer facts and figures 2003,* Atlanta, 2003, The Society.

Arceci R, Ettinger A, Forman E, et al: American Cancer Policy Statement, national action plan for childhood cancer: report of the national summit meetings on childhood cancer, *CA Cancer J Clin* 52(6):377, 2002.

Balch CM, et al: AJCC melanoma staging committee: the new melanoma staging system and factors predicting melanoma survival, *Clin Oncol Updates* 5(3):1, 2002.

Fleming I, Cooper JS, Henson DE, et al: *AJCC cancer staging manual,* ed 5, Philadelphia, 2002, Lippincott Williams & Wilkins.

Jemal A, Murray T, Samuels A, et al: Cancer statistics, 2003, *CA Cancer J Clin* 53 (1):5, 2003.

Jennings-Dozier K, Mahon SM, editors: *Cancer prevention, detection, and control,* Pittsburg, 2002, Oncology Nursing Press.

Krebs LU: Malignant melanoma: etiology, risk factor, sun protection, and the use of sunscreens, *Nurse Investigator* 6(1):21, 2002.

Lamb LA, Hwu WJ: Overview of cutaneous melanoma, *Oncol Nurs* 8(2):1, 2001.

Langhorne M: Skin cancers. In Otto SE, editor: *Oncology Nursing,* ed 4, St. Louis, 2001, Mosby.

Sample D: Cancer vaccines: a new era in cancer management has begun, *Nurse Investigator* 6(1):6, 2002.

Slingluff CL, Hendrix J, Seigler HE: Melanoma and cutaneous malignancies. In Townsend CM Jr, Beauchamp RD, Evers BM, et al, editors: *Textbook of surgery, the biological basis of modern surgical practice,* ed 16, Philadelphia, 2001, WB Saunders.

Smith RA, Cokkinides V, Eyre HJ: American Cancer Society guidelines for the early detection of cancer, 2003, *CA Cancer J Clin* 53(1):27, 2003.

Spahis J: Human genetics: constructing a family pedigree, *Am J Nurs* 102(7):44, 2002.

Cancer Types

19

Pediatric Cancers

I. INCIDENCE
Approximately 9000 new cancer cases will be diagnosed in children younger than 14 years in 2003.

II. MORTALITY
Approximately 1500 cancer-related deaths are expected to occur among children younger than 14 years in 2003, with about one third of those deaths from leukemia. Cancer mortality rates have declined 50% since 1973. However, cancer remains the primary cause of death due to disease for children aged 1 to 14 years.

III. PREVENTION, SCREENING, AND DETECTION
Cancer in children is often difficult to recognize because the symptoms vary and the disease may have a subtle onset. Children should have regular medical checkups, and parents must be alert to and seek medical care for persistent or unusual symptoms. These symptoms include: an unusual mass or swelling; unexplained paleness and lack of energy; sudden tendency to bruise or bleed; a persistent, localized pain, limping, or lack of arm strength; prolonged or unexplained fever; frequent illnesses; headaches, often accompanied by vomiting or

sudden eye or vision changes; and excessive or rapid weight loss.

IV. SURVIVAL

The 5-year survival rates for children vary with the disease site and disease stage at the time of diagnosis. The overall 5-year survival rate for all diseases combined is 77%. The 5-year survival rates for specific sites are:

Bone	73%
Neuroblastoma	69%
Brain/Central Nervous System (CNS)	70%
Wilms' Tumor	90%
Hodgkin's Disease	94%
Acute Lymphocytic Leukemia	85%

V. CANCERS IN CHILDREN

Pediatric cancers are discussed according to occurrence rates for all childhood cancers in children younger than 14 years. Etiologic factors, classification, clinical features, diagnostic evaluation, prognostic factors, and treatment modalities are also discussed.

A. Leukemia (30%)—

Leukemia is the most common cancer in children, representing 30% of all the childhood cancers. Approximately 500 children in the United States will die from this disease in 2003. The cause is unknown, but contributing factors include viruses, radiation, chemical and drug exposure, chromosomal abnormalities, and familial predisposition. The clinical features are dependent on the degree of bone marrow compromised and the extent of extramedullary infiltration. Common presenting signs and symptoms are fever, pain, bleeding, petechiae, purpura, fatigue, pallor, recurrent infection, and lymphadenopathy. These symptoms may have been present for days or weeks (rarely months) before the diagnosis.

The most common types of leukemia occurring in children include acute lymphoblastic (lymphocytic) leukemia, acute myelogenous leukemia, chronic myelogenous leukemia, and juvenile chronic myelogenous leukemia. The diagnoses listed earlier have a similar diagnostic work-up including computed tomography (CT) scans (e.g., brain), lumbar puncture for cerebrospinal fluid (CSF) analysis, bone scans, magnetic resonance imaging (MRI), laboratory studies, and bone marrow aspiration with cytology studies, immunophenotyping, and cytogenetic evaluations. Prognostic information is obtained at the time of the diagnostic work-up and assists clinicians in determining the best courses of therapy for each of the leukemia diseases.

Chemotherapy through intravenous and intrathecal (for CNS prophylaxis) routes is commonly used with various drugs, doses, and schedules depending on the disease and the child's age. Multiple research protocols currently exist for treatment of childhood leukemia. The chemotherapy courses such as induction, CNS treatment, intensification or consolidation therapy, and maintenance therapy, with or without autologous or allogeneic peripheral blood stem cell transplantation (PBSCT), are pursued. Most leukemia disease relapses occur either during treatment or within 2 years after completion of therapy. Treatment of recurrent leukemia remains under clinical investigation, but usually includes combination chemotherapy with or without stem cell transplantation.

B. **Osteogenic Sarcoma (2.7%)**—
Osteogenic sarcoma is a malignant sarcoma of the bone that originates from osteon. The most common sites of occurrence are in the femur, tibia, humerus, fibula, scapula, ileum, radius, mandible, and clavicle. Pain in the affected site, which can be severe, lasts for a short time or months and increases with activity, often resulting in a limp. Other symptoms include tenderness, swelling, and erythema or limited range of motion. Metastatic disease is present in 15% to 25% of patients at time of diagnosis, with 90% occurring in the lungs. Other possible metastasis sites include bone, kidney, and brain. The diagnostic evaluation includes bone and CT scans, MRI, and chest x-ray to provide information regarding extent of the disease and presence of "skip lesions." A biopsy is required to confirm the diagnosis.

Treatment incorporates both surgery and chemotherapy. The extent of the surgery depends on the location and degree of tumor involvement. Amputations are rare (e.g., pathologic fracture or skeletal immaturity) and have been replaced with limb salvage procedures. Limb salvage is possible if a clear margin of 6 to 7 cm can be maintained and the extremity will be functional after surgery. Neoadjuvant (preoperative) chemotherapy is initiated as soon as the biopsy staging studies are completed and continues until approximately 9 to 12 weeks before the surgical procedure. Preoperative chemotherapy provides not only reduction in tumor size before resection, but also evaluation of tumor response allowing for changes in therapy if efficacy is unsatisfactory. Osteosarcoma is highly radioresistant, and radiation therapy is reserved primarily for reduction before surgery or for palliation of unresponsive disease.

C. **Ewing's Sarcoma (1.8%)**—
Ewing's sarcoma is another type of bone cancer, usually diagnosed in the second decade of life, and is rarely seen in patients younger than 5 or older than 30 years. The most common sites of occurrence are the pelvis, tibia, fibula, and femur. Pain with or without swelling at the primary site is the most frequent symptom. Two thirds of the patients have a palpable mass, and one fifth have a fever and leukocytosis, leading to a *misdiagnosis of osteomyelitis*. The duration of symptoms can be days, months, or years (e.g., pelvic tumors). Systemic systems of weight loss and fatigue are most often associated with metastatic disease. The diagnostic work-up includes radiographs of the primary lesion and MRI or CT scan of the primary site for detection of extent of soft tissue involvement. A biopsy with an adequate tissue specimen is needed to confirm the diagnosis. A chest radiograph and bone scan with evidence of the CT scan is necessary to rule out metastatic disease. Bilateral bone marrow aspirate is used to detect bone marrow involvement. The most important prognostic indicator is extent of disease and metastasis.

Treatment modalities include large doses of radiation therapy with 5000 to 6000 cGy to the whole bone and a 1000-cGy dose to boost the primary lesion. Surgery is usually performed if the bone is resectable and expendable or for children in whom radiation therapy will cause unacceptable morbidity. Chemotherapy is often given before surgery and then followed by radiation therapy, surgical resection of the primary lesion, and then further chemotherapy.

D. Neuroblastoma (7.3%)—
Neuroblastoma originates from neural crest tissue anywhere along the craniospinal axis, is the most common malignancy in infancy, and has bizarre behavior that can regress, mature, or rapidly progress. Several genetic abnormalities have been found associated with neuroblastoma and have prognostic implications—for example, the more *N-myc* copies that are present, the poorer the prognosis. The presenting clinical symptoms depend on location of the tumor and disease stage and most often arise in the retroperitoneum, 65% of which present as hard, nontender masses. Other common sites include the mediastinum (15%), pelvis (5%), and neck (<5%). Metastatic extension of neuroblastoma occurs in two patterns, lymphatic and hematogenous, with approximately two thirds of these tumors metastasized at the time of diagnosis. Metastatic sites include bone marrow, cortical bone, lymph nodes, liver, or subcutaneous tissue.

The diagnostic and treatment process includes multiple laboratory studies such as urine catecholamines, CT scans, bone and meta-iodo-benzyl-guanidine (MIBG) scans with radiographic films, MRI, bilateral bone marrow aspirates and biopsies, and a biopsy from the primary tumor site. The treatment varies but can include no surgery, awaiting spontaneous regression; surgery alone; and low-dose chemotherapy. Newer approaches, including autologous and allogeneic PBSCT, are being investigated.

E. Rhabdomyosarcoma (3.4%)—
Rhabdomyosarcoma is a soft tissue sarcoma with almost two thirds of the cases occurring in children 6 years or younger. Rhabdomyosarcoma is included in the family cancer syndrome known as *Li-Fraumeni syndrome*, which is associated with mutations in the *p53* gene. This is a highly malignant tumor that originates from mesenchymal cells, the precursors to striated skeletal muscle, and is included in the category of small, round, blue cell tumors of childhood. The most common presenting symptom is a mass located in any of the following regions: head and neck area (38%), genitourinary tract (21%), extremity (18%),

trunk (7%), and retroperitoneum (7%). Rhabdomyosar-coma most often metastasizes to lung; bone marrow; bone; and, depending on primary tumor site, lymph node, brain, spinal cord, and heart.

The diagnostic work-up and treatment modality are dependent on the site of origin. CT scans, bone scans, skeletal surveys, MRI, ultrasound, and bone marrow aspiration are performed with a biopsy from the primary site to confirm the diagnosis. Surgical removal of the tumor is indicated when it will not compromise function, and radiation therapy is used to eradicate residual cells at the primary site or to reduce bulk. Chemotherapy is used with varying drugs and doses and may be combined with autologous PBSCT.

F. **Retinoblastoma (2.8%)—**
Retinoblastoma is an eye cancer that usually occurs in children younger than 4 years. When detected early, cure is possible with surgery, chemotherapy, or radiation therapy. The diagnostic and treatment processes are similar to that for rhabdomyosarcoma.

G. **Brain and Intraspinal Malignancies (21%)—**
Brain tumors are the most common solid tumors in children and are second in frequency only to leukemia. The greatest incidence rates occur among infants and children 7 years or younger. Approximately 50% of brain tumors in children are astrocytomas; 11% are high grade; 13% are cerebellar astrocytomas; 25% are medulloblastomas; 10% are brainstem gliomas; 9% are ependymomas; and 9% are other subtypes. Both hereditary and environmental factors have been implicated, including parental occupation in the chemical or aircraft industry. Prior radiotherapy is a known cause of brain tumors. The presenting signs and symptoms with a brain tumor depend on the site and size. Symptoms such as headaches, irritability, nausea, vomiting (projectile), blurred or double vision, dizziness, behavior changes, and difficulty in walking or handling objects are common.

Diagnostic evaluation including MRI or CT scans with or without contrast media, lumbar puncture, and gadolinium-enhanced MRI is necessary for detection of dissemination of tumor into the CSF.

Cancer Types

The treatment modalities include surgery to decrease the tumor burden and radiation therapy with total doses from 2000 to 7000 cGy, depending on the tumor's pathology and location and the child's age. Radiosensitizers have been used to increase cellular radiosensitivity, thereby increasing cell death and minimizing host side effects. Chemotherapy protocols that include nitrosoureas, alkylating agents, and vinca alkaloids vary according to the drugs used, route, schedule, and dosing regimens. Autologous PBSCT is being investigated as a method to intensify therapy with high-grade or recurrent tumors.

H. **Non–Hodgkin's Lymphoma (4.0%)—**
Non–Hodgkin's lymphoma (NHL) has a peak incidence in the 7- to 11-year-old age group, a low incidence in adolescence, and a male predominance. Viruses, genetic factors, and radiation have been implicated as causative factors, with an increased risk in those with a primary immunodeficiency syndrome or immunosuppression. An acute onset of symptoms with a rapid progression such as dyspnea; stridor; dysphagia; wheezing; pain; and swelling of the neck, face, and upper extremities is common in children with NHL. Approximately 75% of cases have a mediastinal mass at diagnosis.

The diagnostic and staging evaluation is based on tissue samples from any bulky disease, bone marrow aspirates, and biopsies to evaluate bone marrow involvement with CSF specimen to detect CNS involvement. All children receive chemotherapy, with the exact combination and therapy duration depending on type and extent of disease. The most common sites for disease relapse are the primary site, bone marrow, and CNS. Those who have disease relapse or have resistant disease have a poor survival rate, and autologous or allogeneic PBSCT is often pursued.

I. **Hodgkin's Disease (4.4%)—**
Hodgkin's disease (HD) in children has a similar etiology, biology, natural history, and response to treatment to that in adults. Ninety percent of children with HD have an unusual lump varying in size, fatigue, anorexia, and slight weight loss at examination. Unexplained fever (>38° C oral), weight loss (>10% within previous 6 months), and drenching

night sweats are of prognostic significance. The diagnostic evaluation (very similar to the adult evaluation) includes laboratory studies, CT scans of chest and abdomen, bone scans, bone marrow aspiration, and biopsy of tissue to confirm the diagnosis. The treatment most often used is combination chemotherapy with traditional regimens and may include autologous PBSCT.

J. **Wilms' Tumor (5.9%)**—
Wilms' tumor is an embryonic tumor predominantly occurring in the initial 5 years of life. An association exists between Wilms' tumor and the deletion or inactivation of the short arm of chromosome 11, band 13. Children with Wilms' tumor may have associated congenital anomalies, including hemihypertrophy, cryptorchidism, hypospadias, and congenital absence of iris. Presenting clinical features include hematuria, dysuria, hypertension, abdominal pain, fever, anemia, and malaise.

Diagnostic evaluation includes CT scans of chest and abdomen; MRI, ultrasound; bone marrow aspirate; skeletal survey; chest x-ray; and biologic, genetic, and laboratory studies, with biopsy of the primary site to confirm the diagnosis. Treatment involves chemotherapy, alone or with radiation therapy, depending on the stage and histologic type. Autologous stem cell transplantation is considered for consolidation therapy of high-risk relapsed disease patients who have achieved complete remission.

Bibliography

American Cancer Society: *Cancer prevention and early detection, facts and figures 2003*, Atlanta, 2003, The Society.

American Cancer Society: *Cancer facts and figures 2003*, Atlanta, 2003, The Society.

Arceci R, Ettinger A, Forman E, et al: National action plan for childhood cancer: report of the national summit meetings on childhood cancer, *CA Cancer J Clin* 52(6):377, 2002.

Byers T, Nestle M, McTiernan A, et al: American Cancer Society guidelines on nutrition and physical activity for cancer prevention: reducing the risks of cancer with healthy food choices and physical activity, *CA Cancer J Clin* 52(2):92, 2002.

Brennan MF, Lewis JJ: Soft tissue sarcomas. In Townsend CM Jr, Beauchamp RD, Evers BM, et al, editors: *Textbook of surgery,*

Cancer Types

the biological basis of modern surgical practice, ed 16, Philadelphia, 2001, WB Saunders.

Fleming I, Cooper JS, Henson De, et al: *AJCC cancer staging manual,* ed 5, Philadelphia, 2002, Lippincott Williams & Wilkins.

Jennings-Dozier K, Mahon SM, editors: *Cancer prevention, detection, and control,* Pittsburgh, 2002, Oncology Nursing Press.

Karayalcin G: Hodgkin's disease. In Lanzkowsky P, editor: *Manual of pediatric hematology and oncology,* ed 3, San Diego, 2000, Academic Press.

Oncology Nursing Society: *Cancer chemotherapy guidelines and recommendations for practice,* Pittsburgh, 2001, Oncology Nursing Press.

Otto SE, editor: *Oncology nursing,* ed 4, St. Louis, 2001, Mosby.

Paley C: Rhabdomyosarcoma and other soft tissue sarcomas. In Lanzkowsky P, editor: *Manual of pediatric hematology and oncology,* ed 3, San Diego, 2000, Academic Press.

Redner A: Central nervous system malignancies. In Lanzkowsky P, editor: *Manual of pediatric hematology and oncology,* ed 3, San Diego, 2000, Academic Press.

Redner A: Leukemias. In Lanzkowsky P, editor: *Manual of pediatric hematology and oncology,* ed 3, San Diego, 2000, Academic Press.

Redner A: Malignant bone tumors. In Lanzkowsky P, editor: *Manual of pediatric hematology and oncology,* ed 3, San Diego, 2000, Academic Press.

Redner A: Wilms' tumor. In Lanzkowsky P, editor: *Manual of pediatric hematology and oncology,* ed 3, San Diego, 2000, Academic Press.

Shende A: Neuroblastoma. In Lanzkowsky P, editor: *Manual of pediatric hematology and oncology,* ed 3, San Diego, 2000, Academic Press.

Shende A: Non-Hodgkin's lymphoma. In Lanzkowsky P, editor: *Manual of pediatric hematology and oncology,* ed 3, San Diego, 2000, Academic Press.

Smith RA, Cokkinides V, Eyre HJ: American Cancer Society guidelines for the early detection of cancer, 2003, *CA Cancer J Clin* 53(1):27, 2003.

UNIT III

CANCER TREATMENTS, THERAPIES, AND MANAGEMENT

20
Surgical Oncology

I. APPLICATIONS

A. Establish Cancer Diagnosis—

1. *Incisional Biopsy*—The most expedient method used to obtain large amounts of tissue for diagnosis (sarcomas) or concern in sampling error in diffuse lesions. Homeostasis must be maintained throughout the procedure to avoid hematogenous seeding.

2. *Excisional Biopsy*—Used when it is necessary to remove the entire lesion and is best suited for small lesions.

3. *Core Needle Biopsy (14- to 16-gauge needle)*—Yields fragments of tissue that allow the evaluation of the tumor architecture; this procedure may be combined with mammography (stereotactic biopsy), computed tomography, or ultrasonography. Caution is used with this technique for patients with coagulation disorders because of the potential for bleeding in surrounding tissue if biopsy is obtained from vascular structures, hollow organs, or in the central nervous system.

4. *Cutaneous Punch Biopsy*—Used to obtain tissue from cutaneous lesions by using 2- to 6-mm round surgical blades with full-thickness skin specimens.

5. *Endoscopic Procedure*—This procedure uses a flexible instrument to remove small portions of tumor located in the gastrointestinal, genitourinary, and pulmonary tracts; it allows access to tumors only accessible by laparotomy or thoracotomy with minimal harm to adjacent tissue.

6. *Fine-Needle Aspiration Cytology*—Uses a small-gauge needle (22 to 25 gauge) that can be percutaneously guided to most anatomic sites. Advantage includes sampling of a wide area of the tumor;

Treatment

limitations include inability to obtain a small sample size, lack of information on histology structure that cannot distinguish between in situ and invasive tumors (breast, thyroid), and inability to grade tumor and interpretation of certain immunohistochemical stains.

B. **Staging Work-Up to Determine Extent of Cancer Disease—**

1. *Laparotomy*—Selectively used for staging ovarian and nonseminomatous testicular cancers.

2. *Lymphadenectomy*—Used with certain cancer types, tumor location, or clinical evidence of nodal involvement to discern indication of distant disease development.

3. *Laparoscopy*—Used as a procedure of diagnosis and staging of intraabdominal cancers such as liver, pancreas, stomach, and medullary thyroid. Biopsies can be obtained from solid organs, lymph nodes, or suggestive lesions. This procedure is a sensitive imaging technique used in detection of liver metastasis. Additional uses include combining laparoscopy with ultrasonography for lesions deep into the parenchyma of an organ, as well as tumor invasion in adjacent structures such as major blood vessels.

4. *Mediastinoscopy*—Used in the preoperative staging of bronchogenic cancer and evaluation of mediastinal adenopathy. This procedure is highly sensitive (100%) and specific (90%) in the staging of bronchogenic cancer.

5. *Sentinel Lymph Node Biopsy*—Uses radiolabeled dye, which is injected around the lesion, followed by a radiograph and intraoperative use of gamma probe to discern the suspect node. A second technique involves use of isosulfan blue dye injected intraoperatively around the tumor and allowed to migrate to the lymphatic channels to the first blue or radioactive lymph node. The procedure may involve lymphoscintigraphy to identify certain draining nodal reservoirs.

C. **Surgical Treatments—**

1. *Primary Treatment*—Removal of malignant tissue and having a disease-free normal tissue margin is the primary treatment. The goal is to achieve a

cure by reducing the patient's total body tumor burden (such as melanoma, head and neck, and breast cancers). Surgery is the preferred treatment for tumors that *have low growth fractions, have long cell cycle times, and are confined locally or regionally* (Figure 20-1).

2. *Adjuvant Treatment*—Reduces risk for incidence, progression, or recurrence of cancer such as cytoreductive or debulking; used in ovarian cancer and for neuroblastoma and other childhood cancers. A secondary use is to mark the residual tumor location for many cancers to receive additional treatment with radiation therapy.

3. *Prophylactic Treatment*—The removal of organ/tissue for prevention of diseases that have a high potential or incidence of occurrence, such as the colon (ulcerative colitis). The decision is based on risk associated with patient medical and family history, presence or absence of symptoms, and the degree of difficulty in diagnosing certain cancers. Prophylactic treatment may also include

Treatment

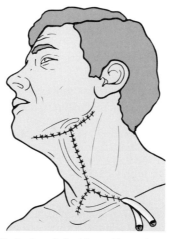

Figure 20-1 Radical neck incision with suction tubing in place. (From Hickey MM, Hoffman LA: Nursing management: upper respiratory problems. In Lewis C, Heitkemper M, Dirkens S, editors: *Medical-surgical nursing*, ed 5, St. Louis, 2004, Mosby.)

cancer prevention with the removal of benign polyps of the cervix, bladder, colon, and stomach and removal of lesions from epithelial surfaces such as skin, oral cavity, and cervix.

4. *Reconstructive Treatment*—Involves the reconstruction of an anatomic defect caused by an extensive cancer surgery. The goal is to improve function and cosmetic appearance, such as facial reconstruction after head and neck cancer surgery, breast reconstruction after mastectomy, superficial tissue repair for skin graft used in treatment of malignant melanoma, and bone grafts or joint prosthesis in osteogenic sarcomas.

5. *Salvage Treatment*—Involves the use of an extensive surgical approach to treat a local disease recurrence such as a mastectomy after initial lumpectomy with radiation therapy for breast cancer.

6. *Palliative Treatment*—Used to alleviate symptoms and to make the patient more comfortable through such treatments as bone stabilization, repair perforation of fistulas, treatment of spinal cord compression, relief of painful or life-threatening obstructions or bleeding, and management of severe and debilitating pain through nerve blocks, cordotomy, neurectomy, or sympathectomy.

D. **Insertion of Therapeutic Hardware and Devices**—Multiple devices are surgically implanted to ease administration of certain therapies or to improve the patient's comfort by alleviating varied symptoms.

1. *Ventricular Reservoir (Ommaya Reservoir)*—Used for the administration of chemotherapy and opioids to allow a more constant and predictable drug delivery into the subarachnoid space and cerebrospinal fluid.

2. *Vascular Access Devices*—Used for intravenous administration of multiple therapies (hydration fluids, chemotherapy, biotherapy, parenteral nutrition, blood and blood products, antimicrobials, antiemetics, and analgesics). They may be connected to ambulatory infusion pumps to allow these therapies to be administered on a continuous or intermittent basis in varied care settings (ambulatory care, home, or hospice) or if the patient will be traveling.

3. *Arterial Catheters*—Used for administration of intraarterial chemotherapy to a specific anatomic site (hepatic or carotid artery); they allow greater levels of drug delivery without concomitant systemic drug toxicity.

4. *Implanted Infusion Pumps*—Used for continuous regional infusion of chemotherapy or analgesics to specific anatomic body sites (hepatic artery or cerebrospinal fluid). It has no external components and is accessed percutaneously. Unique features of this type of pump include "remote programmable changes" through a computer to regulate drug flow rate.

5. *External Feeding Tubes*—Insertion (of gastrostomy and jejunostomy tubes) provides a safe and consistent manner to administer enteral nutrition products.

6. *Malignant Pleural Effusion Shunts*—Inserted into the pleural cavity (internal portion similar to shortened chest tube). The silicone dome shape device near the skin surface is percutaneously accessed to allow drainage of fluid from the pleural cavity.

7. *Tenckhoff Catheters*—Surgical placement aids in the treatment of malignant ascites that occur with lymphomas and cancers of the ovary, colon, or stomach. Insertion of these catheters may also be used for peritoneal dialysis or administration of intraperitoneal chemotherapy.

8. *Ureteral Stents*—Inserted to allow or to improve flow of urine in ureteral obstructive dysfunction.

II. PRINCIPLES

A. Anatomic Location—

The tumor location can prevent or impede access for removal; for example, an adequate margin of healthy tissue cannot be removed or the tumor is attached to vital structures such as the superior vena cava.

B. Histologic Type—

Certain histologic types of cancer are not treated with surgery because the disease is disseminated at the time of diagnosis (small-cell lung cancer, malignant lymphoma).

Treatment

C. **Tumor Size—**
   Smaller sized tumors are less likely to have spread; therefore the patient is more likely to benefit from surgery.

D. **Tumor Cell Kinetics—**
   Well-differentiated, slow-growing tumors consisting of cells with long cell cycles are best suited for surgical resection or removal.

E. **Tumor Invasion—**
   Cells remaining after cancer therapy might have the ability to reproduce and cause disease recurrence; therefore surgery intended to be curative must include the resection of healthy tissue around the tumor to ensure removal of all cancer cells.

F. **Metastatic Potential or Pattern and Extent of Metastatic Spread—**
   Depending on the tumors' metastatic pattern or spread and whether it is early or advanced, tumors can be treated with aggressive surgery. Removal of a tumor-bearing organ and its nearby lymph nodes or tumor resection performed before the patient begins adjuvant courses of chemotherapy, or both, is beneficial to the patient.

III. SELECTED SURGICAL TECHNIQUES

A. **Electrosurgery—**
   Eliminates cancer cells by using the cutting and coagulation effects of a high-frequency electrical current applied by needles, blades, or electrodes.

B. **Cryosurgery—**
   Involves the application of liquid nitrogen through cryoprobe inserted into a tumor for in situ destruction by deep-freezing the intracellular and extracellular structure.

C. **Chemosurgery—**
   The combined use of layer-by-layer surgical resection of tissue and topical application of chemotherapeutic agents (Mohs chemotherapy).

D. **Laser—**
   Process that creates *laser* light (*l*ight *a*mplification by *s*timulated *e*mission of *r*adiation); therapy is used for local excision. The lasers destroy cancer cells by an intense thermal energy therapy and can be used for cancers of the larynx, skin, and female reproductive tract.

E. **Photodynamic Therapy—**
Involves intravenous injection of photosensitizing drug (hematoporphyrin derivative) with uptake by cancer cells, followed by exposure to a *laser light* within 24 to 48 hours of injection. This results in fluorescence of cancer cells and cell death.

F. **Video-Assisted Thoracoscopy—**
Using general anesthesia with single-lung ventilation, the surgeon makes three 1-cm incisions to insert the video-assisted thoracoscopy devices. A rigid telescope and camera are introduced through the first incision, and the endoscopic surgical instrument is introduced into the remaining incisions. Multiple procedures can be performed such as pulmonary wedge resections, diagnosis and treatment of pleural effusions, and biopsy or resection of mediastinal tumors.

G. **Intraoperative Electron Beam Radiation Therapy—**
Tumoricidal doses of radiation are delivered to tumors at the time of surgery while the dose to adjacent healthy tissue is minimized. This therapy is used with preoperative or postoperative external-beam irradiation or neoadjuvant chemotherapy to treat various sites, including the stomach, bile duct, pancreas, retroperitoneum, and rectum.

IV. PATIENT CONSIDERATIONS

A. **Patient's General Health—**
Impacts the ability to undergo the anesthesia and surgical procedure, and is important in assessing the risk for developing postoperative complications.

B. **Host Resistance or Immune Competence—**
Affects the patient's ability to initiate an immunologic response to cancer cells that remain after surgery and to provide resistance to infection.

C. **Patient's Quality of Life—**
Needs to be considered when choosing treatments that may have long-term effects after treatment completion.

D. **Patient's Nutritional Status—**
Protein-calorie malnutrition usually results when there is a decrease in oral intake and an increase in nutritional requirements such as presence of a tumor, intestinal fistulas, or hypermetabolic state. This process contributes to poor wound healing,

anemia, infection, sepsis, increased morbidity, or further malnutrition.

E. **Blood or Coagulation Disorders—**
   Presence of anemia or thrombocytopenia should be addressed before surgery to minimize postoperative bleeding. A hypercoagulability status may result in postoperative deep vein thrombus. Pancreatic, gastric, lung, and brain cancer are the cancers most commonly associated with recurring deep vein thrombus.

F. **Complications of Multimodal Therapy—**
   Combination therapies impact the patient's ability to heal and recover completely from the various side effects of therapy, such as fibrosis and obstructive lymphatic channels from radiation therapy, which interferes with postoperative wound healing. Certain chemotherapy drugs are toxic to specific organ systems (hepatic, renal, respiratory, cardiac) and increase the patient's risk for surgical complications.

G. **Older Patients Have Increased Surgical Risks—**
   For example, there is a greater risk of hypoxemia with general anesthesia. Age, obesity, and preexisting pulmonary disease predispose the patient to hypoxemia development with the potential postoperative complications of pulmonary edema, decreased cardiac output, or aspiration pneumonia.

Bibliography

Aft RL: Principles of surgical oncology. In Govindan R, Arquette MA, editors: *The Washington manual of oncology*, Philadelphia, 2002, Lippincott Williams & Wilkins.

Goedegebuure PS, Eberlein TJ: Tumor biology and tumor markers. In Townsend CM Jr, Beauchamp RD, Evers BM, et al, editors: *Textbook of surgery, the biological basis of modern surgical practice*, ed 16, Philadelphia, 2001, WB Saunders.

Healey JH: Bone tumors. In Townsend CM Jr, Beauchamp RD, Evers BM, et al, editors: *Textbook of surgery, the biological basis of modern surgical practice*, ed 16, Philadelphia, 2001, WB Saunders.

Heizenroth P: Surgery: it's got some nerve, *Nursing* 31(10): 32hn1, 2001.

Joyce M, Houlihan N: Current strategies in the diagnosis and treatment of lung cancer, *Oncol Nurs* 8(1):1, 2001.

Moran AB, Camp-Sorrell D: Maintenance of venous access devices in patients with neutropenia, *Clin J Oncol Nurs* 6(3):126, 2002.

Morrow M, Strom EA, Bassett LW, et al: Standard for the management of ductal carcinoma *in situ* of the breast, *CA Cancer J Clin* 52(5):277, 2002.

O'Brien B: Advances in the treatment of colorectal cancer, *Oncol Nurs* 9(2):1, 2002.

O'Grady NP, Alexander M, Dellinger EP, et al: Guidelines for the prevention of intravascular catheter-related infections. Centers for Disease Control and Prevention, *MMWR Recomm Rep* 51(RR-10):1, 2002.

Otto SE, editor: *Pocket guide to intravenous therapy*, ed 4, St. Louis, 2001, Mosby.

Pfeifer K: Surgery. In Otto SE, editor: *Oncology nursing*, ed 4, St. Louis, 2001, Mosby.

Rosenberg SA: Principles of cancer management: surgical oncology. In DeVita VT Jr, Hellman S, Rosenberg SA, editors: *Cancer principles and practice of oncology*, ed 6, Philadelphia, 2001, Lippincott Williams & Wilkins.

Schrump DS, Nguyen DM: Malignant pleural and pericardial effusions. In DeVita VT Jr, Hellman S, Rosenberg SA, editors: *Cancer principles and practice of oncology*, ed 6, Philadelphia, 2001, Lippincott Williams & Wilkins.

Schwartz SI, Shires GT, editors: *Principles of surgery*, ed 7, New York, 1999, McGraw-Hill.

Slingluff CL, Hendrix J, Seigler HE: Melanoma and cutaneous malignancies. In Townsend CM Jr, Beauchamp RD, Evers BM, et al, editors: *Textbook of surgery, the biological basis of modern surgical practice*, ed 16, Philadelphia, 2001, WB Saunders.

Treatment

21
Radiation Therapy

I. GOALS
Radiation therapy (RT) is a localized treatment that is used alone or in conjunction with other treatments such as chemotherapy and surgery. The radiation dose is recorded as the absorbed energy per unit mass. The Systeme Internationale Unit for radiation dosage is the Gray. The dose of radiation may be reported as gray (Gy) or centigray (cGy). RT has several approaches to treating different cancer diseases or conditions.

A. **Curative—**
   To eradicate the disease and allow the individual to live a normal life span.

B. **Control—**
   To control the growth and spread of the disease, allowing the patient to live for a time without symptoms.

C. **Prevention—**
   To prevent microscopic disease, such as using cranial irradiation for certain types of lung cancers.

D. **Palliation—**
   To improve the quality of life by relieving or diminishing symptoms associated with advanced cancer such as pain from bone metastasis, tumor obstruction around major vessels, or spinal cord compression.

E. **Myeloablative—**
   Leukemic cells are very radiosensitive; and in conjunction with high-dose chemotherapy, total body irradiation is used to reduce the tumor cell volume and provide immunosuppression to prevent the rejection of the blood/stem cell graft.

II. PRINCIPLES
High-energy ionizing radiation destroys the ability of cancer cells to grow and multiply. The ionizing rays or

particles directly damage some cells; other cells are indirectly affected when the particles penetrate the cell's nucleus causing damage to the DNA or chromosomal strands. Immediate cell death may occur at this time or the cell may die at mitosis, when it is unable to repair the damage. The radiosensitivity of cancer cells depends on several factors.

A. **Type of Cell—**
For example, lymphoma, leukemia, and seminoma have high radiosensitivity; squamous cell of oropharynx, bladder, skin, cervical epithelial, and adenocarcinoma of the alimentary tract have a fairly high radiosensitivity; vascular and connective tissue elements of all tumors and astrocytoma have medium radiosensitivity; salivary gland tumors, hepatomas, renal cancer, pancreatic cancer, chondrosarcoma and osteogenic sarcoma have fairly low sensitivity; and rhabdomyosarcoma and leiomyosarcoma have a low radiosensitivity.

B. **Phases of Cell Life—**
Cells in the resting phase are less sensitive to radiation than those in active cellular division.

C. **Division Rate of the Cell—**
Rapidly dividing cells are more sensitive to RT than slowly dividing cells.

D. **Degree of Differentiation—**
Poorly differentiated cells are more sensitive to RT than well-differentiated cells.

E. **Oxygenation—**
Well-oxygenated tissues are more sensitive to RT because oxygen is needed to form the hydroxyl (free) radicals.

III. INNOVATIONS

A. **Three-dimensional Conformal Radiotherapy—**
Combines the use of computed tomography scans or magnetic resonance images with special computer programs to design fields that conform the *radiation dose to the tumor*. This design enables large radiotherapy doses to be delivered to the tumor, thereby increasing cell death and decreasing the metastatic potential of the tumor and morbidity to healthy nearby tissue (prostate, thyroid, and breast).

Treatment

B. **CyberKnife—**
Is a radiosurgical system consisting of a linear accelerator and a robotics arm with the capacity to precisely locate tumors and deliver multiple beams of RT directly to the tumor site while minimizing radiation exposure of surrounding tissue. The CyberKnife has the capacity to treat tumors up to 6 cm in size.

C. **Intensity Modulation RT—**
The design and delivery of nonuniform radiation intensity patterns to maximize dose to tumors and minimize dose to critical structure such as urethra, rectum, and bladder.

D. **High-Dose Rate Brachytherapy—**
Delivers radiation directly into or near the site of tumor or previous site of disease such as pelvis, bronchus, esophagus, head and neck, and breast cancer.

E. **Intraoperative RT—**
Provides direct visualization and treatment of tumors to control local recurrence by using high-dose rate remote afterloading equipment to treat colorectal, gastric, pancreatic, bladder, and cervical cancers and retroperitoneal sarcomas.

F. **Photodynamic Therapy—**
Involves the use of light-sensitive molecules or photosensitizers that are activated by light to form oxygen radicals, which in turn affect cell membrane, the cytoplasm, and the DNA, resulting in cell death. Approximately 48 hours after administration of photosensitizers, laser treatment with the appropriate wavelength is given. It takes approximately 48 hours for the tumor to reach the optimal concentration of porfimer sodium. Photodynamic therapy is used in the treatment of superficial bladder, head and neck, skin, lung, and esophageal cancers, and for bone marrow purging for the treatment of leukemia and lymphoma.

G. **Radiopharmaceuticals—**
Strontium 89 and samarium 153 (administered intravenously [IV]) are used for treating pain from multiple osteoblastic bony metastases from breast, prostate, or lung cancer. Radiopharmaceuticals seek out areas of bone metastases and provide radiation to the bony metastatic site. Pain relief is noted within

1 to 2 weeks and this relief may last for several months.

H. Radioprotectant Drug—
A drug such as amifostine is administered IV approximately 30 minutes before the delivery of RT. Amifostine penetrates the healthy tissue and more slowly penetrates tumor cells, thus providing a vehicle in the delivery of RT treatment to exploit the cell differential effect. This drug also offers a protectant effect on salivary glands, hematopoietic system, mucosal system, and bladder.

I. Radiosensitizers—
Chemical radiosensitizing compounds are used to increase the sensitivity of tumor cells to radiation, thus increasing the lethal effects of radiation, while having minimal or no impact on healthy tissue. Certain chemotherapeutic drugs such as cyclophosphamide or cisplatin are being used not only for their cytotoxic effects but also as radiosensitizers and are given concurrently with RT.

J. Stereotactic Radiosurgery—
This high dose of RT is delivered to a small, well-defined area with the use of a gamma knife, linear accelerator, and heavy beam particles. A head immobilizer with a fixed screw to skull ensures stabilization to perform procedures at precise intracranial locations for purpose of biopsy, to implant antineoplastic drug wafers, or to perform other procedures. Stereotactic radiosurgery is used in the cancer and noncancer patient population in treating astrocytoma, brain metastasis, arterial venous malformations, Parkinson's disease, cluster headaches, and epilepsy.

IV. ADMINISTRATION
A. Treatment Planning—
1. *External Beam Radiation (teletherapy)*—External beam radiation uses a treatment machine placed at some distance from the body. The varied treatment machines deliver the electron energy or gamma rays through linear accelerator or electron beam to the specific tumor site (Figure 21-1).

This process requires a pretreatment planning stage, which uses a simulator to "simulate the actual

Treatment

treatment in its movement and positioning." A variety of radiographic studies such as computed tomography scans, magnetic resonance imaging studies, or nuclear scans are used to define the exact body area requiring treatment and the adjacent organs/tissues that require protection from the radiation dose.

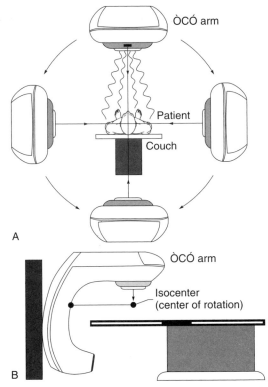

Figure 21-1   Modern linear accelerator. **(A)** Modern linear accelerator can rotate 360 degrees about a single point in space (called the *isocenter*). This allows the isocenter to be placed inside the tumor, at which time the machine can be angled in any direction and will always be treating the region of interest. **(B)** Viewed from the side, the isocentric point can be placed anywhere inside the patient by adjustment of the treatment couch, either up or down, or left or right, toward or away from the gantry.

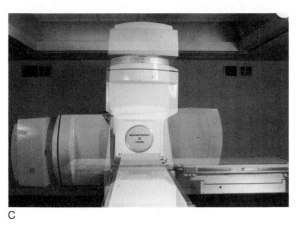

Figure 21-1—cont'd **(C)** An actual high-energy machine photographed in its anterior and right lateral isocentric positions. (From Abeloff MD, Armitage JO, Lichter AS, et al, editors: *Clinical oncology,* New York, 2000, Churchill Livingstone).

Immobilization devices are used to assist the patient in maintaining a precise position during the treatment period. Special shielding blocks are made to minimize radiation exposure of healthy tissue near the treatment area. Marks such as small tattoos are placed on the body of ensure that treatment delivery will be consistent for each dose and time.

B. **Treatment Delivery—**
1. *External RT*—External radiation treatments are usually delivered on a Monday through Friday basis for a period of 2 to 8 weeks. The actual treatment is 2 to 5 minutes for each session. The number of treatments delivered during a treatment course depends on the type and extent of the cancer, the area to be treated, and the dose. The number of treatments is divided into small daily doses called *fractionation. Hyperfractionation* is a treatment dose that is administered two or three times a day with at least 4 to 6 hours between each treatment.
2. *Total Body Irradiation*—Used as a myeloablative therapy in preparation for blood/stem cell transplantation. Doses range from 8 to 14 Gy depending on fractionation.

Treatment

3. *Internal RT*

   a. *Brachytherapy: Sealed Radioactive Sources—* Radiation is delivered by implanting a sealed radioactive source in or near the cancerous site to provide a localized treatment. Commonly used sealed brachytherapy sources include cesium 137, iridium 192, iodine 125, palladium 103, gold 198, and strontium 90. Sealed brachytherapy sources can be placed temporarily (e.g., use of iridium 192 for high-dose rate applications in cervical cancer) or permanently (e.g., use of iodine 125 applications for prostate cancer).

   Brachytherapy is also used in treatment of endometrial cancer through intracavity placement; breast, rectal, and head and neck cancers through interstitial placement; esophageal cancer with intraluminal placement; and bronchogenic cancer with an endobronchial placement. Radioactive sources or implants may be in the form of ribbons, seeds, wires, capsules, catheters, needles, or tubes, which are encapsulated (sealed) to prevent body fluid contamination. These implants may be placed on a temporary or permanent basis depending on tumor type, location, and goal of treatment.

   b. *Brachytherapy: Nonsealed Radioactive Sources—* Commonly used nonsealed brachytherapy sources include iodine 131, phosphorus 32, strontium 89, and samarium 153. Strontium 89 and samarium 153 have demonstrated efficacy in treating pain related to osteoblastic bony metastasis from breast, prostate, or lung cancer. These radioactive isotopes from nonsealed sources are administered IV or are taken orally by the patient. The patient and the body secretions may be radioactive for a period of time. Depending on the type of isotope used, it may be necessary to isolate the patient for 3 to 4 days because of the radioactivity emitted. Instructions before administration of the isotope should include symptom management, how the implant could affect those symptoms, and any activity restriction while the implant is in place.

c. *Radiolabeled   Antibodies*—Joining tumor-specific antibodies with radioactive isotope combines the science of immunology with RT to maximize tumor treatment while minimizing healthy tissue toxicity. These special antibodies are designed to be attracted to specific antigens (e.g., CD20 surface antigen) on certain tumor cells (e.g., B-cell non-Hodgkin's lymphoma) while sparing healthy tissues. They are administered IV to the patient; entering the bloodstream, they seek out the tumor, and the radioactivity attached to the antibody directly treats the cancer cells.

A current treatment for non-Hodgkin's lymphoma uses this therapy, combining it with administration of a monoclonal antibody (e.g., rituximab). The rituximab dose is given before the scheduled dose of ibrituomomab tiuxetan (Indium-111) on day 1 of a 7- to 9-day treatment regimen. Assessments of the biodistribution of the radiolabeled isotope are done at 2 to 24 hours, and a second image is made at 48 to 72 hours. If the biodistribution is acceptable, a second infusion of rituximab is administered on day 7 or 9 and within 4 hours an intravenous injection of 0.4 mCi/kg yttrium 90 is administered. This two-step treatment process using the combination of radiolabeled isotopes with monoclonal antibodies is being used in multiple clinical trials.

V. SIDE EFFECTS
A. Alopecia—
Occurs within the treatment area and depends on the dose and extent of radiation to the scalp.
B. Anorexia—
The result of RT used in combination with other therapies; other contributing factors include inactivity, medications, and inability to completely digest food.
C. Cerebral Edema—
Occurs as tissues around the tumor become inflamed resulting in headache, nausea, vomiting, vision changes, motor disabilities, slurred speech, and changes in mental status. Assessment of these symptoms is crucial; note specific changes or progressive

Treatment

symptoms and immediately report changes to the physician.

D. Cough—
May develop or increase if lung tissue is within the treatment field. Initially the cough is productive and then progresses to a nonproductive cough as the mucosa becomes dry. The character, intensity, and frequency of the cough and the lung sounds need to be monitored on a scheduled frequency to minimize respiratory infection.

E. Cystitis—
Occurs if the bladder is in the treatment field. Symptoms include dysuria, nocturia, decreased bladder capacity, urinary frequency, urgency, and hesitancy; occasionally bleeding occurs.

F. Diarrhea—
Can occur 2 to 3 weeks after starting RT and may last throughout the course of the therapy. Symptoms may include an increased number of stools, loose or watery stools, and abdominal cramping and may progress to chronic enteritis.

G. Esophagitis—
Occurs if part of the esophagus is within the treatment field. Symptoms usually occur 2 to 3 weeks from the beginning of therapy and include pain with swallowing (lump in throat) that ranges from moderate to severe, resulting in treatment delays until the acute symptoms subside.

H. Fatigue—
May result from the tumor breakdown. An increased metabolic rate usually occurs after treatment each day and gradually decreases when treatment is completed.

I. Hair Texture and Color—
Changes in hair color or texture may also occur. The scalp can develop pruritus and can become very dry or peel.

J. Hypopituitarism—
Occurs as a result of decreased secretions of cortisol, thyroxine, and sex hormones. Accompanying signs and symptoms may include fatigue, weakness, weight loss or weight gain, dry skin and hair, decrease in sexual libido, hypoglycemia, alopecia, and muscle weakness. These symptoms may occur within the first year after RT or may be delayed several years after treatment.

K. **Myelosuppression—**
   Occurs when volumes of active bone marrow are in the treatment field (pelvis, spine, sternum, ribs, and metaphyses of long bones). Monitor blood counts on a scheduled frequency.

L. **Osteoradionecrosis—**
   A late and chronic effect of RT that can occur any time after RT and usually occurs in the mandible. Tooth decay, poorly healed infections, and compromised bone structure lead to bone necrosis.

M. **Ovarian Failure—**
   Occurs with small amounts of radiation and produces symptoms associated with menopause such as hot flashes, amenorrhea, decreased libido, and osteoporosis.

N. **Radiation Fibrosis—**
   May occur 6 to 12 months after the radiation treatment to the lung is completed. This consequence of RT is a restrictive disease of the lung. Shortness of breath is the primary symptom.

O. **Radiation Pneumonitis—**
   Can occur approximately 1 to 3 months after RT to the lung. Initial symptoms begin with an unproductive cough that becomes productive accompanied by fever and dyspnea.

P. **Skin—**
   Erythema may range from mild, light pink, to deep and dusk red.

Q. **Stomatitis—**
   Occurs as result of radiation effects on rapidly dividing cells. Symptoms may range from mild to severe. Prudent and frequent mouth care is essential to minimize complications such as bleeding or infection.

R. **Testicles—**
   The testicles are shielded from radiation during therapy; however, if accidental exposure occurs, spermatogenesis will stop and can result in permanent sterility.

S. **Tooth Decay and Caries—**
   Cariogenic bacteria adhere to the teeth and flourish in the acidic environment that is the result of xerostomia. Pre-RT examination with a dentist and use of fluoride is recommended.

Treatment

T. **Xerostomia—**
Usually occurs when the treatment field includes the salivary glands. Dryness of the mouth may occur 1 to 2 weeks into therapy and may result in speaking, eating, and swallowing problems. Ensure prudent mouth care.

VI. PROTECTION MEASURES

A. **Staff Protection—**
Occupational radiation exposure should be kept as low as reasonably achievable. The major agencies and organizations that have regulatory authority (U.S. Nuclear Regulatory Commission, Food and Drug Administration, and the individual states) determine radiation protection standards and regulations. ALWAYS USE the principles of Time, Distance, and Shielding to minimize the nurse's individual radiation exposure.

1. *Time—Minimize time* spent in close proximity to the radioactive source/patient.
2. *Distance—Maximize the distance* from the radioactive material.
3. *Shielding—*When appropriate, *use shielding to decrease exposure* to radiation. With radium or cesium implants, a 1-inch-thick lead shield is positioned next to the bed to diminish radiation exposure.
4. *Monitoring of Personnel—*It is highly recommended that nurses wear an assigned film badge while caring for radioactive patients, change according to agency guidelines, and do not share badges with any other persons.
   a. NEVER touch a dislodged radioactive source. However, if this incident occurs, immediately notify the appropriate RT personnel and the patient's physician.

B. **Patient/Family/Caregiver Protection—**
1. *Place patient in private room* for internal RT.
2. *Instruct patient and patient's family* on all of the procedures and restrictions (visitors, activity, body fluid precautions, linen and dietary requirements).
3. *Provide discharge instructions,* including any further protective measures the patient/family/caregiver will need in the home setting.

4. *Precautions* with pharmaceuticals include:
- Radioactive precautions for body fluids are necessary for approximately 7 days after administration.
- Flush toilet twice after use.
- Wipe up spilled urine with a paper tissue and discard in the toilet before flushing.
- Wash hands after using the toilet.
- Immediately wash linen and clothes that become soiled with urine or blood. Wash these items separately from other laundry.
- If an injury occurs and blood is spilled, wash away any spilled blood with water and a paper tissue and flush the paper tissue in the toilet.

Bibliography

Bradley JD, Perez CA: Fundamentals of patient management in radiation oncology. In Govindan R, Arquette MA, editors: *The Washington manual of oncology,* Philadelphia, 2002, Lippincott Williams & Wilkins.

Bruner DW, Bucholtz JD, Iwamoto RR, et al: *Manual for radiation oncology nursing practice and education,* Pittsburgh, 1998, Oncology Nursing Press.

Dow KH, Bucholtz JD, Iwamoto RR, et al, editors: *Nursing care in radiation oncology,* ed 2, Philadelphia, 1997, WB Saunders.

Hellman S: Principles of cancer management: radiation therapy. In DeVita VT Jr, Hellman S, Rosenberg SA, editors: *Cancer principles and practice of oncology,* ed 6, Philadelphia, 2001, Lippincott Williams & Wilkins.

Hendrix CS, de Leon C, Dillman RO: Radioimmunotherapy for non-Hodgkin's lymphoma with yttrium 90 ibritumomab tiuxetan, *Clin J Oncol Nurs* 6(3):144, 2002.

Iwamoto R: Radiation therapy. In Otto SE, editor: *Oncology nursing,* ed 4, St. Louis, 2001, Mosby.

Murrin J, Glatstein E, Pass HI: Small-cell lung cancer. In DeVita VT Jr, Hellman S, Rosenberg SA, editors: *Cancer principles and practice of oncology,* ed 6, Philadelphia, 2001, Lippincott Williams & Wilkins.

Quinn AM: CyberKnife: a robotic radiosurgery system, *Clin J Oncol Nurs,* 6(3):149, 2002.

Tan SJ: Recognition and treatment of oncological emergencies, *J Infus Nurs,* 25(3):182, 2002.

Wasserman TH, Rich KM, Drzymala RE: Stereotatic irradiation. In Perez CA, Brady LW, editors: *Principles and practice of radiation oncology,* ed 3, Philadelphia, 1998, Lippincott-Raven.

Treatment

Chemotherapy

I. GOALS

A. Cure—
Cure the disease or effect a complete remission of at least 5 years

B. Control—
Provide an extension to patient's survival when cure of the disease is not possible

C. Palliation—
Improve quality of life, and increase comfort by reducing tumor burden or relieving obstruction, pain, or other symptoms

D. Myeloablative—
Provide disease-free bone marrow, create space in marrow, and suppress host immune system in preparation for blood/stem cell transplantation

E. Chemoprevention Agents—
Use varied drugs or nutrients that block the initiation of carcinogenesis or halt the progression of premalignant cells; usually given to individuals at high-risk for certain cancers (such as tamoxifen to women for breast cancer prevention and vitamin E and selenium to men for prostate cancer prevention)

II. USES

A. Adjuvant—
A course of chemotherapy used in conjunction with another treatment (e.g., surgery or radiation therapy). The goals of this therapy are to treat the remaining cancer cells or micrometastasis and to prevent local or distant relapse of the disease.

B. Neoadjuvant—
The administration of chemotherapy given to shrink a tumor before it is removed surgically or treated with radiation therapy.

C. **Primary—**
The treatment of patients who have localized disease. This is also considered as the major treatment source for some diseases.

D. **Induction—**
The initial chemotherapy course used most often in acute leukemia to achieve significant cell death and complete remission of the disease.

E. **Intensification/Consolidation—**
The second course of chemotherapy with different or same drugs or the dose to achieve disease remission for patients with acute lymphoblastic and acute myelogenous leukemia.

F. **Maintenance—**
Chemotherapy therapy given over 1, 2, or 5 years. The treatment goal of maintenance is to prevent the disease from recurring.

G. **Salvage—**
Chemotherapy is used to control the cancer disease or to provide palliation for patients when other treatments were not successful.

H. **Combination Chemotherapy—**
Multiple drugs given in different doses, routes, or schedule. The goal of combination chemotherapy is to enhance the drug(s)' effect on tumor cell death.

Principles used in the selection of drugs for combination chemotherapy include the following:
1. *Verified effectiveness as a single agent*
2. *Results in increased tumor cell death*
3. *Presence of a synergistic action*
4. *Different mechanisms of action*
5. *Varied dose-limiting toxicities*
6. *Prevent or slow development of disease/drug resistance*

III. PRINCIPLES

A. **Cell Generation Cycle—**
A sequence of events that results in replication and distribution of DNA to the daughter cells, produced by cell division. All cells, nonmalignant and malignant, progress through the five phases of the cell cycle.

The disruption of the cell cycle offers numerous opportunities for chemotherapy or radiation therapy

Treatment

to be effective in targeting the cancer cells for increased cell death—for example, by inducing an arrest of G1/S and G2/M phases in *p53*-deficient cells, thereby ultimately damaging the DNA in the cycle and causing cell apoptosis.

1. G_0—Resting or dormant phase when healthy renewable tissue is not actively proliferating. In this phase, the cells perform all functions except proliferation. The nondividing and ressubting cells are included in this phase. During the G_0 phase, cancer cells are resistant to effects of chemotherapy.

2. G_1—Extends the previous cell division and the beginning of chromosome replication by synthesizing the protein (RNA) in preparation for S-phase cycle.

3. S—RNA is synthesized in preparation for DNA synthesis. Cells are most vulnerable to damage from chemotherapy and radiation therapy during this phase of the cell cycle.

4. G_2—DNA synthesis and structural protein enzymes develop the mitotic spindle in preparation for mitosis and cell division.

5. M—Mitosis and cell division occur; duplication of DNA must be complete before the cells enter the mitotic cycle. This phase is further subdivided into four stages: *prophase, metaphase, anaphase, and telophase.*

B. **Cell Kill Hypothesis—**
   A single cancer cell is capable of multiplying and eventually killing the host. Every tumor cell must be killed to cure cancer. With each *course of drug therapy,* a given dose of chemotherapeutic drug kills only a *fraction* or percentage of the cancer cells. Repeated courses of chemotherapy must be used to reduce the total number of cancer cells. Skipper and colleagues established this cardinal rule of chemotherapy—inverse relationship between cell number and curability—in the early 1960s.

C. **Classifications of Chemotherapy Drugs—**
   1. *Cell Cycle Phase: Specific*—Specific drugs are active on cells undergoing a specific phase in the cell cycle. These drugs have the greatest effect on cell death when given in divided doses or as a continuous infusion with a short cycle time.

a. *Antimetabolites*—Exhibits action by blocking the essential enzymes necessary for DNA molecule synthesis leading to strand breaks or premature chain termination.

b. *Vinca Plant Alkaloids*—Exerts a cytotoxic action by binding to tubular proteins during the M phase (metaphase stage) causing mitotic arrest with the cell losing its ability to divide and resulting in cell death.

c. *Miscellaneous Agents*—Act with a variety of mechanisms such as inhibiting protein synthesis, cell proliferation, and inducing apoptosis.

2. **Cell Cycle Phase: Nonspecific**—Nonspecific drugs are active on cells in all phases of the cell cycle and are usually administered through bolus dosing.

a. *Alkylating Agents*—Act to form a molecular bond that interferes with nucleic acid duplication, thus preventing mitosis. They also inhibit DNA and RNA and protein synthesis.

b. *Antitumor Antibiotics*—Disrupt DNA transcription and inhibit DNA and RNA synthesis.

c. *Nitrosoureas*—Inhibit synthesis and replication of DNA and RNA. They also have the ability to cross the blood-brain barrier.

d. *Hormonal Agents*—Alter the environment of the cell by affecting membrane's permeability.

e. *Antihormonal Agents*—provide the ability to neutralize the effect of, or inhibit the production of, natural hormones used by hormone-dependent tumors.

f. *Corticosteroids*—Exert an antiinflammatory effect on body tissues, increase appetite, and promote a feeling of well-being.

D. **Factors Influencing Chemotherapy Selection and Administration**—

1. **Blood-Brain Barrier**—The blood-brain barrier is made up of cellular structures that can inhibit certain substances from entering the brain or central nervous system tumors and acts as a screening device, thereby protecting the brain and cerebrospinal fluid from harmful agents.

2. **Cytoprotectant**—Drugs used to prevent or decrease specific system toxicities such as

hemorrhagic cystitis (mesna) and cardiac toxicity (dexrazoxane).

3. *Liposomes (fat body): "Stealth Technology"*—Drugs that are "packaged" or manipulated and tailored to penetrate specific target tissues, thereby limiting organ toxicity such as with doxorubicin HCL.

4. *Drug Resistance*—A process by which the cancer cell becomes resistant to chemotherapeutic agents. This resistance effect may occur before exposure to the chemotherapeutic agent or may become acquired when the cells have been exposed to the drug with repeated doses. Some malignant cells are resistant to a single drug or can develop multidrug resistance.

5. *Radiosensitizers*—The use of concomitant continuous infusion chemotherapy and radiation therapy in the treatment of a variety of cancers. These compounds enhance the sensitivity of the tumors to the effects of radiation but do not affect healthy tissue. Drugs such as amifostine, cisplatin, gemcitabine, and paclitaxel have been documented and evaluated as radiosensitizers.

E. **Patient Factors Considered in Chemotherapy Drug Selection**—
   1. *Patient's eligibility for chemotherapy* (confirmed diagnosis; previous therapies; age; bone marrow, cardiac, hepatic, respiratory, renal, and nutritional status)
   2. *Cancer cell histology type* (e.g., squamous cell, adenocarcinoma)
   3. *Rate of drug absorption* (e.g., treatment interval, dosages, and routes)
   4. *Tumor location* (many drugs do not cross the blood-brain barrier)
   5. *Tumor burden* (larger tumors are generally less responsive to chemotherapy)
   6. *Tumor resistance to chemotherapy* (tumor cells can mutate and produce variant cells distinct from the tumor stem cell of origin)

F. **Chemotherapy Dosing Listings**—
   1. *Standard-Dose Therapy*—This is the usual adult dose administered for most patients with cancer.

2. **High-Dose Therapy**—An increased drug dose is given to achieve tumor cell death; this therapy results in severe side effects such as myelosuppression in myeloablative therapy for blood/stem cell transplantation.
3. **Dose Intensity**—Specific drugs are administered at a greater dose than standard therapy and at shorter intervals such as every 21 days rather than every 28 days.
4. **Dose Density**—This refers to increased drug doses and combinations of varied drugs and is sometimes stated as *doublet* or *triplet therapy* in cancer protocols.

IV. ADMINISTRATION

A. Drug Dose Calculation—

The drug dosage for chemotherapy is based on body surface area in both children and adults. Some drug dosages are calculated proportionally to the patient's body surface area, which is calculated in square meters (m^2) with a nomogram. An accurate height and weight must be obtained and used in these calculations. All drug calculations should be verified by a second person to ensure dose accuracy.

B. Drug Reconstitution—

Staff involved in chemotherapeutic drug reconstitution should be knowledgeable, skilled, and competent and should use a class II biologic safety cabinet. Aseptic technique must be used in accordance with manufacturer's current recommendations for reconstitution. All syringes or infusion solutions of such drugs should be labeled immediately with the drug's name and dose.

C. Drug Administration Recommendations—

1. *Verify the patient's identification, drug, dose, route, and time of administration* with the prescribing physician's order.
2. *Review drug allergy history* with the patient.
3. *Anticipate and plan for possible side effects or major system toxicity* (Table 22-1).
4. *Verify informed consent* for treatment.
5. *Review appropriate laboratory and diagnostic test results*.

Treatment

Table 22-1 MAJOR SYSTEM TOXICITY OR DYSFUNCTION AND NURSING MANAGEMENT

Toxicity/Dysfunction	Nursing Management
CARDIAC TOXICITY	
Drugs associated with potential for: chlorambucil, cyclophosphamide, dactinomycin, daunorubicin, doxorubicin, mitoxantrone, and high-dose ifosfamide, paclitaxel	Verify baseline cardiac studies (e.g., electrocardiogram, ejection fraction, cardiac enzymes) before drug administration.
	Monitor cardiac status and report symptoms regarding tachycardia, shortness of breath, distended neck veins, gallop heart rhythm, and ankle edema.
	Monitor and record total cumulative dose of drug in the patient's medical record; doxorubicin approximate maximum lifetime dose is 500 mg/m^2.
HEPATIC TOXICITY	
Drugs associated with potential for: asparaginase, busulfan, carmustine, chlorambucil, cytarabine, doxorubicin, 5-fluorouracil, lomustine, mercaptopurine, methotrexate, mitoxantrone, mithramycin, mitomycin, paclitaxel, and streptozocin	Verify physician order for administration of dexrazoxane (Zinecard).
	Monitor liver function studies, such as lactic dehydrogenase (LDH), bilirubin, prothrombin time, and liver function tests (SGOT, SGPT). Report to

the physician signs of jaundice, tenderness over the liver, and urine and stool color changes.

HYPERSENSITIVITY REACTION

Drugs associated with potential for: asparaginase, bleomycin, docetaxel, doxorubicin (local erythema), etoposide, paclitaxel, and teniposide

Review the patient's allergy history.

Monitor for symptoms of hypersensitivity and anaphylaxis, such as agitation, urticaria, rash, chills, cyanosis, bronchospasm, abdominal cramping, and hypotension; onset may be rapid or delayed; advise the patient to report subjective symptoms promptly.

Ensure proper medical equipment is nearby and in good working condition.

Drugs for emergency intervention should be readily available.

When administering a drug with potential for a reaction, give a test dose, monitor vital signs, and observe for allergic response.

If allergic response occurs, stop drug administration and notify the physician immediately.

Continued

Treatment

Table 22-1   MAJOR SYSTEM TOXICITY OR DYSFUNCTION AND NURSING MANAGEMENT—cont'd

Toxicity/Dysfunction	Nursing Management
METABOLIC ALTERATIONS	
Hypercalcemia	Monitor serum level; observe for anorexia, constipation, nausea, vomiting, polyuria, and mental status change.
Hyperglycemia	Monitor serum and urine levels; observe for symptoms of thirst, hunger, glucosuria, and weight loss.
Hyperkalemia	Monitor serum level: observe for symptoms of confusion, complaints of numbness or tingling, weakness, and cardiac arrhythmias.
Hypernatremia	Monitor serum level and weight loss; observe for symptoms of thirst, dry mucous membranes, poor skin turgor, rapid thready pulse, restlessness, lethargy.
Hyperuricemia Potential with treatment of highly proliferative tumors, such as leukemia and lymphoma	Monitor serum and urine levels; daily intake and output. Initiate prescribed drug therapy (e.g., allopurinol) to inhibit the formation of uric acid before administration of chemotherapy drug.

Provide vigorous hydration, such as oral and intravenous (IV) fluid intake (2000–3000 ml), beginning 12–24 hr after initiation of chemotherapy.

Alkalize urine to pH >7 by administration of IV $NaHCO_3$ (sodium bicarbonate).

Report symptoms of pain, chills, fever, and diminished urinary output.

Hypocalcemia

Monitor serum level; observe for symptoms of muscle cramping, tingling of extremities, depression, and tetany.

Hypomagnesemia

Monitor serum level; observe for symptoms of personality changes, anorexia, nausea, vomiting, lethargy, weakness, and tetany.

Hyponatremia

Monitor serum level; observe for symptoms of rales, shortness of breath, distended neck vein, weight gain, edema of sacrum or lower extremity, increasing mental status changes.

Treatment

Continued

Table 22-1   MAJOR SYSTEM TOXICITY OR DYSFUNCTION AND NURSING MANAGEMENT—cont'd

Toxicity/Dysfunction	Nursing Management
NEUROTOXICITY Drugs associated with potential for: ifosfamide, vinblastine, vincristine, high peak plasma levels of etoposide, 5-fluorouracil; high-dose and/or intrathecal administration of cytarabine, carboplatin, cisplatin, and methotrexate	Monitor and report symptoms of weakness, numbness, and tingling sensation of hands, arms, and feet; also monitor and report symptoms of hoarseness, jaw pain, hallucinations, mental depression, decreased or absent deep tendon reflexes, slapping gait or footdrop, severe constipation, and paralytic ileus.
OTOTOXICITY Drug associated with potential for: cisplatin	Verify baseline audiogram. Verify physician order for administration of amifostine (Ethyol). Monitor and report symptoms of tinnitus, hearing loss, and vertigo.
PULMONARY TOXICITY Drugs associated with potential for: bleomycin, busulfan, carmustine	Verify baseline respiratory function. Individuals older than age 70 yr have increased risk.

RENAL SYSTEM TOXICITY

Drugs associated with potential for: carmustine, cisplatin, cyclophosphamide, ifosfamide, methotrexate, mitomycin C, streptozocin, and thiotepa

Monitor respiratory status and report symptoms of dyspnea, dry cough, rales, tachypnea, and fever.

Assess 24-hr urine creatinine clearance before treatment.
Verify baseline renal function.
Verify physician order for administration of amifostine (Ethyol).
Encourage adequate fluid intake, such as 2–3 L for 24 hr before and after therapy.
Monitor intake and output, weight changes.
Report diminished output to physician, e.g., <500 ml in 24 hr.
Administer drug mesna concomitant with ifosfamide, high-dose cyclophosphamide, and thiotepa.

REPRODUCTIVE SYSTEM DYSFUNCTION

Drugs associated with potential for: busulfan, chlorambucil, cyclophosphamide,

Assess for nature and frequency of sexual dysfunction.
Counsel patients regarding avoidance of pregnancy and

Continued

Treatment

Table 22-1   MAJOR SYSTEM TOXICITY OR DYSFUNCTION AND NURSING MANAGEMENT—cont'd

Toxicity/Dysfunction	Nursing Management
REPRODUCTIVE SYSTEM DYSFUNCTION—cont'd	
mechlorethamine, melphalan, thalidomide, thiotepa, vinblastine, and vincristine Antihormonal agents: fenretinide, finasteride, flutamide, goserelin, letrozole, leuprolide, tamoxifen	sperm banking before chemotherapy administration; provide information on contraceptives. Birth control practices are recommended by most practitioners for 2 yr following chemotherapy to provide for evaluation of disease response, avoidance of possible teratogenic drug effects, and in male patients, recovery of spermatogenesis. Inform the patients of potential for temporary or permanent infertility and loss of libido. Women may experience symptoms including amenorrhea, "hot flashes," insomnia, dyspareunia, and vaginal dryness; estrogen therapy may be helpful in management of these symptoms.
HEMATOPOIETIC CHANGES: LEUKOPENIA	
Most myelosuppressive agents produce white blood cell (WBC) nadir 7–14 days after drug	Avoid sources of infection, such as contact with people with bacterial infections, colds, sore throats, flu,

administration; myelosuppression will be severe and prolonged with increased dosages: for example, with cytarabine 3–6 g; busulfan 2–6 g; cyclophosphamide 2–3 g; methotrexate 6–8 g; etoposide 2–3 g.

chickenpox, measles, or cold sores or people recently vaccinated with live vaccines such as measles-mumps-rubella or diphtheria-pertussis-tetanus.

Avoid having fresh fruit, live plants, and flowers at or near bedside.

Avoid eating raw vegetables, fruits, and eggs.

Nursing Intervention

Monitor WBC and differential; change equipment as indicated—for example, O_2 setup, denture cups, IV supplies; teach sexual hygiene.

Avoid cleaning animal litter boxes because feces contain highlevels of bacteria and fungi.

Maintain good personal hygiene—for example, bathe daily, wash hands before eating and preparing food, clean carefully after bowel movements, and keep nails clean and clipped short and straight across; maintain adequate fluid intake.

Conserve energy; get adequate rest and exercise.

Prevent trauma to the skin and mucous membranes.

Avoid elective dental work or surgery.

Avoid enemas, rectal suppositories and temperatures, and catheterizations.

Continued

Treatment

Table 22-1 MAJOR SYSTEM TOXICITY OR DYSFUNCTION AND NURSING MANAGEMENT—cont'd

Toxicity/Dysfunction	Nursing Management
Nursing Intervention—cont'd	Use toothettes or nonabrasive dental cleaning devices. Report signs and symptoms of infection immediately to the physician; for example, report fever of 38°C or greater, cough, sore throat, a shaking chill, painful or frequent urination, or vaginal discharge.
HEMATOPOIETIC CHANGES: THROMBOCYTOPENIA	
Drugs associated with a delayed cumulative effect: mitomycin and all nitrosoureas	Avoid use of straight-edge razor, power tools, and physical activity that could cause injury. Avoid use of drugs containing aspirin. Humidify the air; use lotion and lubricants on skin and lips; use a soft bristle toothbrush.
Nursing Intervention Monitor platelet counts; observe bleeding precautions; apply firm pressure to venipuncture site for 3–5 min; monitor pad count on menstruating females; monitor environment for sharp objects.	Avoid invasive procedures; no intramuscular injections, rectal or vaginal examinations, enemas, suppositories, or the use of rectal thermometers. Discourage bare feet when ambulatory Use sanitary pads instead of tampons.

Immediately report the following signs and symptoms to the physician: bleeding gums, increased bruising, petechiae, purpura, hypermenorrhea, tarry-colored stools, blood in urine, or coffee-ground emesis. Check with the physician before any dental work.

HEMATOPOIETIC CHANGES: ANEMIA

Nursing Intervention

Monitor hematocrit and hemoglobin, especially during drug nadir.

Adjust physical activity to accommodate periods of rest. Report the following signs and symptoms promptly to the physician: fatigue, dizziness, shortness of breath, and palpitations.

From Otto SE, editor: *Oncology nursing* ed 4, St. Louis, Mosby, 2001.

Treatment

6. *Select appropriate equipment and supplies* and ensure that emergent supplies are at or near the patient's bedside.

7. *Calculate the dose and reconstitute the drug using aseptic technique;* also follow safe handling guidelines.

8. *Explain the procedure to the patient* and the patient's family.

9. *Administer antiemetics* or other prescribed medications.

10. *Initiate peripheral intravenous (IV) site,* or prepare venous access device and site.

    Peripheral venipuncture sites must be changed on a scheduled basis to reduce the possibility of phlebitis and infiltration. If vesicant drugs are administered, the peripheral IV access must be changed every 24 hours.

11. *Always use sterile normal saline (0.9%)* to test vein or catheter lumen patency or vein patency and flush the IV access with sterile normal saline *before, between,* and *after* each drug or solution administration.

12. *Administer chemotherapy drugs at the prescribed rate and schedule.*

    a. Monitor the patient and the chemotherapy drug infusion at scheduled intervals throughout the course of drug administration.

    b. *Vesicant drugs administered through bolus technique*—Validate blood return before, during, and after drug administration. Plan verification of blood return checks on a scheduled frequency (e.g., every 2 to 4 hours) for continuous vesicant infusions.

    c. *Nonvesicant drug-administered boluses*—Validate blood return before and after drug administration and on a scheduled frequency (e.g., every 4 hours) for continuous infusion.

    d. *Irritant drug-administered boluses*—Validate blood return before, during, and after drug administration; monitor continuous infusion every 4 hours.

    e. Continuous chemotherapy infusions should be monitored on a scheduled frequency and should be infused through a reliable infusion pump. Observe the desired volume infusing over the scheduled time and make the prescribed rate adjustments.

    f. Dispose of all used supplies and unused drugs in approved, puncture-proof, leak-proof containers outside the patient area.

    g. Document the procedure in the patient's medical record according to agency policy and guidelines.

D. Routes of Chemotherapy Administration—

  1. *Oral Route*—Ensure patient compliance with the prescribed schedule and instruct the patient on the potential diet or oral intake-related requirements.

  2. *Subcutaneous and Intramuscular Route*—Provide injection demonstration and then allow patient/caregiver the opportunity to demonstrate the technique; teach safe handling and disposal of supplies requirements and teach injection site assessment.

  3. *Intravenous:*

    a. *Bolus*—Administer drug into IV access injection port with keep-open IV infusion rate; validate blood return *before, during,* and *after* drug administration.

    b. *Continuous or Intermittent*—Plan scheduled monitoring for drug infusion to include drug/infusion solution, infusion device, venous access site, and potential patient drug-related side effects. Verify that venous access device and infusion tubing solution have secure connection(s).

  4. *Intraarterial*—Drug may be administered through temporary catheter threaded into the brachial, carotid, or femoral artery with use of an infusion pump with designated PSI to overcome resistance of arterial pressure. The catheter is inserted by a physician during fluoroscopy and is connected to a *one-way* valve inserted into the infusion tubing/solution to prevent back flow of blood into the infusate. Premedicate patient before catheter insertion; verify end-point catheter tip placement with the physician before use for chemotherapy. Monitor the patient, drug infusion, infusion pump and catheter site on a scheduled frequency during the temporary arterial catheter placement.

  5. *Intraperitoneal*—Drug and infusion solution should be warmed to body temperature with dry

Treatment

heat before infusion. A sterile procedure is used to cleanse the intraperitoneal catheter connection before chemotherapy infusion solution. Monitor on a scheduled frequency the catheter and catheter patency, infusate, device access, and patient for drug-related side effects.

6. *Intrapleural*—Drug is infused into chest tubes. Provide patient analgesia before drug infusion; monitor vital signs and drug side effects; assist patient in changing body position (side-to-side and side-to-back at least four times after drug injection); and provide analgesia, other comfort measures, or both.

7. *Intrathecal*—Drug is administered through an Ommaya reservoir, lumbar puncture access, or both; it requires *preservative-free diluent for drug reconstitution.* Monitor potential neurotoxicity side effects, potential for infection, and increased intracranial pressure.

8. *Intravesicular*—Skin testing technique is used to inject medication to make a wheal on the inner aspect of the forearm. Monitor site for erythema. This technique is used most often in performing a drug (hypersensitivity) skin test at least 60 minutes before scheduled drug infusion.

9. *Intracavity*—Drug/solution is infused through a Foley catheter into body cavity (bladder). Instill the solution and keep the catheter tubing clamped for a designated period (30 to 60 minutes). Unclamp the catheter and allow drainage; dispose all used supplies (catheter, tubing, drainage bag) and other chemotherapy supplies into chemotherapy disposal containers.

E. **Special Considerations for Administration—**

1. *Anaphylaxis and Hypersensitivity Management*— Anaphylaxis and hypersensitivity are severe reactions that occur from a life-threatening immunologic response to a foreign substance or antigen. Certain chemotherapeutic drugs are known to cause hypersensitivity or anaphylaxis in many patients. These reactions can occur immediately or can be delayed for several hours. Most occur within 30 minutes of drug or solution initiation

(see Chapter 32 for detailed information). Prompt, effective nursing intervention for anaphylaxis reduces complications. Be alert to the signs and symptoms of hypersensitivity and anaphylaxis. All or some of the following symptoms may be present: anxiety, cyanosis, hypotension, urticaria, respiratory distress, abdominal cramping, flushed appearance, and chills.

If the Patient Develops Any of These Symptoms Follow These Guidelines:

a. Immediately stop the drug/infusion solution.
b. Maintain an IV access and infusion line with isotonic saline.
c. Position the patient for comfort to promote perfusion of the vital organs.
d. Notify the physician, nursing agency, or emergency medical services.
e. Maintain the airway and anticipate the need for cardiopulmonary resuscitation.
f. Monitor the patient's vital signs according to agency policy.
g. Administer the appropriate prescribed medications with an approved physician's order.
h. Follow the agency's protocol for follow-up care (e.g., evaluation of the patient by a physician).
i. Document the incident and the interventions in the patient's medical record.
j. Ensure prompt replacement of all emergency drugs and supplies used in the hypersensitivity or anaphylaxis management.

2. *Extravasation Management*—

a. *Pathophysiology*—Extravasation is the accidental infiltration of a vesicant or irritant chemotherapeutic drug from the access device or vein into the surrounding tissue at the IV or venous access site. Vesicant drugs can produce a blister or can cause tissue necrosis or destruction. Irritant drugs are known to cause venous pain at the IV site and along the vein pathway with or without an obvious inflammatory reaction. Injuries that may occur from extravasation include sloughing of tissue, infection, pain, and formation of substantial scar tissue.

Treatment

b. *Risk Factors*—Risk factors include *patient conditions* (small fragile veins, superior vena cava syndrome, peripheral neuropathy, and excessive movement at or near IV access site) and *venous access techniques* (venipuncture and drug administration technique and anatomic placement [wrist or elbow] of venous access device).

c. *Clinical Features*—Clinical features include pain, hyperpigmentation, induration, erythema or tissue discoloration, vesicle (blister) formation, tissue ulceration or sloughing, damage to secondary tissue (tendons and nerves) and necrosis. The degree of tissue damage is related to several factors including drug vesicant potential, drug concentration and amount of drug extravasated, duration of tissue exposure, and venous access insertion technique or type of device.

d. Protocol for Extravasation Management at a Peripheral Site
   - STOP administration of the chemotherapy drug.
   - ENSURE IV access/leave current IV access in place.
   - NOTIFY the physician and OBTAIN orders for drug antidote and treatment.
   - ASPIRATE any chemotherapy drug residual and blood in the IV access.
   - INSTILL the IV/subcutaneous antidote or apply topical antidote.
   - ELEVATE the extremity and APPLY cold or warm compresses as indicated.
   - CONSULT regarding removal of venous access per PHYSICIAN'S ORDER.
   - CONSIDER referral to a plastic surgeon and PHOTOGRAPH SITE according to agency policy and procedure for documentation and follow-up.
   - DOCUMENT all interventions for the drug extravasation. Complete the agency form for documentation of the incident—who, what, when, where, and how.
   - MONITOR the drug extravasation site on a scheduled frequency for pain, erythema, induration, and necrosis and the response to the interventions provided.

    e. *Nurse Practice Issues*—Be knowledgeable of the chemotherapy drugs that have vesicant and irritant potential and know placement of emergent supplies needed to provide the appropriate interventions for drug extravasation.

- *Chemotherapy Drugs with Vesicant Potential:* mechlorethamine hydrochloride, idarubicin, doxorubicin, daunorubicin, mitomycin, dactinomycin, mitoxantrone epirubicin, vincristine, vinblastine, vindesine, vinorelbine, and paclitaxel
- *Chemotherapy Drugs with Irritant Potential:* dacarbazine, ifosfamide, carboplatin, cisplatin, doxorubicin liposome, bleomycin, menogaril, etoposide, and teniposide

G. Safe Handling of Chemotherapy Guidelines—

    1. *Potential Health Risks Associated with Chemotherapy Drugs*—Occupational exposure to chemotherapeutic agents can impact the health/wellness of the nurse and the nurse's offspring. These drugs bind to genetic material in the cell nucleus or interfere with cellular protein synthesis and potentially result in cell death, cell mutation, or cell transformation.

        Conditions associated with occupational exposure to chemotherapeutic drugs include:

    a. *Carcinogenicity*—The carcinogenic drug properties' risk for causing cancer

    b. *Genotoxicity*—The risk for chromosomal changes caused by chemotherapy drugs

    c. *Teratogenicity (fertility impairment)*—The risk from chemotherapy drugs that cause gonadal dysfunction (spermatotoxicity and ovarian follicular destruction)

    d. *Organ Toxicity*—Many chemotherapeutic drugs are known to be toxic to skin, mucous membranes, and cornea.

    e. *Accidental Exposures*—Exposure in a poorly ventilated area can result in symptoms such as dyspnea, headache, eye or throat irritation, and dizziness.

    2. *Safe Handling Guidelines*

    a. Drug Preparation:

- Wash hands before and after drug handling.
- Limit access to drug preparation area.

Treatment

- Keep labeled drug spill kit near preparation area.
- Apply latex gloves, long-sleeve gown with cuff, and snug-fitting goggles before drug handling.
- Prepare drugs using aseptic technique.
- Use Luer-Lok equipment and prime IV drug tubings inside zip-lock bag.
- Label all chemotherapeutic drugs and other drugs administered.
- Clean up any spills immediately.

b. Drug Administration
- Wear protective equipment (latex gloves, long-sleeve gown with cuff, and snug-fitting goggles).
- Inform patient that chemotherapeutic drugs are harmful to healthy cells and that protective measures used by staff minimize their exposure.
- Administer drugs in a safe unhurried environment.
- Place a plastic-backed absorbent pad under infusion tubing and syringes to minimize spills.
- Do NOT dispose of any used supplies in a patient care area.

3. *Disposal of Supplies and Unused Drugs*
   a. Place all supplies and unused drugs into a puncture-proof, leak-proof, labeled container. *The container should not be in the nurse's immediate work area or at the patient's bedside.*
   b. Disposal of containers filled with chemotherapeutic supplies and unused drugs should be in accordance with regulations regarding hazardous wastes.
   c. All hazardous containers should be appropriately labeled.

4. *Management of Chemotherapy Spills*
   a. *Supplies*—Chemotherapy spill kit; disposable protective gown; safety goggles; detergent solution for post-spill cleanup; leak-proof, puncture-proof, labeled container for disposal; dustpan/brush; and eye wash adapters in place at work sink

b. Procedure for Chemotherapy Spill
- Obtain spill kit.
- Apply protective apparel (long-sleeve gown, gloves, and goggles).
- Open disposal bags.
- Restrict area of spill.
- Use absorbent pads to absorb drug spill.
- Cleanse surface after spill.
- Dispose of all supplies in approved container.
- Wash hands.
- Document occurrence.
- If chemotherapy is splashed or sprayed into the eye, immediately flush the eyes with copious amount of water and seek follow-up medical eye examination.
- CLEANSE ALL EXPOSED SKIN (patient/personnel exposed to chemotherapy spill) with soap and water.

5. *Patient Care Issues*—Patient care issues include elimination, linen contamination, and home care issues. During and for 48 hours after chemotherapy administration, agency/hospital personnel must handle ALL patient excreta with chemotherapy protection apparel. Any hospital/agency linen soiled from chemotherapy should be placed in labeled impervious bags to notify laundry regarding special cleaning. Patient-owned linen is double-bagged to send home with the family with instructions to wash the linen separately from all other linen.

Bibliography

Berenblum I: Established principles and unresolved problem in carcinogenesis, *J Natl Cancer Inst* 60:723, 1978.

Brown CA: Safeguarding chemotherapy, *Nursing* 31(5):32hn1, 2001.

Camp-Sorrell D: Surviving the cancer, surviving the treatment: acute cardiac and pulmonary toxicity, *Oncol Nurs Forum* 26(6):983, 1999.

Chu E, DeVita VT Jr: Principles of cancer management: chemotherapy. In DeVita VT Jr, Hellman S, Rosenberg SA, editors: *Cancer principles and practice of oncology*, ed 6, Philadelphia, 2001, Lippincott Williams & Wilkins.

Chu E, Grever MR, Chabner BA: Cancer drug development. In DeVita VT Jr, Hellman S, Rosenberg SA, editors: *Cancer*

Treatment

principles and practice of oncology, ed 6, Philadelphia, 2001, Lippincott Williams & Wilkins.

Cleri LB, Haywood R: *Oncology pocket guide to chemotherapy*, Philadelphia, 2002, Elsevier.

Gahart BL, Nazareno AR: *Intravenous medications*, ed 18, St. Louis, 2002, Mosby.

Ginsberg RJ, Vokes EE, Rosenzweig K: Non-small-cell lung cancer. In DeVita VT Jr, Hellman S, Rosenberg SA, editors: *Cancer principles and practice of oncology*, ed 6, Philadelphia, 2001, Lippincott Wilkins & Wilkins.

Hodgson BB, Kizior RJ: *Saunders nursing drug handbook 2003*, Philadelphia, 2002, WB Saunders.

Holland JF, Frei E III, Bast RC Jr, et al, editors: *Cancer medicine*, ed 5, American Cancer Society, Hamilton, London, 2000, BC Decker.

Intravenous Nurses Society: *Standards of practice*, 23(65) 2000, The Society.

Joyce M, Houlihan N: Current strategies in the diagnosis and treatment of lung cancer, *Oncol Nurs* 8(1):1, 2001.

Murrin J, Glatstein E, Pass HI: Small-cell lung cancer. In DeVita VT Jr, Hellman S, Rosenberg SA, editors: *Cancer principles and practice of oncology*, ed 6, Philadelphia, 2001, Lippincott Williams & Wilkins.

Oncology Nursing Society: *Cancer chemotherapy guidelines and recommendations for practice*, Pittsburgh, Pa, 2001, Oncology Nursing Press.

Oncology Nursing Society: Oncology Nursing Society position, preventing and reporting of medication errors, *Oncol Nurs Forum* 28(1):15, 2001.

Oncology Special Edition: *Annual clinical reference*, New York, 2001, McMahon Publishing Group, oncologyse.com.

Otto SE, editor: *Pocket guide to intravenous therapy*, ed 4, St. Louis, 2001, Mosby.

Otto SE: Chemotherapy. In Otto SE, editor: *Oncology nursing*, ed 4, St. Louis, 2001, Mosby.

Papageorgio C, McLeod HL: Chemotherapy: principles and pharmacology. In Govindan R, Arquette MA, editors: *The Washington manual of oncology*, Philadelphia, 2002, Lippincott, Williams & Wilkins.

Schulmeister L: Chemotherapy medication errors: descriptions, severity, and contributing factors, *Oncol Nurs Forum* 26(6): 1033, 1999.

Sonnevald P: Multidrug resistance in hematological malignancies, *J Intern Med* 247:521, 2000.

SuperGen: *Safe handling of cytotoxic agents*, Pittsburgh, Pa, 2001, Oncology Education Services.

U.S. Department of Labor, Office of Occupational Medicine, OSHA: Controlling occupational exposure to hazardous, CPL 2-2.20B CH-4, Washington, DC, 1995, U.S. Government Printing Office.

Westervelt P, Vij R, DiPersio J: Principles of high-dose chemotherapy and stem cell transplantation. In Govindan R, Arquette MA, editors: *The Washington manual of oncology*, Philadelphia, 2002, Lippincott Williams & Wilkins.

23
Biotherapy

I. OVERVIEW

Biotherapy may be defined as treatment with agents derived from biologic sources or those that affect biologic responses. The subcommittee on Biologic Response Modifiers (BRMs) of the National Cancer Institute Division of Cancer Treatment defines BRMs as "agents or approaches that modify the relationship between tumor and host by modifying the host's biologic response to tumor cells with a resultant therapeutic effect." The continued advances in biotherapy are related to a more thorough understanding of the immune system and the biology of cancer, refinements in technology leading to the development and use of many agents that can affect tumor cell growth, and the product supply availability needed for many disease and treatment regimens.

Although nonspecific immunomodulating agents such as bacillus Calmette Guerin and *C. parvum* are still used, a variety of newer agents such as interferons (IFNs), interleukins, monoclonal antibodies, and hematopoietic growth factors are integrated into multiple therapeutic modalities. Many of these are naturally occurring body substances that act as messengers among cells. A generic term for these messengers is *cytokine*, which refers to protein products from cells that serve as cell regulators. More specifically, *lymphokines* are products of lymphocytes, and *monokines* are products of monocytes. The name *interleukin* refers to proteins that act as messengers among cells.

BRMs have more than one mode of action and can be classified into three major divisions:

- Agents that augment, modulate, or restore the host's immunologic mechanisms
- Agents that have direct antitumor activity (cytotoxic or antiproliferative mechanisms)

- Agents that possess other biologic effects, such as affecting differentiation or maturation of cells, interfering with the ability of a tumor cell to metastasize, or affecting initiation or maintenance of neoplastic transformation

II. DIAGNOSTIC USES
A. Detection of Disease—
Radiolabeled monoclonal targeted antibodies are administered in tracer doses, and using specialized scanners they are able to detect specific tumor cells that express certain antigens.
B. Differential Diagnosis—
Biotherapy agents are able to microscopically identify tumors and recognize cell-surface markers on certain tumor cells such as imaging studies for small-cell and non–small-cell lung cancer and prostate cancer.

III. THERAPEUTIC USES
A. Cure—
Used as a primary or adjuvant therapy to treat diseases such as hairy cell leukemia and melanoma.
B. Control—
Radioimmunotherapies/radiolabeled monoclonal antibodies target tumor cells that express certain antigens (e.g., CD20 surface antigen) delivering cytotoxic drug doses to those cells used in treatment of B-cell non-Hodgkin's lymphoma.
C. Prolong Survival—
IFN is used as a nontransplant treatment for chronic myelogenous leukemia and erythropoietin for treatment of chronic anemia in renal failure.

IV. BIOTHERAPY AGENTS IN USE
A. Interferons—
1. *Mechanism of Action*—Antiviral, antiproliferative, regulates tumor-cell growth, immunomodulator enhances natural kill cell activity, mediates other cytokines, and enhances antigen expression in some tumor types
2. *Generic Products*—IFN-α, IFN-β, and IFN-γ
3. *Clinical Indications*—Hairy cell leukemia, Kaposi's sarcoma, chronic myelogenous leukemia, chronic

Treatment

hepatitis C, chronic hepatitis B, melanoma, and condyloma acuminata

4. *Administration Route/Doses*—Most common administration method is subcutaneously (SC) and intravenously (IV); occasionally given intralesionally and intravesically. Dose range depends on route and goal of therapy—3 to 10 million U/m^2.

5. *Side Effects*—Flulike syndrome (fever [temperature spikes up to 104°F], chills, arthralgia, headache, and fatigue), hair thinning, nausea, vomiting, diarrhea, anorexia, weight loss, mild skin rash, and increased transaminase level. Flulike symptoms may occur within 2 to 4 hours after injection. Chronic side effects relating to these symptoms tend to increase in intensity and maintain that level of intensity for several weeks.

B. **Interleukins—**

1. *Mechanism of Action/Product*—Varies with the specific generic product

   a. *Interleukin-1 (IL-1) Immunoregulation*—Hematopoietic stimulation of early bone marrow precursors; augments T-cell activity, antiproliferative activity, and mediation of inflammatory response

   b. *IL-2 Immunomodulation*—Proliferation of lymphocytes, cytokine production, and enhancement of cell cytotoxicity

   c. *IL-3*—Multilinage stimulator of early bone marrow progenitors (granulocyte, monocyte, erythrocyte); stimulator of cytokine production and enhancer of myeloid cell function

   d. *IL-4*—Regulates B cell growth and antibody isotype expression, stimulates T cell growth and generation of cytotoxic T lymphocytes, regulates growth and differentiation of hematopoietic bone marrow stem cells, and stimulates macrophage function and mast cells

   e. *IL-6*—Provides cofactor for proliferation and differentiation of special populations of cytotoxic T cells, stimulates hematopoiesis (megakaryocyte differentiation), augments IL-3 activity, and regulates B cell growth

    f. IL-12—Facilitates T helper-1 responses, enhances lytic activity of natural kill cells, augments specific cytotoxic T lymphocyte responses, increases secretion of IFN-γ, promotes host resistance to infection, and provides antiangiogenic properties

  2. *Clinical Indications*—Renal cell carcinoma and melanoma; currently is being investigated in many clinical trials.

  3. *Administration Route/Doses*—Most common route is SC. Dose range includes 0.5 to 1.5 mcg/kg per dose over multiple doses and scheduled days of therapy.

  4. *Side Effects*—Fever, rigors, headache, nasal stuffiness, myalgia, and pruritus. Severe side effects such as tachycardia, hypotension, capillary leak syndromes, dyspnea, oliguria, arrhythmia, transient changes in liver function studies, and cardiomyopathy occur when scheduled treatment doses are given as protocol prescribes.

C. Hematopoietic Growth Factors—

  1. *Mechanism of Action/Product*—Varies with the specific generic product

    a. Erythropoietin—Stimulates differentiation of stem cells in bone marrow to increase red blood cell production.

    b. Granulocyte–Colony Stimulating Factor (G-CSF)—Promotes proliferation and differentiation of neutrophils and enhances functional properties of mature neutrophils.

    c. Granulocyte Macrophage-CSF (GM-CSF)—Stimulates production and differentiation of macrophages.

    d. Macrophage-CSF (M-CSF)—Stimulates production and differentiation of macrophages

    e. Oprelvekin (IL-11)—Stimulates proliferation of hematopoietic stem cells and megakaryocyte progenitor cells and induces megakaryocyte maturation resulting in increased platelet production.

  2. *Clinical Indications/Dose/Route*—Varies with the generic product, clinical disease, and goal of therapy

Treatment

> a. *Erythropoietin*—Prevent and treat anemia caused by cancer therapies (chemotherapy and stem cell transplantation) or chronic renal failure. *Usual dosage:* 150 to 300 U/kg three times weekly or 40,000 U as the starting dose.
>
> b. *G-CSF*—Decrease incidence of infection such as febrile neutropenia in patients with non-myeloid cancers who receive myelosuppressive anticancer drugs, and after blood/stem cell transplantation to decrease duration of neutropenia. *Usual starting dosage:* 5 μg/kg per day; dosage varies for blood/stem cell transplantation.
>
> c. *GM-CSF*—Enhance myeloid recovery after autologous blood/stem cell transplantation in patients with Hodgkin's disease, non-Hodgkin's lymphoma, and acute lymphocyte leukemia. *Usual dosage:* 250 μg/m² per day for a series of days.
>
> d. *Multi-CSF*—Stimulates production and differentiation of macrophages. Product is in clinical trials to determine clinical indications, dose, route, and potential side effects.
>
> e. *Oprelvekin*—Prevents severe thrombocytopenia and reduces need for platelet transfusions postmyelosuppressive chemotherapy for patients with nonmyeloid cancers. *Usual dosage:* 50 μg/kg per day SC initiated 6 to 24 hours after chemotherapy.

3. **Side Effects**—Fever, chills, myalgia, headache, bone pain, flushing-like sensation usually at time of product infusion, transient alteration of liver function, and rarely nausea, vomiting, and diarrhea

D. **Monoclonal Antibodies**—

Mechanism of action, product, clinical indications, dose and route, and side effects all vary with the specific product

1. *Satumomab Pendetide (OncoScint)*—Imaging of colon and ovarian cancer

> a. *Drug Information*—1 mg radiolabeled with 5 mCi indium 111 in chloride IV over 5 minutes; possible allergic reaction

2. ***Capromab Pendetide (ProstaScint)***—Imaging of prostate cancer
   a. *Drug Information*—0.5 mg radiolabeled with 5 mCi indium 111 in chloride IV over 5 minutes; possible allergic reaction
3. ***Rituximab (Rituxan)***—Treatment of relapsed or refractory low-grade or follicular, CD20$^+$ B-cell non-Hodgkin's lymphoma
   a. *Drug Information*—DO NOT administer through IV push or bolus; infuse at 50 mg/hr. Pretreatment with acetaminophen and diphenhydramine before each infusion may prevent infusion-related side effects (bronchospasm, hypotension, and increased respiratory secretions). *Usual dosage:* 375 µg/m^2 IV weekly for 4 weeks; initial infusion at 50 mg/hr, with subsequent infusions increased by 50 mg/hr every 30 minutes to a maximum dose of 400 mg/hr.
   b. *Side Effects*—Fever, chills, rigors, urticaria, mucosal congestion, nausea, diarrhea, myalgia, and arthralgia
4. ***Trastuzumab (Herceptin)***—Treatment of patients with metastatic breast cancer whose tumors overexpress the HER2 protein
   a. *Drug Information*—DO NOT administer through IV push or bolus; DO NOT mix with any other medications; DO NOT use dextrose solutions. Requires initial and ongoing cardiac assessment. *Usual dosage:* Initial loading dose 4 mg/kg over a 90-minute infusion, then 2 mg/kg IV weekly over 30 minutes.
   b. *Side Effects*—Fever, chills, nausea, vomiting, pain at tumor site, and *cardiac toxicity*
5. ***Gemtuzumab Ozogamicin (Mylotarg)***
   a. *Drug Information*—DO NOT administer through IV push or bolus. Use a separate intravenous line equipped with a low protein binding 1.2-micron filter. *Usual dosage:* 9 mg/m^2 intravenous infusion over 2 hours.
   b. *Side Effects*—Severe neutropenia, anemia, thrombocytopenia, chills, fever, nausea, vomiting, headache, hypotension, rash, mucositis, and hepatic toxicity

Treatment

6. *Muromonab-CD 3 (Orthoclone Okt-3)*—Treatment of rejection in organ transplant
   a. *Drug Information*—Administer IV push over at least 1 minute. Administer 1 mg/kg methylprednisolone before and 100 mg hydrocortisone 30 minutes after dose to decrease adverse reaction to **first dose.** *Usual dosage:* 5 mg/day for 10 to 14 days.
   b. *Side Effects*—Fever, chills, dyspnea, and malaise; occasional chest pain, nausea, vomiting, diarrhea, and tremor

E. **Retinoids**—
   All-*trans*-retinoic acid, tretinoin
   1. *Mechanism of Action*—Provides a role in vision, growth and reproduction, epithelial cell differentiation, and immune function. Current area of research is use in chemoprevention studies exploring the drug's ability to arrest or reverse the process of carcinogenesis, that is, prevent cancer invasion and metastasis in cancer.
   2. *Clinical Indications/Dose/Route*—Approved for the induction of remission in patients with acute promyelocytic leukemia (APL). All patients should receive standard consolidation or maintenance chemotherapy for APL after completion of induction therapy with tretinoin unless otherwise indicated. *Usual dosage and route:* PO 45 mg/m^2 per day in two evenly divided doses.
   3. *Side Effects*—Temporary change in pigmentation, photosensitivity, and pruritus.

F. **Immunomodulators**—
   1. *Bacillus Calmette Guerin*
      a. *Mechanism of Action*—Nonspecific immunostimulating effect.
      b. *Clinical Indications/Dose/Route*—Localized bladder cancer; bacillus Calmette Guerin can be administered through intravesical instillation, and the dose varies. Additional routes include intralesion, intradermal scarification, and the tine technique.
      c. *Side Effects*—Flulike symptoms (fever, chills, headache, and nausea) and potential hypersensitivity reaction

2. *Levamisole*
  a. *Mechanism of Action*—Anthelmintic; immuno-modulation (immunostimulation, immunosup-pression)
  b. *Clinical Indications/Dose/Route*—Adjuvant treatment of colon cancer. *Usual dosage:* PO 50 mg every 8 hours starting 7 to 30 days after surgery for 2 weeks up to 1 year.
  c. *Side Effects*—Nausea, vomiting, diarrhea, stomatitis, anorexia, abdominal pain, alopecia, pruritus, and myalgia

G. Tumor Necrosis Factor—
  1. *Mechanism of Action*—Induction of cytokines (IL-1, INF-β, IL-6, GM-CSF) currently undergoing clinical investigation to explore drug activity, such as whether they are cytotoxic or cytostatic, are phagocytic, activate lysosomes, generate superoxides, mediate inflammatory response, or augment immune function through activation of leukocytes.
  2. *Clinical Indications/Route/Dose*—Currently under clinical investigation for treatment of varied cancer diseases. It has been administered SC, IV, and IM. The specific drug dose and route have not been established.
  3. *Side Effects*—Currently, clinical investigation reports symptoms found in septic shock (e.g., tachycardia, hypotension, dyspnea, and fever).

H. Gene Therapy—
  Gene therapy is under clinical investigation. Projected outcomes will be to insert a functioning gene into a cell to correct a genetic disorder or introduce a new function to the cell.

I. Vaccines—
  Vaccines are undergoing clinical investigation to explore their potential to stimulate specific immune defenses against tumor-associated antigens (autologous, allogeneic, recombinant, and synthetic). Pivotal phase III clinical trials are currently being conducted in several clinical indications including for metastatic breast cancer, melanoma, and prostate cancer.

Treatment

V. SAFE PRACTICE GUIDELINES

A. Personnel Protection—

Limited data are available regarding the effects of handling biologic agents. Most of the biologic agents do not impact or affect cell DNA and are not considered mutagenic substances. However, the Occupational Safety and Health Administration has identified IFNs as hazardous agents and stresses that they must be handled according to the guidelines for cytotoxic agents (see Chapter 22 for safe handling guidelines.)

B. Drug/Agent Preparation—

1. *Nonradiolabeled Biotherapeutic Agents*
   a. Inject the diluent into the side of the vial rather than directly into the powder to prevent foaming of the product.
   b. Gently swirl the reconstituted agent, and NEVER SHAKE the drug vial—shaking can denature the protein components of the drug.
   c. Note DO NOT FREEZE manufacturer guidelines, indicated for many biotherapy products.

2. *Radiolabeled Biotherapeutic Agents*
   a. A nuclear pharmacist prepares radiolabeled monoclonal antibodies for injection or infusion.
   b. Federal and state laws require that radiation safety warning signs designate areas in which radioisotopes are stored or used.
   c. Precautions for patients administered radiolabeled pharmaceuticals:
      - Radioactive precautions for body fluids are necessary for approximately 7 days after administration.
      - Flush toilet twice after use.
      - Wipe up spilled urine with a paper tissue and discard in the toilet before flushing.
      - Wash hands after using the toilet.
      - Immediately wash linen and clothes that become soiled with urine or blood. Wash these items separately from other laundry.
      - If an injury occurs and blood is spilled, wash away any spilled blood with water and a paper tissue and flush the paper tissue in the toilet.

Bibliography

Amgen, 2002, Aranesp (darbepoetin alfa) and Neulasta (pegfilgrastim). Available at www.amgen.com/

Appel CP: Biotherapy. In Otto SE, editor: *Oncology nursing*, ed 4, St. Louis, 2001, Mosby.

Bender CM, Kramer PA, Miaskowoski C: *New directions in the management of cancer-related cognitive impairment, fatigue and pain*, Ortho-Biotech Oncology, Raritan, N.J., 2002, Scientific Connexions.

Buchsel PC, Forgey A, Grape FB, etal: Granulocyte macrophage colony-stimulating factor: current practice and novel approaches, *Clin J Oncol Nurs* 6(4):198, 2002.

Buchsel PC, Murphy BJ, Newton SA: Epoetin Alfa: current and future indications and nursing implications, *Clin J Oncol Nurs* 6(5):261, 2002.

Camp-Sorrell D: Surviving the cancer, surviving the treatment: acute cardiac and pulmonary toxicity, *Oncol Nurs Forum* 26(6):983, 1999.

Erickson J, Kuck A: biotherapy. In Lin EM, editor: *Advanced practice in oncology nursing*, Philadelphia, 2001, WB Saunders.

Griffin JD: Hematopoietic growth factors. In DeVita VT Jr, Hellman S, Rosenberg SA, editors: *Cancer principles and practice of oncology*, ed 6, Philadelphia, 2001, Lippincott Williams & Wilkins.

Hendrix CS, de Leon C, Dillman RO: Radioimmunotherapy for non-Hodgkin's lymphoma with yttrium 90 ibritumomab tiuxetan, *Clin J Oncol Nurs* 6(3):144, 2002.

Nail LM: I'm coping as fast as I can: psychological adjustment to cancer & cancer treatment, *Oncol Nurs Forum* 28(6):967, 2001.

Oncology Nursing Society: *Cancer chemotherapy guidelines and recommendations for practice*, Pittsburgh, Pa., 2001, Oncology Nursing Press.

Rieger PT: *Clinical handbook for biotherapy*, Boston, 1999, Jones and Bartlett.

Rosenberg SA: Principles of cancer management: biologic therapy. In DeVita VT Jr, Hellman S, Rosenberg SA, editors: *Cancer principles and practice of oncology*, ed 6, Philadelphia, 2001, Lippincott Williams & Wilkins.

Sample D: Cancer vaccines: a new era in cancer management has begun, *Nurse Investigator* 6(1):6, 2002.

Treatment

Bone Marrow and Peripheral Blood Stem Cell Transplantation

I. OVERVIEW

Bone marrow is a soft, spongelike material found inside bones. It contains immature cells called *stem cells* that produce blood cells. The three types of blood cells are (1) white blood cells, which protect the body against infection; (2) red blood cells, which carry oxygen to and remove waste products from organs and tissues; and (3) platelets, which enable the blood to clot and form protection when an injury occurs. Most stem cells are found in bone marrow, but some, called *peripheral blood stem cells* (PBSCs), are found in the bloodstream. An additional source of stem cells is found in the umbilical cord, which contains a small but rich source of stem cells. Stem cells can divide to form more stem cells or they can mature into white blood cells, red blood cells, or platelets.

II. TYPES OF TRANSPLANTATION

Bone marrow transplantation (BMT) and peripheral blood stem cell transplantation (PBSCT) are treatments used to replace the diseased or destroyed bone marrow as a result of high doses of chemotherapy or radiation therapy. There are two major types of transplants: autologous and allogeneic. The type of transplant is identified by the patient's relationship to the marrow/stem cell donor.

A. **Autologous Transplant—**

 The patient receives his or her own stem cells.

B. **Allogeneic Transplant—**

 The patient receives marrow/stem cells from another person. There are three types of allogeneic transplants with each type named according to the donor source.

1. *Syngeneic*—The donor is the patient's identical twin.
2. *Related*—The donor is related to the recipient and is usually a sibling.
3. *Unrelated*—The donor is NOT related to the recipient.

III. SOURCES

A. Autologous Peripheral Stem Cells—

1. *Mobilization*—To collect an adequate number of stem cells in the least number of apheresis sessions, it is necessary to stimulate the production of PBSCs through a process called *mobilization*. Two techniques are typically used to mobilize the PBSCs: administration of granulocyte–colony-stimulating factors (G-CSF) or granulocyte macrophage–colony-stimulating factors (GM-CSF) alone or in combination with chemotherapy drugs. Cyclophosphamide, etoposide, and paclitaxel are the most commonly used chemotherapy drugs.

2. *Apheresis*—A process called *apheresis* is used to obtain PBSCs for transplantation. Approximately 4 to 5 days before the apheresis, the patient is administered medications such as hematopoietic growth factors to increase the number of stem cells released into the bloodstream as described earlier. In the apheresis procedure, PBSCs are removed through a central venous catheter that is connected to a standard commercially available cell separator. The cell separator is programmed to collect either lymphocytes or low-density leukocytes. The remaining blood components are returned to the patient and the collected PBSCs are stored. Apheresis typically takes 3 to 4 hours to complete for each collection period and is performed from 1 to 10 days. Side effects of apheresis are minimal but include transient hypocalcemia from the anticoagulant used in the apheresis process, fatigue, anemia, and thrombocytopenia.

B. Allogeneic Peripheral Blood Stem Cells—

The majority of allogeneic transplantation sources are obtained through PBSC collection. Advantages of this source include quicker engraftment and decreased transplant-related mortality, the ability

Treatment

to obtain a larger number of stem cells, and the possibility of faster reconstitution of the immune system and comparable rates of graft-versus-host disease (GVHD).

1. *Mobilization*—The mobilization process for allogeneic PBSCs collection is similar to the process for autologous PBSCs, with the only exception being that allogeneic PBSC donors are given G-CSF or GM-CSF for mobilization of the stem cells.

2. *Apheresis*—Allogeneic PBSCs are collected through an apheresis process similar to that used for autologous PBSCs. In healthy donors, a peripheral line inserted into the antecubital vein is used for the venous access that is connected to the cell separator. An adequate number of CD34+ cells can be collected in one to two sessions. Occasionally more than one collection period is required to collect the required volume and quality for the transplantation.

C. **Bone Marrow Harvest**—

Bone marrow harvests are used only occasionally for the collection of marrow. In general, the procedure for obtaining bone marrow, which is also called *harvesting*, is similar for both types of BMTs (autologous and allogeneic). The donor is usually administered general anesthesia. Two physicians work simultaneously, one on either side of the patient. Multiple punctures are made with a large-bore needle into the patient's posterior and occasionally anterior iliac crests. Each puncture aspiration obtains approximately 2 to 5 ml bone marrow. The amount of bone marrow collected depends on the size of the recipient and the donor, as well as the type of BMT (autologous or allogeneic). Usually, 10 to 15 ml/kg body weight will yield the required amount of stem cells. This bone marrow collection process takes approximately 2 to 3 hours.

After collection, the marrow is mixed with a heparinized solution and is filtered to remove blood, bone fragments, and fat. At this time the harvested bone marrow can be treated or purged. Purging is the process of removing residual malignant cells from the marrow for the autologous transplant. For an autologous BMT, the collected marrow is combined with a preservative, dimethyl sulfoxide (DMSO), placed in a blood bag, and placed in a liquid nitrogen freezer to keep the stem cells alive until they are needed. This technique is known as *cryopreservation*. Stem cells may be cryopreserved for many years. When an allogeneic BMT is being performed, the marrow is usually immediately transfused into the recipient.

D. **Unrelated Donors—**

The National Marrow Donor Program was established in 1987 and maintains a registry of more than 4 million available bone marrow, PBSC, and umbilical cord donors. All of the donors have completed previous tissue typing and have expressed a desire to donate. The National Marrow Donor Program has developed a directory of participating transplant centers. Each directory includes a description of the center, a summary of the center's areas of expertise, and contact information. The registry search determines which listed donors have compatible typing with the recipient. When chosen, the *patient/recipient* does not know from which donor the bone marrow, PBSCs, or umbilical cord blood came or where the donor resides.

E. **Umbilical Cord Blood—**

Collecting umbilical cord blood is a simple procedure and poses no risk to the donor. After the delivery of the baby, the umbilical cord is clamped and the blood is withdrawn from the umbilical cord using a needle and syringe. The blood is then cryopreserved in the same way as PBSCs or bone marrow.

F. **Human Leukocyte Antigen (HLA) Typing—**

To increase the likelihood of successful transplantation and to minimize potential complications, it is important that the transplanted marrow/stem cells match the patient's own marrow as closely as possible. To determine a person's tissue type, a small amount of peripheral blood is drawn, and antigens on the surface of the leukocytes are analyzed. These antigens make up the human leukocyte–associated system, which has a major role in immune surveillance by constantly identifying "self" from "nonself." There is a pair of antigens at several sites on the white blood cells called *loci*. Three of these

Treatment

loci—HLA-A, HLA-B, and HLA-DR—are important in determining whether a patient is compatible with a potential donor.

The success of allogeneic transplantation depends largely on how closely the HLAs of the donor's marrow match those of the recipient's marrow. The greater the number of matching HLAs, the greater the chance that the patient's body will accept the donor's bone marrow. Close relatives, particularly siblings, are more likely than nonrelatives to have HLA-matched bone marrow. However, only 30% to 40% of patients have an HLA-matched sibling. Because identical twins have the same genes, they also have the same set of HLA antigens; therefore the recipient's body readily accepts this donated marrow.

Mixed lymphocyte culture testing, in which donor and recipient lymphocytes are grown in culture together to assess their reaction, was considered important in determining HLA-DR antigen compatibility, but often the results were difficult to analyze or reproduce. The advent and use of DNA technology has replaced the mixed lymphocyte testing procedure.

IV. INDICATIONS

Bone marrow and stem cell transplantation is used to treat several malignant and nonmalignant diseases. The type and stage of disease, patient's age, performance status, and donor availability determine the type of transplant that can be performed and the recipient's chances for survival. Allogeneic transplant is used for the treatment of patients with hematologic malignancies, bone marrow failure, severe combined immunodeficiency syndrome, and some inherited metabolic disorders. Autologous transplant is used primarily for the treatment of diseases in which the patient's own marrow contains an adequate marrow/stem cell supply that can eventually generate functioning white blood cells, red blood cells, and platelets.

Marrow/stem cell transplantation is used in the treatment of the following clinical diseases:

A. **Hematologic Malignancies—**
   Acute lymphocytic leukemia, acute myelogenous leukemia, chronic myelogenous leukemia, Hodgkin's

and non-Hodgkin's lymphoma, myelodysplastic syndrome, and multiple myeloma

B. **Solid Tumors—**
Breast cancer, neuroblastoma, Ewing's sarcoma, malignant melanoma, rhabdomyosarcoma, testicular cancer, Wilm's tumor, and ovarian cancer

C. **Nonmalignant Diseases—**
Aplastic anemia and severe combined immunodeficiency syndrome.

V. TRANSPLANTATION PROCESS

A. **Pretreatment Workup—**
An extensive evaluation is performed on the BMT/ PBSCT recipient before the transplant occurs (Box 24-1). This process is performed to establish the recipient's physical and psychosocial status. For the allogeneic transplant, the marrow/stem cell donor is also thoroughly evaluated (Box 24-2). The assessment process is completed on an outpatient basis and includes a variety of tests, procedures, and consultations. Multiple and sequential diagnostic tests are performed, as well as consultations from professionals in designated interdisciplines such as psychology, social work, surgery, chaplaincy, radiology, and nursing and medicine.

B. **Conditioning Regimens—**
The conditioning regimen is the process of preparing the patient to receive bone marrow or stem cells. Its purpose is to *obliterate* the malignant cancer cells, *destroy* the patient's preexisting immunologic state, and *create space* in the marrow cavity for the proliferation of transplanted marrow or stem cells. On completion of the "conditioning regimen" it is crucial that the patient receives the transplantation product of marrow/stem cells. Without this transfusion product, the patient will incur consequential side effects and will die.

The conditioning regimen consists of high-dose chemotherapy treatment with or without total body irradiation (TBI). Drugs selected for use in high-dose chemotherapy treatment include cyclophosphamide, carmustine, etoposide, busulfan, and cytarabine. The drug dose, route, and schedule are dependent on the patient's disease type, clinical condition, and weight/height/total body surface area. In addition, other factors for the specific

Treatment

Box 24-1
PRETRANSPLANT EVALUATION OF THE PATIENT

Pretreatment testing and evaluation of the patient undergoing hematopoietic stem cell transplantation includes the following:

- History of current illness, including presenting signs and symptoms, previous therapies, initial diagnosis, pathology and staging, complications, relapses or progressions, current disease status, transfusion history
- Medical history, including major illnesses, chronic illnesses, recurring illnesses, surgical history, childhood illnesses, and infectious disease exposure; for women, should also include menarche, onset of menopause or date of last menstrual period, pregnancies and outcomes
- Current medications
- Allergies
- Social and family history
- Performance status
- Current laboratory studies, including liver function tests, renal function, complete blood count
- Infectious disease serologies, including HIV, hepatitis B and C, cytomegalovirus, herpes simplex virus, HTLV-1, Epstein-Barr virus, toxoplasma titer, ABO and Rh typing
- HLA typing and DNA procurement for future engraftment studies (allogeneic transplant patients only)
- Chest radiograph
- Electrocardiogram
- MUGA scan
- Pulmonary function tests, including DLco
- 24-hour urine for creatinine clearance
- CT scans of chest and sinuses, if there are symptoms or a history of repeated infections
- Disease restaging, including CT scans, nuclear medicine scans, bone marrow aspirate and biopsy, cytogenetics, molecular diagnostics, and measures of minimal residual disease

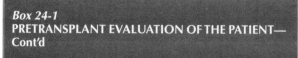

Box 24-1
**PRETRANSPLANT EVALUATION OF THE PATIENT—
Cont'd**

- Dental evaluation, including full-mouth
  radiographs and cleaning
- Sperm/fertilized embryo banking
- Autologous stem cell backup if undergoing
  unrelated or mismatched transplantation
- Informed consent for treatment, transfusion
  support, clinical trials
- Nutritional evaluation, if appropriate
- Consultations with radiation therapy, infectious
  disease, pulmonary, cardiology, or renal
  services, if clinically indicated
- Financial screening
- Psychosocial evaluation

Source: Lin EM, editor: *Advanced practice in oncology nursing,
case studies and review*, Philadelphia, 2001, WB Saunders.
CT, Computed tomography; *HIV,* human immunodeficiency
virus; *HLA,* human leukocyte antigen; *HTLV,* human T-
lymphotropic virus; *MUGA,* multiple gated acquisition.

Box 24-2
**EVALUATION OF THE HEMATOPOIETIC STEM CELL
DONOR**

Pretreatment testing and evaluation of the
  hematopoietic stem cell donor usually includes
  the following:

- History and physical examination, noting
  history of serious or chronic illnesses, history of
  hematologic problems (including bleeding
  tendencies, cancer history, and transfusion
  history), current medications, allergies, and
  pregnancy history for females
- The presence of any risk factors for HIV or viral
  hepatitis infection is noted
- Physical examination for any abnormalities and
  an assessment of the adequacy of peripheral veins

Treatment

Continued

> ### Box 24-2
> ### EVALUATION OF THE HEMATOPOIETIC STEM CELL DONOR—Cont'd
>
> - Complete blood count with differential, chemistries, liver and renal function tests, coagulation studies, ABO and Rh typing, pregnancy test
> - Confirmatory HLA typing; DNA procurement for future engraftment studies (allogeneic donors only)
> - Infectious disease serologies, including VDRL, HIV, hepatitis B and C, cytomegalovirus, herpes simplex virus, HTLV-1, Epstein-Barr virus, toxoplasma titer

Source: Lin EM, editor: *Advanced practice in oncology nursing, Case Studies and Review,* Philadelphia, 2001, WB Saunders.
HIV, Human immunodeficiency virus; *HLA,* human leukocyte antigen; *HTLV,* human T-lymphotropic virus; *VORL,* Venereal Disease Research Laboratory (test for syphilis).

regimen chosen depend on the amount and response to previous radiation or chemotherapy.

VI. TRANSPLANTATION OF MARROW AND STEM CELLS

On completion of the conditioning regimen, the bone marrow or stem cells must be infused. If the regimen included chemotherapy as the last treatment given, a rest period of 24 to 72 hours is scheduled before the transplant. This rest period is necessary because of the drug's half-life. For autologous BMT, the frozen marrow or stem cells are brought to the patient's room. The bag of cells is thawed in a normal saline bath before infusion through a central venous catheter. The entire process takes 45 to 60 minutes depending on the volume of cells being transplanted. Patients usually experience mild dyspnea and nausea and vomiting from the preservative DMSO. The DMSO also gives off a garliclike odor as it is eliminated through the patient's respiratory system.

For allogeneic BMT, the marrow or stem cells are usually infused on the same day as they are collected. This procedure resembles a red blood cell transfusion in that the bag of marrow or stem cells is transfused through a central venous catheter. *Unfiltered blood tubing must be used to prevent the stem cells from being trapped and not being infused.*

The total infusion time lasts from 1 to 4 hours. Potential side effects that may occur are similar to those of a blood transfusion (chills, fever, chest pain, hypotension, and dyspnea). Patients are usually premedicated with diphenhydramine, hydrocortisone, or both to minimize these reactions.

In both transplant procedures, emergency equipment is always available at the patient's bedside. The physician is also available throughout the entire transplant infusion process. Nursing staff is responsible for closely monitoring vital signs, signs and symptoms of a reaction, and the stem cell/marrow infusion process.

VII. MINITRANSPLANT

A "minitransplant" is a type of allogeneic transplant that is being investigated in clinical trials for the treatment of several types of cancers, including leukemia, lymphoma, multiple myeloma, melanoma, and kidney cancer. A minitransplant uses lower, less toxic doses of chemotherapy and TBI for the conditioning regimens. The use of low chemotherapy doses and TBI eliminates some, but not all, of the patient's bone marrow; it also reduces the number of cancer cells and suppresses the patient's immune system to prevent rejection of the transplanted marrow or stem cells.

Unlike traditional BMT or PBSCT, bone marrow cells both from the donor and the patient may exist in the patient's body for some time after the minitransplant. When the bone marrow cells from the donor begin to engraft, they may cause what is called a *graft-versus-tumor effect* and may work to destroy the cancer cells that were not eliminated by the chemotherapy drugs or TBI. To boost the graft-versus-tumor effect, the patient may be given an infusion of the donor's white blood cells. This procedure is called *donor lymphocyte infusion*. This process is performed to induce the state of host-versus-graft tolerance, thereby giving donor-derived T-lymphocytes the opportunity to recognize and eradicate host-derived tumor cells as anti-GVHD prophylaxis.

Treatment

VIII. ENGRAFTMENT PERIOD

On entering the bloodstream, the transplanted stem cells/marrow travel to the bone marrow, where they begin to produce new white blood cells, red blood cells, and platelets in a process known as *engraftment*. Engraftment usually occurs within 2 to 3 weeks after transplantation and is monitored by an ongoing process of blood counts on a frequently scheduled basis. Patients receiving PBSCs engraft as early as 5 days and on average 11 to 16 days after the stem cell transplantation. Cord blood takes an average of 26 days but as long as 42 days to engraft.

During the initial process of recovery after the transplantation, the patient experiences severe pancytopenia and immunosuppression. Multiple interventions are provided to prevent and treat conditions such as infection and bleeding, thus allowing the patient's immune system to recover. Complete recovery of the immune function takes as long as several months for the autologous transplant recipient and 1 to 2 years for the allogeneic transplant recipient. Evaluations regarding recovery of the immune system and the status of the bone marrow will be monitored through bone marrow aspiration studies.

Supportive care is provided to the patient through blood transfusions; administration of antibiotics, antifungals, and antiviral drugs to minimize or treat infections; hematopoietic growth factors to boost the marrow; aggressive antiemetic regimens; analgesia for pain relief; and nutrition intervention to maintain a proper nutritional balance.

IX. COMPLICATIONS

Patients receiving transplantation experience multiple and varied complications as the result of the pretreatment regimens, transplantation infusion, posttransplantation therapies, and the sequential side effects incurred from all of these therapies. The type, severity, and number of complications are related to the transplantation type (autologous versus allogeneic), the recipient's age, concomitant clinical conditions, and performance status.

The significant transplantation complications are graft failure, infection, interstitial pneumonia, venoocclusive disease, and GVHD (Table 24-1). GVHD is the result of T cells in the donor graft recognizing host antigens as foreign and is a complication associated with

Text continued on p. 254

Table 24-1 MAJOR COMPLICATIONS AFTER TRANSPLANT

Complication	Appearance	Signs/Symptoms	Management
Graft Rejection	1–4 wk	Absent/prolonged neutropenia	Administer blood component therapy.
		Partial marrow recovery	Consider retransplantation.
		Hypoplasia	
		Hemolysis	
Infection			
Bacterial	1–5 wk	Fever	Maintain protective environment.
Fungal	1–5 wk	Dry, nonproductive cough	Provide good hygiene.
Viral		Change in breath sounds	Monitor vital signs frequently.
Herpes virus	1–3 mo	Erythema—oropharynx/catheter site	Perform frequent head-to-toe systems
CMV	3 mo	Diarrhea	assessments.
Varicella-zoster virus	1st yr	Shortness of breath, fever	Administer colony-stimulating factors.
		Lesions—skin or mucous membranes	Ensure CMV-negative blood products.
		Hypotension	Administer broad-spectrum antibiotics.
			Administer acyclovir and/or ganciclovir.

Continued

Treatment

Table 24-1   MAJOR COMPLICATIONS AFTER TRANSPLANT—cont'd

Complication	Appearance	Signs/Symptoms	Management
Infection—cont'd			Administer intravenous (IV) immunoglobulins.
Venoocclusive Disease	1–3 wk	Weight gain Ascites Hepatomegaly Right upper quadrant pain Bilirubin level > 2 mg/dl	Maintain intravascular volume. Administer RBCs and IV fluids. Frequent physical assessments. Weigh twice daily. Measure abdominal girth daily. Administer low-dose dopamine, heparin, and/or recombinant tissue plasminogen activator.
Pneumonitis Interstitial Toxic	1–4 mo 1–6 mo	Fever Dry, nonproductive cough Shortness of breath	Ensure CMV-negative blood products. Ensure leukocyte-poor blood products. Administer colony-stimulating factors.

	Tachypnea interstitial changes on x-ray film	Administer ganciclovir. Administer IV immunoglobulins.
Acute GVHD		
3–14 wk	Maculopapular skin rash Nausea, vomiting uncontrollable diarrhea Jaundice Elevated liver function tests Hepatomegaly	Provide immunosuppression with cyclosporine, steroids, methotrexate, and/or tacrolimus (Prograf). Provide symptomatic treatment of skin, gastrointestinal tract, and/or liver.
Chronic GVHD Skin	Months–years	Hyperpigmentation or hypopigmentation, patchy erythematous scaling, thickening/hardening resembling scleroderma, hair loss in involved areas	Provide immunosuppression with cyclosporine, steroids, azathioprine (Imuran), and/or thalidomide (investigational).

Continued

Treatment

Table 24-1   MAJOR COMPLICATIONS AFTER TRANSPLANT—cont'd

Complication	Appearance	Signs/Symptoms	Management
Chronic GVHD—cont'd			
Mouth		White striae and erythema on mucosa, decreased salivary flow with dryness of mouth	Manage symptoms of affected organ or system.
Eyes		Dryness, redness, itching/burning; corneal thickening	
Sinuses		Chronic sinusitis, predisposition to gram-positive infections	
Gastrointestinal tract		Difficulty swallowing, retrosternal pain, abdominal discomfort, diarrhea	
Pulmonary		Productive cough, progressive dyspnea, wheezing, pneumothorax	
Vagina		Inflammation, dryness, stenosis	
Muscle		Occasional polymyositis, proximal weakness	
Genitourinary tract		Cystitis, mild nephrotic syndrome	
Hematopoietic		Eosinophilia, thrombocytopenia,	

			Treatment
Lymphoid		hypoplastic marrow, marrow fibrosis	
		Hypocellularity and atrophy of lymph tissues, functional asplenia	
Endocrine		Decreased growth rates, delayed pubertal development, autoimmune hyperthyroidism	
Nervous system		Entrapment neuropathy, peripheral neuropathy, myasthenia gravis	
Late Effects			
Cataracts	1–6 yr	Loss of vision	Consider surgical intervention.
		Dryness	
Gonad dysfunction	Variable	Infertility	Administer replacement sex hormones.
		Menopause	Refer for psychosexual counseling.
Growth failure	Variable	Impaired growth of facial skeleton and dentition (<6 yr old)	Administer supplemental growth hormone.
		Absent growth spurts	Administer replacement sex hormones.
		No height changes	

Continued

Table 24-1 MAJOR COMPLICATIONS AFTER TRANSPLANT—cont'd

Complication	Appearance	Signs/Symptoms	Management
Late Effects—cont'd			
Hypothyroidism	1–15 yr	Dry skin Hoarse speech Lethargy/apathy Weight gain with appetite loss Increased susceptibility to cold	Administer replacement hormones.
Secondary malignancy	Months–years	Specific to disease	Determine by type and extent of disease and patient's physical and psychological status.
Recurrence	Months–years	Signs/symptoms of original disease	Determine by extent and patient's physical and psychological status.

Source: Otto SE, editor: *Oncology Nursing,* ed 4, St. Louis, 2001, Mosby.
CMV, cytomegalovirus; *GVHD,* graft-versus-host disease.

Table 24-2   ACUTE GRAFT-VERSUS-HOST DISEASE SEVERITY GRADING

Stage	Skin	Liver	Gastrointestinal Tract
+	Maculopapular rash over <25% of body surface	Bilirubin 2–3 mg/dl	Diarrhea >500 ml/day
++	Maculopapular rash over 25–30% of body surface	Bilirubin 3–6 mg/dl	Diarrhea >1000 ml/day
+++	Generalized erythroderma	Bilirubin 6–15 mg/dl	Diarrhea >1500 ml/day
++++	Generalized erythroderma with bullous formation (>2-cm vesicle) and desquamation	Bilirubin >15 mg/dl	Severe abdominal pain with or without ileus

Source: Otto SE, editor: *Oncology nursing, ed 4,* St. Louis, 2001, Mosby.

Treatment

allogeneic transplantation. The target organs for GVHD are the liver, gastrointestinal tract, and the skin. Two types of GVHD have been identified: acute (defined as occurring less than 100 days after BMT) and chronic (defined as occurring more than 100 days after the transplant) (Table 24-2).

Bibliography

American Association of Blood Banks: *Technical manual*, ed 14, Bethesda, Md, 2001, American Association of Blood Banks.

Buchsel PC, Kapustay PM: *Stem cell transplantation: a clinical textbook*, Pittsburgh, Pa, 2000, Oncology Nursing Press.

Camp-Sorrell D: Surviving the cancer, surviving the treatment: acute cardiac and pulmonary toxicity, *Oncol Nurs Forum* 26(6):983, 1999.

Childs RW: Allogeneic stem cell transplantation. In DeVita VT Jr, Hellman S, Rosenberg SA, editors: *Cancer principles and practice of oncology*, ed 6, Philadelphia, 2001, Lippincott Willliams & Wilkins.

Chu E, DeVita VT Jr: Principles of cancer management: chemotherapy. In DeVita VT Jr, Hellman S, Rosenberg SA, editors: *Cancer principles and practice of oncology*, ed 6, Philadelphia, 2001, Lippincott Williams & Wilkins.

Cooper DL, Seropian S: Autologous stem cell transplantation. In DeVita VT Jr, Hellman S, Rosenberg SA, editors: *Cancer principles and practice of oncology*, ed 6, Philadelphia, 2001, Lippincott Williams & Wilkins.

Hadaway LC: Vascular access devices: meeting patients' needs, *Medsurg Nurs* 8(5):296, 1999.

Harmening DM: *Modern blood banking and transfusion practices*, ed 4, Philadelphia, 1999, FA Davis.

Keller C: Bone marrow and stem cell transplantation. In Otto SE, editor: *Oncology Nursing*, ed 4, St. Louis, 2001, Mosby.

Mitchell SA: Hematopoietic stem cell transplantation. In Lin EM, editor: *Advanced practice in oncology nursing*, Philadelphia, 2001, WB Saunders.

Moran AB, Camp-Sorrell D: Maintenance of venous access devices in patients with neutropenia, *Clin J Oncol Nurs* 6(3):126, 2002.

National Marrow Donor Program on line: Available at http://www.marrow.org/

Oncology Nursing Society: *Cancer chemotherapy guidelines and recommendations for practice*, Pittsburgh, Pa, 2001, Oncology Nursing Press.

Westervelt P, Vij R, DiPersio J: Principles of high-dose chemotherapy and stem cell transplantation. In Govindan R, Arquette MA, editors: *The Washington manual of oncology*, Philadelphia, 2002, Lippincott Williams & Wilkins.

25

Pharmacologic and Infusion Therapies

I. ANTIEMETICS

Antiemetic research has had a profound effect on the treatment of chemotherapy-induced nausea and vomiting. The incidence of these side effects is related to the emetic potential of the chemotherapy drug, dose, route, schedule and duration, and combination of drug administration (see Table 25-1 for the emetogenic potential of some chemotherapy drugs).

The combination of antiemetic drugs with different mechanisms, around-the-clock administration, and greater dosages has proved more effective than single-agent dosing and as-needed schedules. Several agents currently used as single agents or in combination are metoclopramide, haloperidol, dexamethasone, lorazepam, and prochlorperazine. Many of these drugs act on the chemoreceptor trigger zone in the brain by blocking dopamine receptors. Although these antiemetics have demonstrated their effectiveness, they are associated with undesirable side effects including sedation, extrapyramidal reactions, anxiety, mood changes, and diarrhea.

With the development and use of the serotonin (5-HT$_3$) antagonists (dolasetron, granisetron, ondansetron, and tropisetron), new strides have been made in effective antiemetic therapy. The side effects are mild and include headache, constipation, and transient increase of liver enzymes. All four of these agents have demonstrated effectiveness as oral agents and have designated doses for children and adults in intravenous and oral routes (see Tables 25-2 and 25-3 for selected antiemetic regimens for adults).

Treatment

Table 25-1 EMETOGENIC POTENTIAL OF SELECTED CHEMOTHERAPY DRUGS

Minimal	Low	Moderate	High
bleomycin	amifostine 200 mg/m^2	aldesleukin	amifostine >740 mg/m^2
busulfan PO <4 mg/kg/day	asparaginase	altretamine PO	carboplatin
chlorambucil PO	cepecitabine	amifostine 340–500 mg/m^2	carmustine <250 mg/m^2
cladribine	cytarabine <1 g/m^2	cyclophosphamide IV	cisplatin <50 mg/m^2
corticosteriods	docetaxel	>750 mg/m^2	cyclophosphamide
fludarabine	doxorubicin <20 mg/m^2	cyclophosphamide PO	750–1500 mg/m^2
hydroxurea	etoposide	doxorubicin 20–60 mg/m^2	cytarabine >1g/m^2
imatinib mesylate	5-fluorouracil <1g/m^2	epirubicin <90 mg/m^2	dacarbazine >500 mg/m^2
melphalan PO	gemcitabine	idarubicin	dactinomycin <1.5 mg/m^2
mercaptopurine	methotrexate >50 mg or	ifosfamide	daunorubicin
methotrexate <50 mg/m^2	<250 mg/m^2	methotrexate 250–1000	doxorubicin >60 mg/m^2
tamoxifen	mitomycin	mg/m^2	irinotecan
thioguanine PO	paclitaxel	mitoxantrone <15 mg/m^2	lomustine >60 mg/m^2
tretinoin	pegaspargase	oxaliplatin	mechlorethamine
vinblastine	teniposide		melphalan IV
vincristine	thiotepa		methotrexate >1 g/m^2
vinorelbine	topotecan		mitoxantrone >15 mg/m^2
			pentostatin
			procarbazine PO
			streptozocin

IV, intravenously; PO, per os (by mouth).

Table 25-2 ANTIEMETIC DRUGS: AVAILABILITY AND DOSAGE SCHEDULE

Drugs	Availability	Dosage Schedule
Chlorpromazine (Thorazine)	10, 25, 50, 100, 200 mg tablets; 75, 150 slow release (SR) capsules	Give 30–75 mg in 2–4 h in divided doses; give 1 hr before chemotherapy administration, then every 4–6 hr PRN.
Dolasetron (Anzemet)	50, 100 mg tablets	Give 100 mg 30–60 min before chemotherapy administration.
Dronabinol (Marinol)	2.5, 5, 10 mg SR capsules	Give 1–3 hr before chemotherapy administration; then 4–6 doses per day every 2–4 hr (maximum 15 mg/m^2 per dose).
Granisetron (Kytril)	1, 2 mg tablets	Give initial 1 mg dose 1 hr before chemotherapy administration and next dose 12 hr after first.
Haloperidol (Haldol)	0.5, 1, 2, 5, 10, 20 mg tablets	Give 0.5–5 mg 2 to 3 times a day Maximum dose 100 mg/day.
Ondansetron (Zofran)	4, 8, 24 mg tablets	Give initial 8 mg dose 30 min before chemotherapy (maximum dose 3 times per day for 2–3 days).

Continued

Treatment

Table 25-2   ANTIEMETIC DRUGS: AVAILABILITY AND DOSAGE SCHEDULE—cont'd

Drugs	Availability	Dosage Schedule
Prochlorperazine (Compazine)	5, 10, 25 mg tablets; 10, 15 mg SR capsules	Give 10–25 mg 1 hr before chemotherapy administration, then 15–30 mg SR capsules. Every 12 hr repeat *one* of above doses every 3–4 1/2 hr.
Promethazine (Phenergan)	12.5, 25, 50 mg tablets	Give 25–50 mg 1 hr before chemotherapy administration, then 12.5–25 mg 4 times per day.
Thiethylperzaine (Torecan)	10 mg tablets	Give 10 mg Q 4 to 6 hr max dose 40 mg/24 hr.
Trimethobenzamide (Tigan)	100, 250 mg capsules	Give 250 mg 1 hr before chemotherapy administration, then 250 mg 4 times per day.
Tropisetron (Navoban)	5 mg	Give 5 mg IV 30 min before chemotherapy followed by 5 mg PO every 6 to 24 hr on subsequent days.

Data from *Physician drug reference*, Montvale, NJ, Medical Economics Data, Medical Economic Co, 2003, and *American Hospital Formulary Service*, Bethesda, MD, 2003.
Adapted from Otto SE, editor: *Oncology nursing*, ed 4, St. Louis, 2001, Mosby.

Table 25-3   PARENTERAL ANTIEMETIC REGIMENS (ADULTS)

Drug	Dosage	Schedule
Metoclopramide (Reglan)	1–3 mg/kg IV	30 min before and 90 min after chemotherapy, then every 4 hours PRN as necessary
Dexamethasone (Decadron)	20 mg IV	30–40 min before chemotherapy
Lorazepam (Ativan)	1.5 mg/m² IV	30 min before chemotherapy
Diphenhydramine (Benadryl)	50 mg IV	30 min before chemotherapy
Dolasetron (Anzemet)	1.8 mg/kg IV	30 min before chemotherapy
	100 mg orally	60 min before chemotherapy
Granisetron (Kytril)	10 mcg/kg IV	30 min before chemotherapy
	2 mg orally	60 min before chemotherapy
Ondansetron (Zofran)	0.15 mg/kg IV infused over 15–30 min	30 min before chemotherapy, then at 4 and 8 hr after initial dose
Tropisetron (Navoban)	5 mg IV	30 min before chemotherapy

Data from *American Society of Hospital Pharmacists*, Bethesda, MD, 2003.
Adapted from Otto SE, editor: *Oncology nursing,* ed. 4, St. Louis, 2001, Mosby.

Treatment

A recent development regarding antiemetic guidelines has been established by a variety of professional organizations—American Society of Clinical Oncologists, American Society of Health System Pharmacists, the Multinational Association of Supportive Care in Cancer, and the National Comprehensive Cancer Network. The goals of this merged professional group included the following:

A. **Practical Approach**—
   The creation of a practical approach to the use of antiemetics in preventing chemotherapy-induced emesis by unifying and clarifying the previous guidelines and producing a single, simple practical document that can be used in everyday practice (Koeller et al., 2002).

B. **Emetic Risk Categories**—
   Four emetic risk categories were created, which encompass both the acute and delayed potential of chemotherapy: High (>90% risk for acute and delayed emesis), Moderate (30% to 90% acute emesis risk and some risk of delayed emesis), Low (10% to 30% [low] risk for acute and delayed emesis), and Minimal (<10% for acute or delayed emesis risk) (see Table 25-1).

C. **Treatment Options**—
   Treatment options were developed for each of the emesis risk categories by the category and route of drugs used.

   1. *High Risk*—The group suggests a 5-HT_3 receptor antagonist plus dexamethasone for the acute management and dexamethasone plus either metoclopramide or 5-HT_3 given orally for the delayed management.

   2. *Moderate Risk*—The group recommends a 5-HT_3 receptor antagonist plus dexamethasone for acute management and other alternatives for the moderate-risk category.

   3. *Low Emesis Risk*—The group suggests a single agent could be recommended for acute emesis management.

   4. *Other Risk Categories*—The antiemetic dosing recommendations regarding the specific drug, dose, or combination of drugs were discussed, but a consensus was not reached for all doses and all categories.

II. BLOOD AND BLOOD PRODUCTS TRANSFUSION THERAPIES

A. Blood Product Transfusion Overview—

Blood transfusions are a major factor in restoring and maintaining quality of life for patients with cancer, hematologic disorders, and trauma-related injuries and for those who have undergone major surgical procedures. The therapeutic goal of a blood transfusion is to increase oxygen delivery according to the physiologic need of the recipient, to replace the blood components required for the homeostasis of the coagulation process, or both. Guidelines for blood transfusions have been issued by several organizations including the National Institutes of Health, American Association of Blood Banks, and the American College of Physicians. The transfusion of blood or blood components has inherent risks; therefore an informed consent (a discussion of benefits, risks, and alternatives between the physician and the patient) is mandatory. Blood and blood components should be administered by competent, experienced, and skilled personnel following the guidelines of the accrediting organizations and agencies providing blood component therapy.

B. Indications for Transfusion—

1. *Whole Blood*
   a. Treatment of acute massive hemorrhage
   b. Should be synonymous with multiple transfusions
   c. Patients with active bleeding who have lost more than 25% of total volume
   d. Patients with a symptomatic deficit in oxygen-carrying capacity combined with hypovolemia of such a degree as to be associated with shock
2. *Red Blood Cells*
   a. Hemoglobin level less than 8 g/dl
   b. Tachycardia, hypotension with adequate volume replacement
   c. Tissue hypoxia
3. *Platelets*
   a. Thrombocytopenia
   b. Decreased production as a result of chemotherapy for cancer

Treatment

   c. Invasive procedures or serious hemorrhage (disseminated intravascular coagulation [DIC] < 50,000 mm^3)

4. *Volume Expanders*—Volume expanders such as Hespan, dextran, and Plasmanate provide expansion to the plasma volume and may be used in conjunction with blood product infusions for the management of shock or impending shock from hemorrhage or sepsis.

5. *Leukoreduced Blood Products*—Leukoreduced blood products have approximately 99.9% of the WBCs removed and are recommended for the following patients:

   a. Patients undergoing autologous and allogeneic peripheral blood stem cell transplantation (PBSCT)

   b. Patients for whom crossmatch-compatible blood is difficult to obtain

   c. Patients who should receive cytomegalovirus (CMV)-negative blood, RBCs, and platelets but for whom CMV-seronegative products are unavailable

   d. Patients who would benefit from a reduced number of febrile events, reduced CMV, and prevention of alloimmunization

6. *Irradiated Blood Products*—Viable lymphocytes (cells capable of division) present in all cellular transfusion products, including stored RBCs, are thought to be capable of triggering graft-versus-host disease (GVHD). This rejection reaction of the graft against seemingly "foreign" host tissues can occur in patients receiving both allogeneic and autologous transplantation. GVHD can occur in human leukocyte antigen (HLA)-matched siblings and patients receiving allogeneic PBSCT, and it is seen more often with lesser degree of matches. Using irradiated blood products can avert GVHD produced by blood product transfusion. A measured amount of radiation to blood products renders the donor lymphocytes incapable of replication. The usual recommended radiation dose is between 1.5 and 3.0 Gy of gamma radiation.

   Irradiated blood products are used to prevent GVHD in immunocompromised patients who are receiving blood components containing viable

WBCs. Irradiation destroys the ability of donor lymphocytes to engraft in the patient. Patients susceptible to transfusion-associated GVHD are those with Hodgkin's or non-Hodgkin's lymphoma, aplastic anemia, acute leukemia, and patients undergoing PBSCT.

Transfusion-associated graft-versus-host disease (TA-GVHD) can occur with directed blood donations (family to patient). Although a rare occurence, the mortality rate for TA-GVHD approaches 100%. The high mortality rate is associated with bone marrow transplantation failure. TA-GVHD has been associated most frequently with directed donations from first-degree relatives such as parents or siblings. TA-GVHD occurs when the transfusion recipient has two nonidentical HLA haplotypes and the transfusion (lymphocyte) donor is homozygous (identical) for either of the HLA haplotypes of the recipient. The recipient is unable to recognize the donor lymphocytes as "non-self." The lymphocyte reaction is essentially the same as seen after allogeneic marrow transplantation. Because of the potential for TA-GVHD after directed donation, it is recommended that all blood components from first-degree relatives be irradiated before transfusion.

C. **Blood and Blood Product Administration Guidelines—**
1. *Verify prescribing physician's order* for the specific blood component and the specific date of the transfusion administration.
2. *Obtain the patient's transfusion history* regarding previous transfusion reactions.
3. *Obtain the patient's informed consent* for blood component transfusion.
4. *Establish venous access site* or prepare venous access device for transfusion administration.
5. *Select all of the appropriate blood component transfusion supplies* (blood tubing, normal saline [0.9%]), and appropriate filter (leukoreduced-RBC or leukoreduced-platelet) (Table 25-4).
6. *Verify blood component product* (blood identification number and donor's ABO and Rh type) with the patient/recipient's identification number on wristband and recipient's ABO and Rh type.

Treatment

Table 25-4   BLOOD COMPONENT THERAPY

Component	Indications	Special Considerations
Packed Red Blood Cells (PRBCs)		
	Hemoglobin is <8.0 g. Patient is symptomatic. Active bleeding occurs.	Type and cross-match procedure is necessary. Infuse over 2–4 hr. Monitor for transfusion reaction (fever, chills, urticaria).
Leukocyte-poor PRBCs: leukocytes are removed during transfusion.	Patient has experienced febrile transfusion reactions. Patient is at risk for alloimmunization.	Infuse through a special filter (Pall).
Washed PRBCs: blood is washed with 1000 ml normal saline and repacked before transfusion.	Patient has known severe allergic reaction to plasma and leukocytes.	Infuse at 20–30 gt/min until completion of unit. Unit expires within 24 hr of washing.
Platelet Concentrates		
	Platelet count is <20,000. Active bleeding occurs.	ABO compatibility is preferred but not necessary.

	Platelets are given before minor procedures or surgery.	1-hr or 24-hr posttransfusion increments are monitored to determine effectiveness. Splenomegaly, disseminated intravascular coagulation, fever, and sepsis may increase demand. Monitor for transfusion reactions. Prophylaxis is done with diphenhydramine, acetaminophen, and hydrocortisone.
Random-donor platelets (RDPs): several units (6–10) harvested from whole blood are pooled into one bag.	Patient has had no prior transfusions. Patient has had no reactions or alloimmunization.	Units expire about 4 hr after pooling.
Leukocyte-poor RDPs: leukocytes are removed before or during transfusion.	Patient is at risk for alloimmunization. Patient has experienced febrile transfusion reactions.	Units is either centrifuged and leukocytes mechanically trapped (Leukotrap) or a special filter (Pall) is used for infusion.

Continued

Treatment

Table 25-4 BLOOD COMPONENT THERAPY—cont'd

Component	Indications	Special Considerations
Single-donor platelets (SDPs): platelets are collected by pheresis from one donor.	Patient is refractory to RDPs. Patient is at risk for alloimmunization.	Try to match ABO/Rh of patient. Usually transfuse with special filter (Pall). Unit expires within 24 hr of collection.
Human leukocyte antigen (HLA)-matched platelets: platelets are collected by pheresis from a donor whose HLA typing closely matches patient's type.	Patient is refractory to RDPs and SDPs. Patient is at risk for alloimmunization.	Patient must have been HLA typed. Unit expires within 24 hr of collection.
Resuspended platelets: plasma is removed from pooled units, and an equivalent amount of normal saline is added.	Patient has experienced severe reaction to platelet concentrates despite prophylaxis.	Prophylaxis is usually needed.

Fresh Frozen Plasma

	Patient has had multiple PRBC transfusions. Abnormal coagulation factors are evident.	Provide ABO-compatible component. Transfuse immediately after thawing.

Irradiated Components

Gamma radiation delivered to blood components inactivates lymphocytes within product.	Severely immunocompromised patients are at risk for graft-versus-host disease.	Component is not radioactive.
		Component should be labeled as being irradiated. RBCs and platelets are not affected.

Source: Otto SE, editor: Oncology nursing, ed 4, St. Louis, 2001, Mosby.

Treatment

7. *Verify the expiration date* on the blood component product.
8. *Ask the patient/recipient to verify self* by giving complete name; verify this information on the patient/recipient's wristband.
9. *Inspect the blood component* for any abnormalities.
10. *Inform the patient of potential adverse effects* (Table 25-5).
11. *Obtain the patient's baseline vital signs* (blood pressure, temperature, pulse, and respirations).
12. *Prime the blood tubing and filter,* taking care to cover the entire filter.
13. *Initiate the blood component product slowly* (5 ml/min for initial 15 minutes). Readjust the transfusion rate after 15 minutes to the desired rate.
14. *Obtain the patient's vital signs* on a scheduled frequency throughout the transfusion process.
15. *Document status in the patient's medical record* and on the agency's blood product required forms.
16. **NOTE that steps 6, 7, 8, and 15 require two licensed professionals to verify information and the required documentation of the blood product component form.**

III. VASCULAR ACCESS DEVICES

Vascular access devices have been the mainstay for vascular access in patients with cancer who require multiple infusates (chemotherapy, analgesics, antimicrobials, blood products, and nutritional support). These devices also provide venous access to obtain blood samples for multiple laboratory tests. The device can vary in design, insertion site, end-point placement, and duration of placement (see Figure 25-1 for examples; see Table 25-6 for catheters used for venous access).

Certain guidelines are required for catheter insertion and maintenance (O'Grady et al 2002).

A. **Site of Catheter Insertion—**

Insertion site is based on catheter type and goal of therapy. Consider the patient's lifestyle, body image changes, and the ability to care for the device.

Table 25-5 **TRANSFUSION REACTIONS**

Type of Reaction	Signs and Symptoms	Interventions
Hemolytic	Fever, chills, low back pain, substernal tightness, dyspnea, circulatory collapse, urticaria, flushing, vomiting, diarrhea, hemoglobinuria, renal shutdown, bleeding diathesis	Prevent by proper identification of patient and blood for transfusion. Discontinue the transfusion; send to blood bank and obtain urine and blood specimens per hospital policy for transfusion reaction work-up. Administer saline diuresis, furosemide, and mannitol to prevent acute renal tubular necrosis.
Allergic	Urticaria, itching, bronchospasm, anaphylactoid reactions, no fever	Elicit history of prior allergic reactions. Premedicate with diphenhydramine and/or corticosteroids. If reaction occurs, stop the transfusion; follow hospital policy for suspected transfusion reaction; for anaphylactoid reaction, administer epinephrine, maintain airway and perfusion; administer additional emergency measures as needed.

Continued

Treatment

Table 25-5 **TRANSFUSION REACTIONS—cont'd**

Type of Reaction	Signs and Symptoms	Interventions
Febrile (leukocyte antigens)	Fever with or without rigors, tachycardia, tachypnea, hypotension, cyanosis, fibrinolysis, leukopenia, headache	Elicit history of febrile reactions. Premedicate with acetaminophen. If reaction occurs, stop the transfusion and follow hospital policy for suspected febrile reaction. Consider leukocyte-poor RBCs (filtered, saline-washed or frozen) if fever occurs more than once.
Bacterial (gram-negative organisms and endotoxin release)	Fever, rigors, circulatory collapse, mental confusion, septic shock	Maintain proper blood storage and administration conditions. Stop the transfusion immediately. Obtain blood for cultures; return blood to laboratory for culturing. Administer emergency treatment as needed. Administer antibiotics as ordered.

Source: Otto SE, editor: *Oncology nursing,* ed 4, St. Louis, 2001, Mosby.

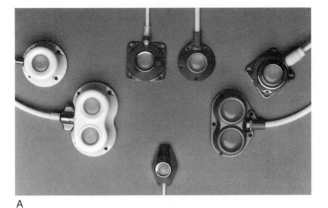

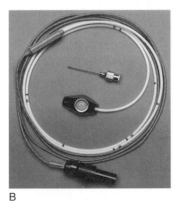

Figure 25-1 **A,** Examples of a number of different implantable infusion devices. **B,** Peripheral access catheter for placement of small port in forearm. (From Ableoff MD, Armitage JO, Lichter AS, et al, editors: *Clinical oncology,* ed 2, New York, 2000, Churchill Livingstone.)

B. Type of Catheter Material—
Most tunneled catheters and implantable port catheter lumens are constructed of Silastic or other silicone material. Peripherally inserted central catheters (PICCs), midline catheters, and peripheral devices are composed of biocompatible silicone elastomer, Teflon, or radiopaque polyurethane materials.

C. Hand Hygiene and Aseptic Technique—
Good hand hygiene can be achieved through the use of either a waterless, alcohol-based product or

Table 25-6   CATHETERS USED FOR VENOUS ACCESS

Catheter Type	Entry Site	Comments
Peripheral venous catheters	Vein of hand or forearm	Requires 72–96 hr site rotation. Phlebitis with prolonged use. Designed for placement <7–10 days.
Midline catheters	Proximal basilic or cephalic; antecubital fossa	Peripheral end-point placement. Anaphylactic reactions reported with catheters made with elastomeric hydrogel. Duration of placement usually is in terms of days.
Peripherally inserted central venous catheters (PICCs)	PICCs inserted antecubital basilic, cephalic, or brachial, or external jugular vein end-point placement superior vena cava	Duration of placement is >14 days to weeks.
Tunneled central venous catheters	Implanted into the subclavian usual end-point placement superior vena cava	Dacron cuff inhibits migration of organisms into the catheter tract. Duration of placement is 1–2 or more years.
Totally implantable ports	Tunneled beneath skin and have a subcutaneous port accessed by Huber needle end-point placement superior vena cava	Duration of placement is more than 2 years.

antibacterial soap and water with adequate rinsing. Maximum sterile barrier precaution (cap, mask, sterile gown, and large sterile drape) should be used for central venous catheters (CVCs) during the insertion procedure. Occupational Safety and Health Administration requires that gloves be worn as the standard precaution for the prevention of blood-borne pathogen exposure. **All CVCs and PICCs that have an end-point placement in a central vein (subclavian, superior vena cava) must have end-point placement verified by radiograph before use.**

D. **Skin Antisepsis—**
Products that have been approved for site preparation include 2% tincture chlorhexidine, 10% povidone-iodine, and 70% alcohol.

E. **Catheter Site Dressing Regimens—**
Transparent, semipermeable polyurethane dressings reliably secure the device, permit continuous visual inspection of the catheter site, permit patients to bathe and shower without saturating the dressing, and require less frequent changes than standard gauze and tape dressings.

F. **In-Line Filters—**
In-line filters reduce the incidence of infusion-related phlebitis; however, no data support their efficacy in preventing infection associated with intravascular catheters and infusion systems.

G. **Antimicrobial/Antiseptic Impregnated Catheters and Cuffs—**
Certain catheters may be coated or impregnated with antimicrobial or antiseptic agents to decrease the risk for infection. Types of coatings include chlorhexidine, silver sulfadiazine, minocycline, platinum, silver, or silver cuffs.

H. **Antibiotic/Antiseptic Ointments—**
Povidone-iodine ointment applied at the insertion site of the CVC is not recommended.

I. **Anticoagulants—**
Anticoagulant flush solutions (heparinized saline) are widely used to maintain catheter patency. This heparinized solution may vary by ml/lumen, heparin concentration 10 U to 100 U/ml, and frequency of heparinization (daily, weekly, monthly) and is dependent on the device (PICC, CVC, or implantable port).

Text continued on p. 281

Table 25-7   CENTRAL VENOUS CATHETERS: RECOMMENDED NURSING MANAGEMENT

Type	Heparinization*	Dressing	Blood Sampling
ADULT			
Central Venous Catheters, Short-Term Use, Subclavian			
Single/dual/triple-lumen	After each use, flush each lumen with 5 mL normal saline (N/S), then heparinized saline 2 ml (100 U/ml). For catheter *not* in use, flush each lumen with heparinized saline 2 ml (100 U/ml) *every 12 hours.*	Daily sterile dressing change at the site for duration of catheter placement. Gauze dressing change every 24 hours. Change Luer-Lok injection caps *every 72 hours.*	Shut off all IV lines for *1 to 3 minutes.* Withdraw 5 ml blood. Discard. Withdraw blood sample. Flush lumen with 5 ml N/S, then heparinize or resume IV line. *Total parenteral nutrition (TPN): Shut off IV line for 10 minutes.*
Peripherally Inserted Central Venous Catheters	After each use, flush lumen with 2 ml N/S, then heparinized	Sterile dressing change after first 24 hours; then every 72 hours. Change	Shut off all IV lines for 1 to 3 minutes. Withdraw 1.5 ml blood. Discard.

Long-line PICC+ Single/dual-lumen (Use gentle pressure on syringe plunger for PICCs.)	saline 1 ml (100 U/ml). For catheter *not* in use, flush lumen with heparinized saline 1 ml (100 U/ml) every 12 hours.	Luer-Lok injection caps every 72 hours.	Withdraw blood sample. Flush lumen with 2.5 ml N/S, then heparinize or resume IV line. *TPN: Shut off IV line for 10 minutes.*
Tunneled Catheters, Long-Term Use Hickman Quinton/Raaf Single/dual/triple-lumen	After each use, flush *each* lumen with 5 ml N/S, then heparinized saline 2 ml (100 U/ml). For catheter *not* in use, flush *each* lumen with heparinized saline 2 to 5 ml (100 U/ml) daily/biweekly.	Daily sterile dressing change at exit site for initial 14 days. Gauze dressing change every 24 hours. Thereafter, cleanse exit site daily (Betadine/alcohol). Optional daily clean dressing. Change Luer-Lok injection caps *weekly*.	Shut off all IV lines for *1 to 3 minutes*. Withdraw 5 ml blood. Discard. Withdraw blood sample. Flush lumen with 5 ml N/S, then heparinize or resume IV line. *TPN: shut off IV lines 10 minutes.*
Groshong Single/dual-lumen	Does not require heparin to maintain catheter	Daily sterile dressing change at exit site for	Shut off all IV lines for *1 to 3 minutes*. Withdraw 5 ml

Continued

Treatment

Table 25-7   CENTRAL VENOUS CATHETERS: RECOMMENDED NURSING MANAGEMENT—cont'd

Type	Heparinization*	Dressing	Blood Sampling
ADULT—cont'd			
Groshong Single/dual-lumen—cont'd	patency. *Use force when flushing.* Flush each lumen with 5 ml N/S after each use, except for TPN, then flush with 30 ml N/S. For catheter *not* in use, flush with 5 ml N/S weekly.‡	initial 14 days. Gauze dressing change every 24 hours. Thereafter, cleanse exit site daily (Betadine/alcohol). Optional daily clean dressing. Change Luer-Lok injection caps weekly.	blood. Discard. Withdraw blood sample. Flush lumen with 30 ml N/S vigorously, then resume IV line or apply injection cap.‡ *TPN: shut off IV line 10 minutes.*
Implantable Vascular Access Devices Davol Port Infuse-A-Port Port-A-Cath	After each use, flush each port with Huber needle: 10 ml N/S, followed by heparinized saline (100 U/ml).§ For port	Sterile bio-occlusive dressing when port accessed. Steri-strips at new incision site for 3 days. When incision site healed and port not	Shut off all IV lines for *1 to 3 minutes.* Withdraw 5 ml blood. Discard. Withdraw blood sample. Flush with 20 ml N/S, followed by 3 to 10 ml heparinized saline

not in use, flush each port with 3 to 10 ml heparinized saline (100 U/ml) every *30 days* (venous placement). Intermittent flush >1/day use N/S and/or low-dose/low-volume heparin.‖	accessed, no dressing required. When port is accessed for continuous infusion, change needle and extension tubing every 5 to 7 days.	(100 U/ml)‡ or resume IV line. *TPN: shut off IV line 10 minutes.*
PEDIATRIC *Short-Term Use, Subclavian* Single-lumen or multilumen		
After each use, flush *each* lumen with 2 ml N/S, followed by 1 ml heparinized saline solution, 10 U/ml, after each use or at least twice a day	Daily sterile dressing change at site for duration of catheter placement. Gauze dressing change every 24 hours. Change Luer-Lok injection caps every 24 hours.	Shut off all IV lines for *1 to 3 minutes.* Withdraw 3 ml blood. Dicard. Withdraw blood sample. Flush lumen with 2 ml N/S, then heparinize or resume IV line. *TPN: shut off IV line 10 minutes.*

Continued

Treatment

Table 25-7   CENTRAL VENOUS CATHETERS: RECOMMENDED NURSING MANAGEMENT—cont'd

Type	Heparinization*	Dressing	Blood Sampling
PEDIATRIC—cont'd			
Peripherally Inserted Catheters Long-line PICC[†] Single/dual lumen (Use gentle pressure on syringe plunger for PICCs.)	After each use, flush lumen: *Pediatrics:* 2 ml N/S in 5-ml syringe or larger, followed by 1 ml heparinized saline (10 U/ml) after each use or at least twice a day. *Special care nursery (neonates):* 0.5 ml N/S, preservative free, in 5 ml syringe or larger, followed by 0.5 ml heparinized saline (4 U/ml). Intermittent flush schedule every	Sterile dressing change after first 24 hours, then every 72 hours. Change Luer-Lok injection caps every 72 hours.	Shut off all IV lines for *1 to 3 minutes.* Withdraw 1.5 ml blood. Discard. Withdraw blood sample. Flush lumen with 2.5 ml N/S, then heparinize or resume IV line. *TPN: shut off IV line 10 minutes.*

	4 to 8 hours: consult with physician's orders.		
Tunneled Catheters, Long-Term Use Broviac	After each use, flush lumen with 2 ml N/S, then heparinized saline 1 ml (10 U/ml). For catheter *not* in use, flush lumen with heparinized saline 1 ml (10 U/ml) daily.	Daily sterile dressing change at exit site for initial 14 days. Gauze dressing change every 24 hours. Thereafter, cleanse exit site daily with Betadine. Apply sterile 2 × 2. Change Luer-Lok injection caps *weekly.*	Shut off all IV lines for *1 to 3 minutes.* Withdraw 3 ml blood. Discard. Withdraw blood sample. Flush lumen with 2 ml N/S, then heparinize or resume IV line. *TPN: shut off IV line 10 minutes.*
Implantable Vascular Access Devices Port-A-Cath	After each use, flush the port with Huber needle, 5 ml N/S, followed by 2 ml heparinized saline (100 U/ml). For port *not* in use, flush port	Sterile bio-occlusive dressing when port accessed. Steri-strips at new incision site for 3 days. When incision site healed and port not accessed, no dressing	Shut off all IV lines for *1 full minute.* Withdraw 3 to 5 ml blood (depending on size of child). Discard. Withdraw blood sample. Flush with 5 ml N/S, then heparinize or resume

Continued

Treatment

Table 25-7 CENTRAL VENOUS CATHETERS: RECOMMENDED NURSING MANAGEMENT—cont'd

Type	Heparinization*	Dressing	Blood Sampling
PEDIATRIC—cont'd	with 2 ml heparinized saline (100 U/ml) *every 30 days* (venous placement).	required. When port is accessed for continuous infusion, change needle and extension tubing every 5 to 7 days.	IV line. *TPN: shut off IV line 10 minutes.*

*Heparinization of central venous catheters varies in frequency, volume of solution, concentration of the heparin dilution, type of device, and patient's age and weight. Confirm with physician managing patient's care and agency/institution for nursing management protocol regarding heparinization of central venous catheters/implantable ports.

Consider patients with an alteration in coagulation factors and/or heparin allergy/intolerance with frequency of use of intermittent device. Potentially these patients may require low-concentration (e.g., 10 U/heparin/mL) and/or alternative flushing solution (e.g., sodium citrate, 1.4% solution).

**Some oncologists use 2 to 5 mL of heparinized saline (100 units/ml).

†Use 5 mL or larger syringes when flushing and/or blood sampling from PICC.

‡Selected oncologists use 2 to 5 mL heparinized saline (100 U/mL).

§Check manufacturer's specific recommendations regarding volume. Oncologists use heparin, 10 mL (100 U/mL).

||Assess patient, disease, platelet count with frequency/volume/concentration of heparinization schedule.

Source: Otto SE, editor: *Pocket guide to intravenous therapy,* ed 4, St. Louis, 2001, Mosby.

J. Catheter Replacement—
Because phlebitis and catheter colonization have been associated with an increased risk for catheter-related infections, short-peripheral catheter sites are commonly rotated at 72- to 96-hour intervals. Midline catheters have remained in place a median of 7 days but for as long as 49 days; recommendations suggest these catheters can be changed when there is a specific indication.

K. Replacement of Administration Sets—
Intravenous administration sets should be replaced at least every 72 hours or more frequently for certain products (blood/blood components with each volume unit, and lipid emulsions and parenteral nutrition at least every 24 hours). Needleless devices used in infusion therapy should be changed at least every 72 hours or if contaminated.

See Table 25-7 for examples of heparinization, dressing, and blood sampling procedures.

Bibliography

American Association of Blood Banks: Association Bulletin #99-7 RE: Leukocyte Reduction, Bethesda, Md, 2002, American Association of Blood Banks.

American Association of Blood Banks: *Technical manual*, ed 14, Bethesda, Md, 2001, American Association of Blood Banks.

Carlson RH: Catheters: peripherally inserted central ones no safe that central venous, *Oncol Times* 25(1):18, 2003.

Goodnough LT: Blood transfusion in the practice of oncology. In Govindan R, Arquette MA, editors: *The Washington manual of oncology*, Philadelphia, 2002, Lippincott, Williams & Wilkins.

Gahart BL, Nazareno AR: *Intravenous medications*, ed 18, St. Louis, 2002, Mosby.

Gonzales JA, Adams CS: Antiemetic agents in cancer chemotherapy, *Oncology Special Edition* 4:87, 2001, Available at http://www.oncologyse.com/

Hadaway LC: Vascular access devices: meeting patients' needs, *Medsurg Nursing* 8(5):296, 1999.

Hadaway LC: How to decrease catheter-related infections, *Nursing* 32(9):46, 2002.

Harmening DM: *Modern blood banking and transfusion practices*, ed 4, Philadelphia, 1999, FA Davis.

Hodgson BB, Kizior RJ: *Saunders nursing drug handbook 2003*, Philadelphia, 2003, WB Saunders.

Intravenous Nurses Society, *Standards of practice*, 23(65), 2000, The Society.

Treatment

Koeller JM et al: *Antiemetic guidelines, creating a more practical approach*, Huntington Valley, Pa, 2002, Atlas Multimedia.

LITE: Management of catheter occlusion with cathflo activase, *Spectrum* 13(4):1, 2001.

Moran AB, Camp-Sorrell D: Maintenance of venous access devices in patients with neutropenia, *Clin J Oncol Nurs* 6(3): 126, 2002.

O'Grady NP, Alexander M, Dellinger EP, et al: Guidelines for the prevention of intravascular catheter-related infections, *MMWR Recomm Rep* 51(RR-10):1, 2002.

Oncology Nursing Society: *Cancer chemotherapy guidelines and recommendations for practice*, Pittsburgh, Pa, 2001, Oncology Nursing Press.

Otto SE: *Pocket guide to intravenous therapy*, ed 4, St. Louis, 2001, Mosby.

Otto SE: *Oncology nursing*, ed 4, St. Louis, 2001, Mosby.

Ponec D, Irwin D, Hair WD, et al: Recombinant tissue plasminogen activator (alteplase) for restoration of flow in occluded central venous access devices: a double-blind placebo-controlled trial—the cardiovascular thrombolytic to open occluded lines (cool) efficacy trial, *J Vasc Interv Radiol* 12(8):951, 2001.

Physician's desk reference (PDR), ed 57, Montvale, NJ, 2003, Medical Economics.

Ross VM: Uncertainty about the clinical detection of sepsis, *J Infus Nurs* 26(1):23, 2003.

Rudnicke C: Transfusion alternatives, *J Infus Nurs* 26(1):29, 2003.

Complementary and Alternative Therapies and Herbal Medicines

I. OVERVIEW

Complementary or alternative therapy may be described as treatments or supportive methods that are used by patients with cancer as their only therapy or to complement or add to their standard or mainstream conventional-type medical treatments. Standard, mainstream, and investigational therapies such as chemotherapy, radiation therapy, biotherapy, and so on follow a scientific method of study using approved research designs, methods, implementation strategies, and evaluations. Not all of the complementary or alternative therapies have completed such a rigorous research process. Some of these therapies are often promoted as potential cures for cancer as independent treatments to be received in settings outside of the medical mainstream arenas. Sufficient data to document their efficacy are not widely known or available.

II. TREATMENT AND THERAPY DEFINITIONS

A. **Standard or Conventional Treatments—**
   Mainstream medical treatments that have been tested following a strict set of guidelines.

B. **Investigational Treatments—**
   Treatments studied in clinical trials or research projects to determine if they are safe and effective.

C. **Alternative Therapy—**
   Treatments that are unproven because they have not been scientifically tested or found to be effective (for example, using a special diet to treat cancer instead of undergoing surgery, radiation, or chemotherapy

that has been recommended by a conventional health care practitioner).

D. **Complementary Therapy—**
   Supportive methods that are used to complement or "add to" mainstream treatments, such as meditation, relaxation, acupuncture, biofeedback, and music therapy. An example of complementary therapy is the use of biofeedback to help lessen a patient's discomfort after surgery.

E. **Integrative Therapy—**
   Combined offering of mainstream and complementary methods.

F. **Quackery—**
   Treatments that are without proven use, offered by people who make claims that are untrue.

G. **Other Terms—**
   Examples include the following: questionable, unorthodox, unconventional, new age, holistic, natural, or herbal.

III. TYPES AND DESCRIPTIONS

Multiple types of products, drugs, and methods are used in complementary and alternative therapies. Following is a brief list describing the types of products or methods used and their descriptions.

A. **Diet and Nutrition—**
   1. *Macrobiotics*—Macrobiotics is a combination of diet, spirituality, and social philosophy intended to promote healing and healthful living. The Yin-Yang concept assigns opposite values to every component of life and nature (**Yin:** *female, dark, passive;* **Yang:** *male qualities*). The macrobiotic diet is based on a unique concept of human physiology and disease. It requires special methods of food selection and preparation (e.g., copper and aluminum may not be used, and gas stoves but not electric ranges may be used).
   2. *Macrobiotic Diet*—This diet derives 50% to 60% of calories from whole grains, 25% to 30% from vegetables, and the remainder (~10% to 20%) from beans, seaweed, and soups; a small amount of fish may be allowed. Foods not allowed include coffee, dairy products, eggs, sugar, meats, and processed foods.

    3. *Metabolic Therapies and Detoxification*—Treatments are composed of a low-salt diet, high-potassium diet with coffee enemas, and a gallon of fruit and vegetable juice daily. The specific therapy varies in each clinical setting.

    4. *Megavitamin Therapy*—Megadoses of vitamins and minerals are self-administered or self-managed.

    5. *Nutritional Supplements*—A variety of products are self-administered to enhance dietary intake.

B. Mind/Body Techniques—

    1. *Art Therapy*—The use of art media to lead an individual toward a neutralization state to deal with issues of conflict.

    2. *Biofeedback*—Prescribed or self-administered technique in which sensors are placed on the body for the purpose of measuring body responses such as heart rate, muscle, and sweat responses. Information is provided through audio or visual tapes to improve health function such as pain relief, high blood pressure reduction, and anxiety relief.

    3. *Hypnotherapy*—Selective attention used to induce a specific altered state (trance) for purposes of memory retrieval, relaxation, weight loss, and smoking cessation.

    4. *Imagery*—Use of vivid descriptions or figures of speech in speaking or writing to produce mental images to promote healing. This physiologic healing change is effective in major body systems such as respiration and heart rate, blood pressure, gastrointestinal mobility and secretion, sexual function, immune response, cortisol, and blood lipids.

    5. *Meditation*—Prescribed or self-administered methods through audio tapes, books, music, and spiritual study/reflection to promote a sense of control, tranquility, and peace for the body, mind, and spirit. It is used to prevent chronic pain, anxiety, and nausea/vomiting associated with some chemotherapy drugs.

    6. *Music Therapy*—Music used in an active or passive role has been shown to help some people express or communicate feelings; reduce stress, anxiety, and pain; enhance relaxation; and improve socialization.

Treatment

7. *Relaxation and Distraction Techniques*—A prescribed or self-administered technique through which music, videotapes, audio tapes, and imagery are used to enhance mind and body relaxation. These techniques have been used in management of stress, anxiety and panic disorders, and chronic illnesses such as headaches, hypertension, and musculoskeletal pain/joint disorders.

8. *Spiritual Healing and Prayer*—Prayers are offered to a higher being or authority to promote healing, reduce stress, and promote a sense of tranquility and peace for the body, mind, and spirit.

9. *Yoga*—A prescribed system of exercises practiced to promote control of the body and mind; a discipline aimed at training the consciousness for a state of spiritual insight and tranquility. Yoga techniques have been effective in regulating heart rate, blood pressure, circulation, and digestion and in healing chronic back pain, respiratory disease, and carpal tunnel syndrome.

C. **Magnetic Field Therapy**—
Uses the low-frequency portion of the electromagnetic spectrum to produce magnetic fields; for example, magnets can be purchased as arm, leg, wrist, or body bands; shoe inserts; or a bed mattress. Common physiologic responses include vasodilation, analgesia, antiinflammatory action, accelerated healing, and antiedemic activity.

D. **Traditional and Folk Remedies**—
Systems of healing that include remedies or strategies that have a strong mind/body component and rely on the concept that human physiology and diseases are interwoven. Techniques may include yoga, body cleanings, acupuncture, acupressure, herbal tea, or other medicinal remedies.

E. **Pharmacologic and Biologic Preparations**—
May include antineoplastics, phenylacetate, shark cartilage, flower essences, phytotherapy (use of plants), hyperthermia (use of various heating methods), enzyme therapy (use of enzymes to catalyze chemical reactions), and chelation therapy. These techniques involve the use of intravenous infusion of a chelating agent, synthetic amino acid ethylenediaminetetraacetic acid of metal, toxins, lead, mercury,

nickel, copper, cadmium, and plaque for the purpose of treating certain diseases such as toxic chemicals in the body.

F. **Manual Healing Methods—**
May include a variety of touch and manipulation techniques, for example, therapeutic touch, Reiki therapy, reflexology, and hands-on massage.

G. **Herbal Medicine—**
1. *Products Included in Herbal Remedies*—May consist of such products as essiac (four elements of herbs: burdock, turkey, rhubarb, sorrel, and slippery elm), iscador (derivative of mistletoe), cat's claw, chaparral tea, comfrey, hot red peppers, willow tea, garlic preparations, multiple types of spice products commonly used in baking or cooking, varieties of dried root (single or combinations), and St. John's wort preparations. (See Table 26-1 for a list of herbal therapies/interactions.)
2. *Suggested Guidelines for Purchase or Use of Herbal Medicine or Remedies*
   • Investigate before you buy.
   • Check with your doctor before your try/take an herbal product.
   • DO NOT take an herbal remedy instead of the prescribed medicine.
   • AVOID herbal remedies if you are pregnant or breast-feeding.
   • DO NOT depend on herbal medicine to cure cancer or other diseases.

IV. QUESTIONS TO ASK
   • What claims are made for the treatment to cure the cancer or to enable the evidence-based treatment to work better? Will the treatment relieve the symptoms or the side effects?
   • What are the credentials of those supporting the treatment? Are they recognized experts in cancer treatment? Have they been published in trustworthy journals?
   • How is their method(s) promoted (mass media, books, magazines, television and talk radio versus scientific journals)?
   • How much does the therapy cost? Is the request for payment made before the treatment?

Text continued on p. 303

Treatment

Table 26-1   HERBAL THERAPIES—INTERACTIONS

Name	Purported Benefit	Interactions	Precautions
Aloe	*Topical:* Promotes burn/wound healing, treatment of cold sores. *Oral:* Laxative, cathartic.	*Topical:* None. *Oral:* May increase risk for side effects with cardiac glycosides, antiarrhythmics, diuretics.	*Topical:* None. *Oral:* Abdominal pain, diarrhea, reduced potassium levels.
Astaxanthin	*Oral:* Treatment for macular degeneration, Alzheimer's, Parkinson's disease, stroke, cancer, hypercholesterolemia. *Topical:* Heals sunburn.	None known.	May cause visual disturbances.
Bilberry	*Topical:* Soothes mild inflammation of mouth/throat. *Oral:* Relief of acute diarrhea, increased visual acuity, angina, atherosclerosis.	May require adjustment of antidiabetic drugs (reduces glucose effect).	May decrease glucose, triglycerides.

Black cohosh	Treatment of menopausal symptoms, pre-menstrual syndrome, dysmenorrhea, nervous tension, dyspepsia. Acts as a mild sedative.	None known.	Side effects: nausea, dizziness, visual changes, migraine.
Capsicum	*Topical:* Relief for pain of shingles; postherpetic, trigeminal, diabetic neuralgias; HIV-associated peripheral neuropathy.	None.	Burning, urticaria, irritation to eyes, mucous membranes.
Cat's claw	*Oral:* Diverticulitis, ulcers, hemorrhoids, colitis, gastritis.	Antihypertensives may increase effect.	Headache, vomiting, hypotension (get up slowly to avoid dizziness).
Catnip	*Topical:* Helps arthritis, hemorrhoids. *Oral:* Treatment for insomnia, migraine, cold, flu, hives, indigestion, cramping, flatulence.	May be additive with other CNS depressants.	Headache, malaise, vomiting (large doses).

Continued

Table 26-1 HERBAL THERAPIES—INTERACTIONS—cont'd

Name	Purported Benefit	Interactions	Precautions
Chamomile	Antispasmodic, sedative, anti-inflammatory, astringent, antibacterial.	May increase bleeding with anticoagulants. May increase sedative effect with benzodiazepines.	Anaphylactic reaction if allergic; avoid use if allergic to chrysanthemums, ragweed, or asters; delays absorption of medications.
Chastberry	*Oral:* Control of menstrual irregularities, painful menstruation.	May interfere with oral contraceptives, hormone replacement therapy, dopamine antagonists (e.g., antipsychotics).	GI disturbances, rash, itching, headache, increased menstrual flow.
Coenzyme Q-10	*Oral:* Treatment for CHF, angina, diabetes, hypertension; reduces symptoms of chronic fatigue; stimulates immune system in those with AIDS.	May decrease effect of warfarin. Statins may decrease effect.	Reduced appetite, gastritis, nausea, diarrhea.

Cranberry	**Oral:** Prevention, treatment of urinary tract infections; urinary deodorizer.	May increase absorption of vitamin B_{12} in those taking proton pump inhibitors (e.g., Prevacid).	Large doses may cause diarrhea.
DHEA	Slows aging, boosts energy, controls weight.	None.	Side effects: May increase risk for breast/prostate cancer. Women may develop acne, hair growth on face/body.
Dong quai	Menstrual cramps, irregularity, menopausal symptoms. Manage high blood pressure, ulcers, constipation. Prevent/treat allergic reactions. Treat psoriasis.	May increase effects of warfarin.	Diarrhea, photosensitivity; skin cancer; avoid in pregnancy/lactation; essential oil may contain the carcinogen safrole.
Echinacea	Prevents/treats colds, flu, bacterial and fungal infections; an immune system stimulator; aids	May interfere with immunosuppressive therapy.	Not to be used with weakened immune system (e.g., HIV/AIDS, tuberculosis, multiple sclerosis).

Continued

Treatment

Table 26-1   HERBAL THERAPIES-INTERACTIONS—cont'd

Name	Purported Benefit	Interactions	Precautions
Echinacea—cont'd	wound healing.		Habitual or continued use may cause immune system suppression (should only be taken for 2–3 mo or alternating schedule of every 2–3 wk).
Emu oil	*Oral:* Hypercholesterolemia, weight loss, cough syrup. *Topical:* Relief from sore muscles, aching joints, pain, inflammation, carpal tunnel syndrome.	None known.	None reported.
Evening primose oil	*Oral:* Relief of PMS, symptoms of menopause (e.g., hot flashes), psoriasis, rheumatoid arthritis.	Antipsychotics may increase risk of seizures.	Indigestion, nausea, headache; large doses may cause diarrhea, abdominal pain.

Feverfew	Relieves migraine; treatment of fever, headache, menstrual irregularities.	May increase bleeding time with aspirin, dipyridamole, warfarin.	Side effects: headache, mouth ulcers abdominal pain, indigestion, diarrhea, nausea, vomiting, flatulence; should be avoided in pregnancy (stimulates menstruation), nursing mother, infants <2 yr of age.
Fish oils	*Oral:* Treatment for hypertension, hyperlipidemia, coronary artery disease, rheumatoid arthritis, psoriasis.	May increase risk for bleeding with antiplatelets, anticoagulants. Additive effect with anti-hypertensives.	Belching, heartburn, nosebleeds; large doses may cause nausea, diarrhea.
Garlic	Reduces cholesterol, LDL, triglycerides, increases HDL, decreases B/P, inhibits platelet aggregation. May also possess antibacterial,	May increase bleeding time with aspirin, dipyridamole, warfarin.	Side effects: taste, offensive odor; large doses may cause heartburn, flatulence, other GI distress.

Continued

Treatment

Table 26-1   HERBAL THERAPIES-INTERACTIONS—cont'd

Name	Purported Benefit	Interactions	Precautions
Garlic—cont'd	antiviral, antithrombotic activity.		
Ginger	Relieves nausea, effective treatment for motion sickness, antiinflammatory for arthritis, nausea/vomiting associated with pregnancy. Possesses ability to decrease platelet aggregation; antithrombotic properties.	May increase risk of bleeding with anticoagulants, antiplatelet medications.	Avoid during pregnancy when bleeding is a concern. Large overdose could potentially depress the CNS, cause cardiac arrhythmias.
Ginko	Boosts mental prowess by improving memory. Sharpens concentration, patient may think more clearly. Overcomes sexual dysfunction occuring with SSRI antidepressants. May	May increase bleeding time with aspirin, dipyridamole, warfarin.	Avoid when patient is taking blood thinners or those hypersensitive to poison ivy, cashews, mangos. Side effects: GI disturbances, headache, dizziness, vertigo.

	be able to slow progress of Alzheimer disease and, improve intermittent claudication.	
Ginseng	Boosts energy, sexual stamina; decreases stress, effects of aging.	May affect platelet adhesiveness/blood coagulation. Use caution with anticoagulants. May increase hypoglycemia with insulin. Avoid in patients receiving anticoagulants, medications that increase B/P. Side effects: breast tenderness, nervousness, headache, increased B/P, abnormal vaginal bleeding.
Glucosamine and chondroitin	Osteoarthritis.	No known interactions but monitor anticoagulant effects. Nausea, heartburn, diarrhea/constipation.
Golden-seal	**Topical:** Treatment for eczema, itching, acne. **Oral:** Treatment for UTI,	May interfere with antacids, sucralfate, H₂ antagonists, proton pump inhibitors. Constipation, hallucinations; large doses may cause nausea, vomiting, diarrhea,

Continued

Treatment

Table 26-1   HERBAL THERAPIES-INTERACTIONS—cont'd

Name	Purported Benefit	Interactions	Precautions
Golden-seal—cont'd	hemorrhoids, gastritis, colitis, mucosal inflammation.		CNS stimulation, respiratory failure.
Goldenrod	*Oral:* Diuretic, anti-inflammatory, antispasmodic; prevents urinary tract inflammation, urinary calculi, kidney stones.	May interfere with diuretics.	Allergic reactions.
Grape seed extract	Improves circulation, decreases tissue injury, hemorrhoids. Used as antioxidant to treat hypoxia from atherosclerosis, inflammation.	May increase risk of bleeding with wafarin.	None reported.
Green tea	*Oral:* Improves cognition function; treats nausea, vomiting, headache, weight loss.	May increase risk for bleeding with antiplatelets.	GI upset, constipation.

Hawthorn	Cardiovascular conditions (e.g., atherosclerosis), GI conditions (diarrhea, indigestion, abdominal pain), sleep disorders.	Cardiovascular drugs, digoxin may potentiate or interfere; additive effect with CNS depressants.	Nausea, GI complaints, headache, dizziness, insomnia, agitation.
Kava kava	Reduces stress, muscle relaxant; relieves anxiety; induces sleep and counters fatigue.	Increases CNS depression with alcohol, sedatives.	Side effects: GI disturbances; temporary discoloration of skin, hair, nails. Do not use in pregnancy, lactation, endogenous depression. Large doses cause muscle weakness. Chronic use may cause scaly skin resembling psoriasis (reversible). Causes pupil dilation affecting vision (avoid driving, operating heavy machinery). Store in cool, dry place (excess heat/light will alter contents).

Continued

Treatment

Table 26-1 HERBAL THERAPIES-INTERACTIONS—cont'd

Name	Purported Benefit	Interactions	Precautions
Licorice	*Oral:* Treatment for inflammation of upper respiratory tract, mucous membranes, ulcers, expectorant.	May decrease effect of antihypertensives. Thiazides may increase potassium loss.	Large doses may cause pseudoaldosteronism (hypertension, headache, lethargy, edema).
Ma huang (Ephedra)	Controls weight; boosts energy; treatment of colds, allergies, appetite suppressant.	Increases toxicity with beta-blockers, MAOIs, caffeine, theophylline, decongestants, St. John's wort.	Linked to high B/P, headache, seizures; can cause confusion, insomnia, dizziness, sweating, fever, nausea, vomiting.
Melatonin	Aids sleep; prevents jet lag.	Decreases effects of antidepressants.	Side effects: headache, confusion, fatigue does not lengthen total sleep time.
Milk thistle	Hepatoprotective, antioxidant, liver disorders, including poisoning (e.g., mushroom), cirrhosis, hepatitis.	None.	Mild allergic reactions, laxative effect.

MSM (methylsulfonyl methane)	*Oral/topical:* Treatment for chronic pain, arthritis, inflammation, arthritis, osteoporosis, muscle cramps/pain, wrinkles; protection against wind or sun burn.	None known.	May cause nausea, diarrhea, headache, pruritus increase in allergic symptoms.
Omega 6 fatty acid	*Oral:* Treatment for coronary artery disease; decreases total cholesterol LDL; increases HDL.	None.	Increases triglycerides.
Red clover	*Oral:* Treatment for menopausal symptoms; hot flashes; prevention of cancer, indigestion, asthma. *Topical:* Treatment for skin sores, burns, chronic skin disease (e.g., eczema, psoriasis).	May increase anticoagulant effects of warfarin. May interfere with hormone replacement therapy, oral contraceptives, or tamoxifen.	Rash, myalgia, headache, nausea, vaginal spotting.

Treatment

Continued

Table 26-1 HERBAL THERAPIES-INTERACTIONS—cont'd

Name	Purported Benefit	Interactions	Precautions
SAMe	*Oral:* Treatment for depression, heart disease, osteoarthritis, Alzheimer's disease, Parkinson's disease, slows aging process.	May increase adverse effects with antidepressants.	Nausea, vomiting, diarrhea, flatulence, headache.
St. John's wort	Relieves mild to moderate depression; heals wounds.	May cause "serotonin syndrome" (confusion, agitation, chills, fever, sweating, diarrhea, nausea, muscle spasms or twitching), hyperreflexia, tremor with antidepressants, yohimbine.	Side effects: dizziness, dry mouth, increased sensitivity to sunlight; report symptoms of "serotonin syndrome."
Saw palmetto	Eases symptoms of large prostate (frequency, dysuria, nocturia).	None.	Side effects: upset stomach, headache, erectile dysfunction. Does not reduce

			size of enlarged prostate. Obtain baseline PSA levels before initiating. Large doses can cause diarrhea.
Shark cartilage	***Oral:*** Treatment for cancer, arthritis, psoriasis, wound healing.	None.	Nausea, vomiting, constipation, dyspepsia, bad taste in mouth.
Soy	Treatment for menopausal symptoms; prevents osteoporosis and cardiovascular disease in postmenopausal women; hypertension, hyperlipidemia.	May decrease effects of estrogen replacement therapy.	Constipation, bloating, nausea, allergic reaction.
Valerian	Aids sleep, relieves restlessness and nervousness. Does not decrease night awakenings.	May have additive therapeutic effect and adverse effects with medications with sedative properties.	Side effects: heart palpitations, upset stomach, headache, excitability, uneasiness. May cause increased morning drowsiness.

Continued

Treatment

Table 26-1   HERBAL THERAPIES-INTERACTIONS—cont'd

Name	Purported Benefit	Interactions	Precautions
Wild yam	**Oral:** Alternative for estrogen replacement therapy, postmenopausal vaginal dryness, premenstrual syndrome, osteoporosis, increase energy/libido, breast enlargement.	None known.	Large amounts may cause vomiting (tincture).
Yohimbine	Male aphrodisiac. Used to treat impotence, erectile dysfunction, orthostatic hypotension.	Decreases effects of antidepressants, antihypertensives, St. John's wort.	Large doses linked to weakness, paralysis, excitation, tremor, isomnia, anxiety, nausea, vomiting, dizziness.

AIDS, acquired immune deficiency syndrome; BP, blood pressure; CHF, congestive heart failure; CNS, central nervous system; GI, gastrointestinal; HDL, high-density lipoprotein; HIV, human immunodeficiency virus; LDL, low-density lipoprotein; MAOI, monoamine oxidase inhibitor; PMS, premenstrual syndrome; PSA, prostate-specific antigen; UTI, urinary tract infection.
Source: Hodgson BB, Kizior RJ: Saunders Nursing Drug Handbook 2004, Philadelphia, 2004, Saunders.

- Is the method(s) widely available for use within the healthcare community, or is it controlled with limited access to its use?
- If used in place of standard therapies or clinical trials, will the ensuing delay affect any chances for cure or advance the cancer disease stage?
- Is the treatment based on an unproven or proven theory?
- Is there a claim made for harmless, painless, or nontoxic treatment?

V. INTERNET RESOURCES

Alternative Medicine Foundation:
www.AMFoundation.org

American Cancer Society Complementary & Alternative Methods:
www.cancer.org/alt_therapy/index.html

American Botanical Council:
www.herbalgram.org

ConsumerLab.com:
www.consumerlab.com

Healthfinder:
www.healthfinder.gov

Medwatch:
www.fda.gov./genherbinfo/herbref.html

Memorial Sloan-Kettering Cancer Page:
www. mskcc.org/aboutherbs

Mindbodytravel.com:
www.mindbodytravel. com

National Center for Complementary and Alternative Medicine:
www.altmed.od.nih.gov/nccam

National Medicines Comprehensive Database:
www.naturaldatabase.com

Treatment

Bibliography

Cade M: Reflexology, *Kansas Nurse* 77(5):5, 2002

Cassileth BR: Complementary and alternative cancer medicine, *J Clin Oncol* 17(11s):44, 1999.

Decker GM, editor: *An introduction to complementary & alternative therapies,* Pittsburgh, Pa, 1999, Oncology Nursing Press.

Decker GM, Myers J: Commonly used herbs: implications for clinical practice, *Clin J Oncol Nurs* 5(2):13, 2001.

Hite AL: Recommendations for herbal supplements and the perioperative patient, *Kansas Nurse* 77(5):3, 2002.

Gullatte MM, Otto SE: Cancer clinical trials. In Otto SE, editor: *Oncology nursing,* ed 4, St. Louis, 2001, Mosby.

Guthrie D: Diabetes: complementary and alternative care, *Kansas Nurse* 77(5):1, 2002.

Hodgson BB, Kizior RJ: *Saunders nursing drug handbook,* Philadelphia, 2003, Saunders.

National Center for Complementary and Alternative Medicine, *Cancer facts, complementary and alternative medicine.* Available on-line at http://www.cis.nci.nih.gov/fact9_14.htm. Accessed December 3, 2002.

Oncology Nursing Society: Oncology nursing position on the use of complementary and alternatives in cancer care, *Oncol Nurs Forum* 27(5):749, 2000.

Shaller J, Rivera-Smith C: Music therapy with adolescents experiencing loss, *Forum* 28(5):1, 2002.

Sinna A: Art of healing, *Cure cancer updates, research and education* 1(3):46, 2002.

Stanley KJ: The healing power of presence: respite form the fear of abandonment, *Oncol Nurs Forum* 29(6):935, 2002.

Tedesco P, Cicchetti J: Like cures like: homeopathy, *Am J Nurs* 101(9):43, 2001.

Tucker SM: Complementary and alternative medicine and contemporary nursing practice. In Thompson JM, McFarland GK, Hirsch JE, et al., editors: *Mosby's clinical nursing,* ed 5, St. Louis, Mosby, 2002.

Watson E: Using art as a therapeutic tool, *Forum* 28(5):10, 2002.

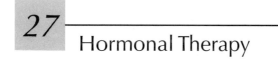

27 Hormonal Therapy

I. OVERVIEW

Hormonal therapy has a history of use of more than 200 years. It remains one of the selected therapies for approximately 30% of patients with hormone-dependent cancers. Cancers of the breast, prostate, and endometrium are among the best known of the hormone-dependent tumors. Additional cancers that are responsive to endocrine manipulation to some degree include Kaposi's sarcoma and renal, liver, ovarian, and pancreatic cancer. Breast and prostate cancers have specifically designed hormonal therapies related to cancer prevention and treatment; therefore the following information regarding such therapies will be restricted to these two cancer types (O'Shaughnessy 2002).

II. BREAST CANCER

The effects of estrogen and progesterone on human breast cancer cells are mediated by steroid receptors known as estrogen receptors (ERs) and progesterone receptors (PRs). Both healthy cells and cancer cells have these receptors, but they are frequently overexpressed in breast cancer. These receptors are located in the nucleus or on the surface of the cell and bind to the circulating steroid hormones; the receptor/hormone complex then works within the cell nucleus to promote cellular growth and division. A biochemical or immunohistochemical analysis of breast cancer cells removed at the time of tissue diagnosis can quantify the presence of these receptors in noninvasive or invasive breast cancers. Patients are said to be positive or negative for ER and PR based on the level of binding receptors that are present. Approximately 60% to 65% of primary breast cancers are ER-positive, and fewer are PR positive. The presence of ERs and PRs in the breast cancer tissue is a predictor of responsiveness to hormonal therapy and adjuvant therapy and of survival.

Treatment

For patients with metastatic breast cancer whose disease is ER-positive, PR-positive, or both and is not rapidly progressive, immediately life-threatening, or highly symptomatic, the sequential use of hormone therapies represent optimal care. Patients whose disease responds to a hormonal agent by achieving stability for a minimum of 6 months have approximately a 40% to 50% chance of achieving clinical benefit from a subsequent hormonal therapy and a 25% chance with a third-line therapy. The five major categories of hormonal therapies used in breast cancer disease management are as follows (O'Shaughnessy 2002):

A. **Estrogens—**

Estrogens were initially introduced in the 1940s for the treatment of advanced breast cancer. The most commonly prescribed drug in this classification was diethylstilbestrol, which binds to the ER, making it less responsive to the endogenous estrogen. Currently, estrogens are not used in the treatment of metastatic breast cancer because of their side effects and the development of multiple other hormonal agents that are more efficacious and less toxic to the patient. The undesirable side effects of estrogens include nausea and vomiting, depression, increased risk for thromboembolic complications, fluid retention, urinary incontinence, vaginal bleeding, congestive heart failure, and a tumor flare reaction.

B. **Androgens—**

The mechanism of action of androgens is not completely clear, but it appears to be directed at the ER, where it disrupts the stimulating effects of endogenous estrogens. Virilization (e.g., facial hair, voice deepening, acne, increased libido, and clitoral hypertrophy) is the most common side effect of androgen therapy. Tumor flare (temporary increased pain at tumor site) and hypercalcemia are also common occurrences.

C. **Progestins—**

Progestins suppress the release of leuteinizing hormone from the anterior pituitary by inhibiting the pituitary function, thus regressing the tumor size. Commonly reported side effects include hypertension, vaginal bleeding, fluid retention, thromboembolism, and weight gain. Currently, with the development of more effective selective estrogen receptor modulators (SERMs), progestins are used as a third- and fourth-line therapy.

D. **Aromatase Inhibitors—**

In about 7 out of 10 cases of breast cancer, the cancer cells have areas on their surface called *receptors* to which hormones such as estrogen and progesterone attach, thus providing fuel for the cells' growth into a tumor. Nonsteroidal antiestrogen agents (e.g., tamoxifen) and aromatase inhibitors (AIs) (e.g., anastrozole and Femara) both interfere with cancer cells' use of hormones to help them grow, but these drugs work in different ways. Nonsteroidal antiestrogens interfere directly with the cancer cells' ability to use estrogen for fuel. AIs block the action of a substance called *aromatase*, which helps the body to produce estrogen. This interference at the cellular level inhibits the breast cancer cell of estrogen, thereby depriving the tumor of estrogen and resulting in cancer cell death. Reported side effects for AIs include nausea, headache, mild hot flashes, and musculoskeletal pain (back, arm, and leg).

E. **Selective Estrogen Receptor Modulators—**

SERMs block estrogen action by interfering with the estrogen binding site on the cell receptor, thus preventing estrogen from gaining access. SERMs have been used in multiple studies with healthy women to reduce the incidence of menopausal symptoms of atrophic vaginitis, hot flashes, and mood swings. Additional functions of SERMs include use in breast cancer chemoprevention studies and in the treatment of metastatic breast cancer. Tamoxifen is the standard SERM currently used in breast cancer adjuvant therapy. It binds to the ER site in breast cancer cells, thereby blocking the uptake of estrogen necessary for cell proliferation.

Side effects of SERMS experienced by women include hot flashes, nausea, vomiting, change in menstrual period, genital itching, vaginal discharge, and endometrial hyperplasia/polyps. Side effects reported by men include headache, nausea, vomiting, rash, bone pain, weakness, and sleepiness (Table 27-1; Hawkins 2002).

Treatment

Table 27-1   COMMON HORMONAL AGENTS USED IN BREAST AND PROSTATE CANCER TREATMENT

Hormonal Agents	Cancer	Route(s)	Dose	Side Effects
Aminoglutethimide (Cytadren)	Breast, prostate	PO	500–1000 mg daily	Nausea, hypotension, fever, hypoglycemia or hyperglycemia, rash, masculinization
Anastrozole (Arimidex)	Metastatic breast cancer	PO	1 mg daily	Nausea, peripheral edema, headache, hot flashes, constipation, back pain, weight gain, anemia, diarrhea
Bicalutamide (Casodex)	Metastatic prostate cancer	PO	50 mg daily	Gynecomastia, hot flashes, nocturia, impotence, dizziness, insomnia, diarrhea, constipation
Corticosteroid (dexamethasone [Decadron], hydrocortisone [Solu-	Used in many pretreatment protocols before varied	PO, IV, IM	Varies with protocol	Fluid and electrolyte disturbances, neuromuscular imbalances, weight gain, changes in appetite or energy; may

	drug administration			require glucose/insulin dose adjustments
Cortef], methylprednisolone [Solu-Medrol], Prednisone)				
Extremestan (Aromasin)	Advanced breast cancer	PO	25 mg daily	Sweating, fatigue, hot flashes, anxiety, swelling, dizziness, headache, nausea, vomiting, abdominal pain
Finasteride (Proscar)	Prostate	PO	5 mg daily	Impotence, decreased libido, gynecomastia
Flutamide (Eulexin)	Prostate	PO	250 mg TID	Nausea, diarrhea, gynecomastia, hot flashes, impotence, decreased libido, anxiety, headache
Fulvestrant (Faslodex)	Metastatic breast cancer	IM	250 mg every month	Headache, pain, nausea, vomiting, constipation, loss of appetite, peripheral edema, dizziness, sweating, increased cough

Continued

Treatment

Table 27-1   COMMON HORMONAL AGENTS USED IN BREAST AND PROSTATE CANCER TREATMENT—cont'd

Hormonal Agents	Cancer	Route(s)	Dose	Side Effects
Goserelin (Zoladex)	Breast, prostate	IM, SC	3.6 mg every 28 days	Postmenopausal symptoms, sexual dysfunction, decreased erections, gynecomastia, hot flashes, transient-increased bone pain
Letrozole (Femara)	Metastatic breast cancer	PO	2.5 mg daily	Mild hot flashes, vaginal dryness, headache, nausea, weight gain
Leuprolide (Lupron)	Prostate	IM,SC	SC: 1 mg daily IM: 7.5 mg every 28 days	Impotence, hot flashes, gynecomastia, nausea, vomiting, insomnia, peripheral edema, joint and bone pain
Megestrol (Megace)	Breast, prostate	PO	40 mg four times daily	Menstrual changes, hot flashes, nausea, headache, fluid retention, weight gain, breakthrough bleeding

Nilutamide (Nilandron)	Metastatic prostate cancer	PO	300 mg × 30 days; 150 mg/day	Alcohol intolerance, hot flashes, dyspnea, nausea, hypertension, visual disturbances (adapt to darkness)
Raloxifene (Evista)	Metastatic breast cancer; Chemoprevention Trial	PO	60 mg daily	Menstrual irregularities, hot flashes, weight gain, vaginitis, blurred vision, change in vision
Tamoxifen (Nolvadex)	Metastatic breast cancer; Chemoprevention Trial	PO	20–40 mg daily	Menstrual changes, hot flashes, weight gain, vaginitis, myalgia, nausea
Toremifene (Fareston)	Metastatic breast cancer	PO	60 mg daily	Hot flashes, nausea, vaginal discharge, sweating, bone pain, dry eyes

IM, intramuscularly; *IV*, intravenously; *PO*, orally (by mouth); *SC*, subcutaneously; *TID*, three times daily.

Treatment

III. PROSTATE CANCER

Hormonal or androgen deprivation therapy is used in multiple settings for the patient with prostate cancer. In general, androgen deprivation induces a remission in 80% to 90% of men with advanced cancer and results in a median progression-free survival of 12 to 33 months. Multiple strategies have been used to induce castrate serum levels of testosterone or interfere with its function. Medical castration was initially accomplished by the administration of exogenous estrogen such as diethyl-stilbestrol, but it is now more commonly accomplished by the administration of leuteinizing hormone–releasing hormone (LHRH) agonists. Hormonal therapy is used in conjunction with external beam radiation therapy, brachytherapy, and radical prostatectomy for the treatment of prostate cancer, and is used in chemoprevention studies for prostate cancer prevention. The three major categories of hormonal therapies used in prostate cancer disease management are as follows:

A. **LHRH Agonists—**

Leuteinizing hormone is normally released from the anterior pituitary in response to the pulsatile release of LHRH, which is synthesized in the hypothalamus. The presence of LH results in the testicular secretion of a physiologic level of testosterone with corresponding spermatogenesis. Medically induced continuous LHRH stimulation, however, results in desensitization of the pituitary gland and inhibits LH production. Within the initial 5 to 8 days of treatment, there is an initial increase in testosterone levels resulting from the increased LH production induced by the LHRH agonist. This initial increase corresponds with a disease flare and may exacerbate bone pain or result in obstructive urinary symptoms. Examples of LHRH agonists' are leuprolide and goserelin. LHRH agonists side effects include hot flashes, bone pain, peripheral edema, fatigue, osteopenia (decreased bone density) with osteoporosis (excessive calcification of bone), and increased risk for fracture in men who have been on prolonged androgen suppression (O'Rourke 2001).

B. **Antiandrogens—**

Steroidal antiandrogens inhibit LH secretion from the pituitary gland and block androgens at the receptor level. Because testosterone levels are affected by this mechanism, these agents are associated with decreased libido and erectile dysfunction. The most commonly prescribed steroid antiandrogen is megestrol acetate.

C. **Nonsteroidal Antiandrogens—**
Nonsteroidal antiandrogens such as bicalutamide, flutamide, and nilutamide interfere with the binding of testosterone and dihydrotestosterone to the androgen receptor. Usually these drugs are not used as a single agent in the treatment of advanced prostate cancer. Reported side effects include hot flashes, loss of libido, impotence, diarrhea, generalized pain, nausea, and nocturia (see Table 27-1).

Bibliography

Erlichman C, Loprinzi CL: Hormonal therapies. In DeVita VT Jr, Hellman S, Rosenberg SA, editors: *Cancer principles and practice of oncology,* ed 6, Philadelphia, 2001, Lippincott Williams & Wilkins.

Goldberg NJ: Nursing perspective on selective estrogen receptor modulators in the prevention and treatment of breast cancer, *Clinical Oncology Updates* 1(4):1, 2001.

Hawkins R: Hormone therapy in cancer, *Oncology Nursing Patient Treatment and Support* 9(3):1, 2002.

Hellerstedt BA, Pienta KJ: The current status of hormonal therapy for prostate cancer, *CA Cancer J Clin* 52(3):154, 2002.

Hodgson BB, Kizior RJ: *Saunders nursing drug handbook,* Philadelphia, 2003, WB Saunders.

O'Rourke ME: Genitourinary cancers. In Otto SE, editor: *Oncology nursing,* ed 4, St. Louis, 2001, Mosby.

O'Shaughnessy JA: Recent advances in the treatment of metatastic breast cancer, *Clinical Oncology Updates* 5(2):1, 2002.

Treatment

28
Nutrition

I. OVERVIEW

Nutritional assessment is an integral component for the nutritional care of the patient with cancer. This assessment includes an estimate of body composition such as fat, skeletal muscle protein, and visceral protein. The information provided will determine the patient's risk for cancer disease or cancer treatment–induced malnutrition.

Secondarily, the required cancer therapies can have a major impact on the nutritional status of the patient, such as the following:

A. **Surgery—**

Increases stress on the body, thereby increasing the body's metabolic requirements; extra calories and proteins are needed for healing and repair.

An altered gastrointestinal (GI) system related to surgery, procedures, or effects of combined therapies results in nothing by mouth status or presence of tubes or drains, thereby depleting the nutritional stores.

B. **Radiation Therapy—**

Exerts its effects on the "healthy cells" and the cancer cells in the radiation treatment fields. Specific side effects are related to the anatomic site in the treatment field, such as dry mouth, diarrhea, nausea and vomiting, difficulty in chewing or swallowing, and altered taste. Additional conditions such as fatigue, anorexia, and myelosuppression increase the patient's potential for infection or decreased nutritional intake and may influence the scheduled radiation treatment plan.

C. **Biotherapy, Chemotherapy, Blood/Stem Cell Transplantation—**

The goals of these therapies are to destroy or stop abnormal growth of cancer cells, incur rapid cellular destruction in the bone marrow, or create space in the bone marrow for new infused cells. Many of the drugs or agents used have multiple and varied side effects, such as nausea, vomiting, fatigue, myelo-suppression, weight loss or weight gain, diarrhea, constipation, stomatitis, and mucositis. Severe nutritional compromises can occur related to the patient's side effects, thereby increasing the potential complications to include severe enteritis, dehydration, and malnutrition. Secondary protein and calorie stores are depleted, which may result in treatment delay, interruption, or stoppage.

D. **Specific Nutritional Deficits—**
1. *Weight Loss Cycle*—An unintentional weight loss of 10% or more of usual body weight within the previous 6 months may signal a nutritional deficit.
2. *Malnutrition*—An unintentional weight loss of greater than 10% of body weight associated with a serum albumin less than 3.5 g/dl are predictors of muscle wasting, loss of muscle strength, or depletion of fat stores. Malnutrition conditions may be described as *kwashiorkor* (protein deficiency), *marasmus* (energy deficiency), and *marasmic-kwashiorkor* (protein and energy deficiency).
3. *Anorexia-Cachexia Syndrome*—This is a complicated physiologic state that is associated with increased morbidity and mortality rates. This severe condition, present in up to 80% of patients with cancer, is characterized by wasting, weight loss, weakness, fatigue, poor performance status, and impaired immune function.

II. PATIENT ASSESSMENT PARAMETERS

Patient assessment parameters comprise a significant proportion of data that will determine the patient's clinical nutritional deficits and will assist in designing the appropriate interventions. A thorough and detailed assessment is crucial to obtain all of the required information. Consider other factors such as patient age (older patient), psychosocial issues such as the home environment, and the ability to purchase certain food products.

The components include the following:

A. **Physical History and Assessment—**
1. *Type of cancer and date of diagnosis*

2. *Type(s) and duration of cancer therapy*
3. *Concurrent medications*
4. *Concomitant medical conditions* (e.g., cardiac disease or diabetes)
5. *Allergies*
6. *Alterations in nutrition and elimination*
7. *Condition of mouth, gums, teeth or dentures, hair texture, skin turgor*

B. **Anthropometric Data—**
   1. *Height and current weight compared with ideal body weight*
   2. *Weight change (percentage of weight change over specific time period)*
   3. *Triceps skin fold*
   4. *Midarm muscle circumference*
   5. *Subscapular skinfold thickness*

C. **Dietary History—**
   1. *24-Hour recall of intake*
   2. *Food preferences and allergies*
   3. *Changes in diet or eating habits or patterns*
   4. *Use and type of dietary supplements*

D. **Laboratory Tests—**
   1. *Serum albumin (3.5–5.0 g/dl)*
   2. *Serum creatinine (0.7–1.4 mg/100/ml)*
   3. *Serum transferrin (<200 mg/dl)*
   4. *Total lymphocyte count (2000/mm³)*
   5. *Hemoglobulin (12.5–18 gm/dl)*
   6. *Hematocrit (37–52%)*
   7. *Prealbumin (10–45 mg/dl)*
   8. *Blood urea nitrogen (8–21 mg/dl)*
   9. *Skin test (such as T cell–mediated immunocompetence)*

III. MANAGEMENT OF NUTRITIONAL ALTERATIONS

Creative and timely strategies are needed to provide the interventions specific to the symptom or nutritional alteration. If one approach does not resolve the problem, be creative and willing to try different methods to increase the patient's nutritional intake.

A. **Altered Taste—**
   Try different seasonings (lemon juice, herbs, spices, flavor additives) in food preparation; use tart foods to stimulate taste, use nonsweetened mints or candies,

and substitute fish or chicken for beef or pork meat preparations. Marinate meats in sweet fruit juices, wines, salad dressing, barbecue sauce, or sweet and sour sauces. Chilled or frozen food typically is more acceptable than warm food. Use plastic utensils if food tastes metallic. Brush teeth before and after each meal.

B. Anorexia—

Use smaller plates with more frequent meals; use high nutrient supplements such as Ensure, Boost Plus, or Carnation Instant Breakfast; eat with family and friends; and try new foods or recipes.

C. Constipation—

Increase fiber, fruits, and vegetables in diet; increase fluid intake to at least eight 8-ounce assortments of liquids in 24 hours; increase daily activity; and avoid cheese or concentrated foods.

D. Diarrhea—

Avoid greasy and spicy foods, gas-producing foods, foods high in fiber (raw vegetables or fruits, nuts), alcohol, tobacco, and caffeine products; eat bland or cool foods (soups, macaroni and cheese).

E. Dry Mouth—

Try thickened liquids, practice good oral hygiene, use artificial saliva and nonsweetened candies or mints, and apply lip protectant such as petroleum jelly.

F. Dysphagia—

Encourage a soft, more liquid diet with easy-to-swallow foods, use nutritional supplements, eat small frequent servings, and consult with a speech therapist for special swallowing techniques.

G. Early Satiety—

To avoid a "feeling of being too full" when only small amounts of food or fluid have been consumed, eat small and frequent meals and liquids on an around-the-clock basis, practice good oral hygiene to cleanse the palate, and participate in mobility or activity to increase GI stimulation.

H. Nausea and Vomiting—

Drink clear liquids or broths; advance diet as tolerated; avoid sweet, rich, or fatty foods; try cool foods or easily digested foods (rice, baked potato, cooked cereal); avoid food with noxious odors; and try dry foods (crackers, toast, dry cereal products).

Treatment

I. **Radiation Esophagitis—**
Eat soft bland foods; use cream-based soups; eat foods that are cool and soothing to swallow (milk shakes, frozen yogurt or custards); avoid eating tart and acidic fruit and juices; and avoid use of alcohol, tobacco, or caffeine products.

J. **Sore Mouth and Throat—**
Eat foods that are moist and easy to swallow or chew such as casseroles and omelets; use sauces or gravies in meat preparations; take nutritional supplements; and try enriched liquids such as ice cream or dry nutrition products added to milk.

K. **Too Tired to Eat—**
Eat with family or friends, alternate scheduled rest and activity periods throughout the 24 hours, and use distraction or relaxation methods (music, movies).

L. **Xerostomia—**
Relieving an abnormal, excessive dryness in the mouth requires short- and long-term interventions; avoid use of alcohol, tobacco, and caffeine products; increase fluid intake in diet and drink fluids on a planned frequency around the clock; eat bland, moist foods; try nonsweetened candies or mints; and use artificial saliva products.

IV. NUTRITIONAL SUPPLEMENTS

Multiple nutritional supplements are available for oral nutrition support. The supplements can be taken between meals or used when patient travel is necessary. Most of the liquid products "taste better" when the product is cold and served in a glass rather than in the original container. Using the dry prepackaged soups, custards, and puddings provide snacks that are convenient and nutritious. Some of the products have a milk base or fruit base, contain more fiber, or are lactose-free.

Such products include:
- 2 Calorie High Protein
- Boost High, Boost Plus
- Carnation Instant Breakfast
- Ensure, Ensure Plus, Ensure Fiber
- Nutri-shake
- Resource
- Slim Fast Ultra
- Scandi-Shake (lactose-free is available)

V. ENTERAL AND PARENTERAL NUTRITION

When the normal GI digestive system is functioning abnormally or the medical condition or treatment requires alternative methods for calorie intake, enteral or parenteral nutrition methods are selected. The enteral route is preferable when the GI system is intact and functional. Parenteral nutrition is indicated for patients who have totally nonfunctioning GI tracts, who require bowel rest, or who are intolerant of enteral therapy. See the Appendix for enteral and parenteral nutrition information.

Bibliography

ASPEN Board of Directors: Standards for home nutrition support, *Nutr Clin Pract* 14:151, 1999.

Byers T, Nestle M, McTiernan A, et al: American Cancer Society Guidelines on nutrition and physical activity for cancer prevention: reducing the risks of cancer with healthy food choices and physical activity, *CA Cancer J Clin* 52(2):92, 2002.

Body JJ: The syndrome of anorexia-cachexia, *Curr Opin Oncol* 11:255, 1999.

Gahart BL, Nazareno AR: *Intravenous medications,* ed 18, St. Louis, 2002, Mosby.

Hodgson BB, Kizior RJ: *Saunders nursing drug handbook,* Philadelphia, 2003, Saunders.

Javier CC: Nutritional support for the cancer patient. In Govindan R, Arquette MA, editors: *The Washington manual of oncology,* Philadelphia, 2002, Lippincott Williams & Wilkins.

Koeller JM, et al: *Antiemetic guidelines, creating a more practical approach,* Huntington Valley, Pa, 2002, Atlas Multimedia.

Sacher RA, McPherson, Campos JM: *Widmann's clinical interpretation of laboratory tests,* Philadelphia, 2000, FA Davis.

Schulmeister L: Nutrition. In Otto SE, editor: *Oncology nursing,* ed 4, St. Louis, 2001, Mosby.

Sherry VW: Taste alterations among patients with cancer, *Clin J Oncol Nurs* 6(2):73, 2002.

Treatment

I. OVERVIEW

Nurses have a significant role in symptom management for the patient/family with cancer. Sequential and frequent assessments with an evaluation of the interventions are essential to determine if the pertinent symptom has resolved or has progressed to a more compromised state. At the initial contact and at the assessment and status evaluation times, determine the "chief complaint" or what is problematic to the patient. Include the following queries: current/previous **medications**, **therapies**, and **blood counts** (white blood cells [WBCs], nadir, red blood cells [RBCs], and platelets); **presence or absence** of the following symptoms: pain, nausea and vomiting (N&V), fever/chills, alteration(s) in elimination, bleeding, and dyspnea;, and changes in weight status and skin integrity. **Consider** the patient's age, performance status, ability to report symptomology, resources for self-care in the home, and the cancer disease treatment goal (cure, control, and palliation). Many of these symptoms can have treatment dose-limiting effects that result in life-threatening circumstances if the symptom is not assessed and intervention is not provided in a prompt and astute manner.

Patient/family/caregiver **education** is an ongoing process from the time of the initial cancer diagnosis and throughout the disease and treatment continuum. Use every opportunity to teach, reinforce, reassure, and discern knowledge deficits regarding self-care for symptom intervention and reporting pertinent information to the healthcare team. Strategies such as demonstration with return-demonstration; keeping a log of medications, pain, and fatigue reports; and review of concepts with the patient/family/caregiver paraphrasing key points will enhance the learning process.

Be sensitive to and incorporate materials with respect to the patient's cultural, language, and spiritual needs. Use simple, everyday language that is easy for the patient to understand.

Keep the instructions simple and specific to what you want the patient to know or to perform. Following are common symptoms that occur as the result of the cancer disease or cancer treatment process, including the symptom definition and etiologic factors, along with assessment and intervention strategies (see Chapter 25 for discussion of pharmacologic and infusion therapies).

A. **Alopecia—**

    1. *Definition/Etiologic Factors*—Alopecia is the temporary or permanent loss of hair as the result of chemotherapy drugs or radiation therapy. Hair loss occurs within 10 to 21 days after drug administration; hair loss is usually temporary and regrowth may take 3 to 5 months after the cytotoxic therapy is completed. Hair loss may occur spontaneously or during shampooing or hair grooming. Cancer therapies, nutritional status, certain medical conditions (aging and hypothyroidism), and poor hair condition also contribute to hair loss.

        a. *Chemotherapy Related*—Consider the *type* of chemotherapy drug, such as those presenting greatest risk for hair loss: daunorubicin, cyclophosphamide, doxorubicin, etoposide,

Treatment

ifosfamide, and paclitaxel; the *dose* of chemotherapy drug(s), such as high-dose therapy vinblastine; and *combination* of certain chemotherapy drugs. With hair thinning the hair becomes very thin and dull looking; this is related to drugs used, for example, bleomycin, floxuridine, and vincristine.

b. *Radiation Therapy*—Alopecia that occurs within the treatment area depends on the dose and extent of radiation to the scalp, for example, 4000 cGy radiation may result in permanent hair loss, whereas 3000 to 3500 cGy may result in a temporary hair loss. Changes in hair texture and color may also occur. Pruritus can develop on the scalp causing it to become very dry or to peel.

2. *Interventions*
   a. Instruct the patient to avoid using curling irons or hair curlers, hair dryers, permanent waves, coloring agents, harsh shampoos, and frequent shampooing.
   b. Encourage the patient to select a comfortable wig, cap, scarf, or turban to wear before hair loss occurs.
   c. Encourage the patient to keep the head covered in summer to prevent severe sunburn and in winter to prevent heat loss.
   d. Instruct the patient to use gentle shampoo products and gentle drying techniques.
   e. Encourage participation in the American Cancer Society "Look Good—Feel Better Program."

B. **Ascites**—
   1. *Definition/Etiologic Factors*—Ascites is an abnormal accumulation of fluid in the abdominal cavity that is not absorbed into the systemic circulation. The cancer disease–related factors include ovarian, breast, endometrial, colon, gastric, and pancreatic cancers and often are associated with liver metastasis. Treatment-related factors include previous radiation to the abdomen or a surgical procedure with modification of the venous or lymphatic channels. The patient experiences abdominal discomfort and distention, anorexia,

decreased bladder capacity, bowel obstruction, electrolyte imbalance, weight gain, infection, edema, and respiratory compromise. Life expectancy is a few months; therefore the treatment should focus on palliative care measures.

2. *Interventions*
    a. Potential removal of fluid from the associated body cavity with shunting devices
    b. Nutrition interventions including small frequent feedings on an around-the-clock basis to diminish "early satiety" (feeling too full when only bits of food have been eaten)
    c. Proper oral hygiene to cleanse the palate and mobility or activity to increase gastrointestinal (GI) stimulation
    d. Skin care with careful attention to skin folds at breast, perineum, and underarms
    e. Change in position from side to side and side to back; position support with pillows, cushions, and wedge-type devices
    f. A powered air-fluidized bed or device that uses circulation of filtered air through silicone-coated ceramic beads creating the characteristic of fluid to aid in comfort and position and to minimize skin breakdown
    g. Pharmacologic medications such as analgesics, diuretics, and sedatives
    h. Nonrestrictive cotton clothing that is soothing to the skin surfaces

C. **Constipation—**
    1. *Definition/Etiologic Factors*—Constipation is the infrequent passage of hard stool, associated with abdominal and rectal pain. It usually results from decreased physical activity; low-fiber diet; pharmacologic agents such as analgesic opiates, chemotherapy (vinca alkaloids), anticonvulsants, and antihistamines; bowel obstruction; spinal cord compression; metabolic effects (hypercalcemia, hypokalemia, hypothyroidism); or lack of time or privacy for defecation.
    2. *Assessment*—Assess change in usual patterns of bowel elimination; current medications that potentiate constipation; date of last bowel movement; history of constipation and laxative use;

Treatment

GI-related symptoms such as N&V, anorexia, and cramping; and history of rectal fissures or abscesses.

3. *Interventions*
   a. Establish a daily bowel program—note amount/frequency of bowel movement.
   b. Initiate a prophylactic bowel regimen such as by prescribing natural laxatives such as senna (Senokot) twice daily and titrate (up to 4 tablets twice daily) until regular bowel routine is established. Additional options include the following: 1 tablespoon milk of magnesia can be added to senna, docusate sodium, mineral oil, or bisacodyl. Enemas and suppositories are not recommended because they can inadvertently cause rectal mucosal injury that may lead to inflammation or infection in an immunocompromised patient.
   c. Modify diet to include high-fiber foods, fresh fruits, and vegetables, and avoid cheese or concentrated foods.
   d. Maintain and or increase activity level.

D. Diarrhea—
   1. *Definition/Etiologic Factors*—Diarrhea is an increase in the quantity, frequency, or fluid content of stool that is different from the usual pattern of bowel elimination. It may be related to cancer therapies such as the following:
      a. *Biotherapy Drugs*—Interferons, interleukin-2
      b. *Chemotherapy Drugs*—Irinotecan, 5-fluorouracil topotecan, paclitaxel, dactinomycin, dacarbazine, fludarabine, and cytarabine
      c. *Radiation Therapy*—Diarrhea can occur 2 to 3 weeks after starting radiation therapy and may last throughout the course of the therapy. Symptoms may include an increased number of stools, loose or watery stools, and abdominal cramping and may progress to chronic enteritis.
      d. *Postallogeneic Transplantation*—Gut-related graft-versus-host disease (GVHD)
   2. *Assessment*—Assess disease-related factors such as intestinal bacteria or virus and bowel obstruction, gut-related GVHD, treatment related to bio-

therapy, chemotherapy, and radiation therapy. Query the patient regarding the following:

  a. Current medications such as antibiotics, antacids, or laxatives
  b. Current nutritional therapies such as dietary supplements or tube feedings
  c. Lifestyle stresses, alcohol and tobacco use, food products such as milk or dairy products, lactose intolerance, spicy foods, fruit juices (prune, orange), or high-fiber food

3. Interventions

  a. Initiate antidiarrheal or antispasmodic medications such as Kaopectate, octreotide acetate, loperamide, kaolin-pectin, bismuth subsalicylate, and diphenoxylate hydrochloride with atropine sulfate. See the Appendix for more information.
  b. Avoid greasy and spicy foods, gas-producing foods, and foods high in fiber (raw vegetables or fruits, nuts); avoid use of alcohol, tobacco, and caffeine products; and eat bland or cool foods (soups, macaroni and cheese).

E. Fatigue—

1. Definition/Etiologic Factors—Cancer-related fatigue is a condition or energy deficit related to the cancer disease or treatment that affects the patient's psychological, physical, social, and spiritual well-being. The fatigue interferes with the patient's ability to get adequate rest, sleep, or participate in the routine activities of daily living (ADLs). Fatigue is the most frequently experienced symptom of cancer and usually precedes or accompanies most malignancy diagnoses. Subjective symptoms include being excessively tired, lack of ability to concentrate, decreased socialization, lethargy, insomnia, depression, and declining interest in social and spiritual activities. Cancer treatment–related factors such as chemotherapy cause fatigue that generally peaks 3 to 4 days after the drug nadir and administration of biotherapy drugs such as interferon, interleukin-2, and monoclonal antibodies. Radiation therapy has an impact on fatigue in almost 100% of patients because of the ionizing radiation

Treatment

on cells and the cumulative dose over the treatment course. Surgical procedures, especially when added to other interventions, can have a prolonged effect on the patient's recovery process. Additional factors influencing the patient's fatigue level include poor nutrition, pain, stress, infection or fever, and immobility.

2. *Assessment*
   a. Assess various patterns of fatigue onset, duration, timing, and impact on ADLs.
   b. Assess the patient's individual symptoms, for example, mobility, mood, sleeping, or hygiene.
   c. Assess for use of caffeine, alcohol, or recreational drugs.
   d. Assess for benefits and use of complementary therapies that facilitate rest or sleep.
   e. Determine whether the fatigue has altered the patient's ability to perform ADLs, role functions, shopping, errands, social and religious activities, hobbies, or leisure activities.
   f. Determine whether the fatigue has affected the patient's mental abilities such as memory or concentration.
   g. Determine what *factors* make the fatigue better or worse and what interventions facilitate fatigue.

3. *Interventions*
   a. Discuss the potential of fatigue at the time of diagnosis and treatment (e.g., biotherapy, chemotherapy, radiation therapy, and surgery issues).
   b. Encourage the patient/family to discuss fatigue and its impact on ADLs.
   c. Explore intervention strategies to conserve energy: pace/plan/prioritize needs and keep a regular schedule for sleep, rest, or scheduled activities.
   d. Encourage relaxation or distraction opportunities such as hobbies, tapes, music, and reading.
   e. Plan and balance energy expenditures with rest intervals; encourage adequate sleep and rest.
   f. Encourage adequate nutrition to promote ideal body weight.
   g. Encourage the patient to keep a fatigue/energy log to identify patterns.

  h. Encourage the patient to ask for help with personal and social responsibilities.
  i. Encourage the patient to participate in energy-enhancing activities such as meditation, yoga, aerobic exercises, or short walks.
  j. Explore use of assessment tools such as Brief Fatigue Inventory, Functional Assessment of Chronic Illness Therapy, Cancer-Related Fatigue Distress Scale, or Visual Analog Scales that are helpful in discerning fatigue assessment with intervention strategies.
F. **Hemorrhagic Cystitis—**
  1. *Definition/Etiologic Factors*—Hemorrhagic cystitis is an inflammatory disorder in which mucosal damage to the bladder occurs as the result of drug metabolites or byproducts. This condition is highly associated with intravenous infusions of cyclophosphamide and ifosfamide. The severity of symptoms is related to the specific drug and drug dose: standard or low dose less than 1000 mg cyclophosphamide is associated with a 10% incidence, and high dose of at least 120 mg/kg is associated with a 40% incidence. Ifosfamide is associated with up to 30% incidence of frank hematuria. Previous radiation therapy to the pelvis or bladder area also increases the risk. Clinical features include dysuria, increased frequency, burning during urination, nocturia, oliguria, microscopic or frank hematuria, and fever and chills.
  2. *Assessment*—Assess the amount, frequency, duration, and changes related to dysuria and hematuria.
  3. *Interventions*
    a. Before drug infusions (mentioned earlier), administer a bladder protection mesna.
    b. Encourage frequent voiding, at least every 2 hours, day and night.
    c. Encourage patient to drink fluids—a minimum of eight 8-ounce glasses of water each day; if unable to drink fluids, provide parenteral hydration.
    d. Administer IV preparations of drugs mentioned previously early in the day.
    e. Catheterize the patient if unable to void.

f. Provide patient (or have patient self-medicate) with analgesics and other prescribed pharmaceuticals.

g. Instruct patient to take oral chemotherapy medications before 4 PM each day to allow the drug to pass through the bladder before bedtime.

h. Instruct the patient to promptly report increased severity of symptoms.

G. **Myelosuppression (Anemia, Neutropenia, Thrombocytopenia)—**

1. *Definition/Etiologic Factors*—Myelosuppression refers to the suppression of bone marrow resulting in a decreased number of WBCs, RBCs, and platelets. Cancer treatments such as chemotherapy and radiation therapy are the most common causes of myelosuppression and often have dose-limiting toxicities with life-threatening consequences. The chemotherapy drugs and radiation therapy treatments destroy the rapidly dividing healthy hematopoietic cells, which results in a decreased production and maturation of the healthy WBCs, RBCs, and platelets. Combination therapy or high-dose therapy associated with blood/stem cell transplantation can result in an extreme marrow suppression condition. Cancer diseases associated with myelosuppression include leukemia, multiple myeloma, lymphoma, and invasion of tumor cells into the bone marrow.

Secondary causes of myelosuppression may be disease-related, such as aplastic anemia, idiopathic/thrombocytic thrombocytopenia purpura, hypocoagulation disorders (liver disease, vitamin K deficiency), hypercoagulation disorders (disseminated intravascular coagulation), slow or persistent blood loss (GI bleed, neoplasm, peptic ulcer, esophageal varices), medication use (nonsteroidal antiinflammatory drugs, aspirin), primary malignancies of the marrow/tumor, invasion of the marrow/red cell deficiencies (thalassemia) causing decreased quantity and quality of RBCs, impaired absorption (celiac disease, postgastrectomy), inadequate intake or decreased use of iron, folic acid, and vitamins K and B_{12}.

Additional factors that impact myelosuppression include nutritional status, age, certain medications (aspirin, heparin, and digitalis), endotoxins from a bacterial infection, and biotherapy agents that alter the immune system.

Terms associated with myelosuppression include the following:

a. *Anemia*—A decrease in the hemoglobin (Hgb) level or circulating erythrocytes

b. *Thrombocytopenia*—A decreased number of circulating platelets or thrombocytes

c. *Neutropenia*—An absolute decrease in the number of circulating neutrophils (ANC), usually less than $1000/mm^3$ (e.g., an ANC $<500/mm^3$ describes profound neutropenia).

d. *Granulocytopenia*—A reduction of the absolute granulocyte complement

e. *Leukopenia*—A reduction or depletion of the total leukocyte complement

f. *Pancytopenia*—A deficiency of all the cell elements of the blood (erythrocytes, platelets, neutrophils, eosinophils, basophils, monocytes, macrophages, and lymphocytes)

g. *Nadir*—After chemotherapy, the point at which the lowest blood cell count is reached. The nadir usually occurs 7 to 10 days after treatment and depends on the type, dose, and number of chemotherapy agents. The **WBCs** and **platelets** are usually the **first to drop in number** and usually are the **first to appear** in the cell count recovery process.

Anemia, thrombocytopenia, and neutropenia are the most pertinent myelosuppressive conditions and are discussed in the following section.

2. *Clinical Features, Assessment, and Interventions*

a. *Anemia*—The normal role of RBCs is to transport oxygen from the capillaries of the lungs to the systemic capillaries of the tissues and to carry carbon dioxide from the tissues to the lungs. The typical life span of the RBC is 120 days; therefore when losses or deficits occur, replacement of the RBCs is necessary to maintain homeostasis. Normal values: RBC 4 to

Treatment

6 million; Hgb: 12 to 16 g/dl; hematocrit (Hct): 37% to 52%.

Clinical Features—Clinical features include pallor, tachycardia, tachypnea, dyspnea at rest and on exertion, exercise intolerance, fatigue, sensitivity to cold, headache, dizziness, difficulty sleeping and with concentration, menstrual problems, male impotence, and anorexia.

Assessment

- Assess patient's disease and treatment goal status.
- Assess presence or absence of active/passive bleeding.
- Compare current and previous RBC, Hgb, and Hct laboratory values.
- Determine contributing factors (treatment, disease, and nutrition).
- Identify underlying cause(s) of patient's anemia.

Interventions

- Administer prescribed therapies (epoetin alfa, blood, or blood products).
- Administer oxygen if oxygen saturation is less than 90%.
- Educate patient/caregiver regarding energy conservation measures.
- Instruct patient/caregiver regarding signs and symptoms of anemia and when to report certain events to the physician or nurse.
- Explore consultation with dietitian regarding nutrition interventions.
- Teach patient/caregiver mechanisms to cope with the side effects related to anemia (fatigue, dyspnea, and rest/energy expenditures).

b. *Thrombocytopenia*—Platelets facilitate the coagulation process when an injury or assault occurs (e.g., chemotherapy); defined as a platelet count less than 100,000 (normal platelet count is 150,000 to 400,000/mm^3).

Clinical Features—Clinical features include petechiae (small, purple-red dots); ecchymoses (bruises); overt bleeding from nose, gums, wounds, around tubes/catheters, GI and urinary tracts; oozing from puncture sites: occult blood in stool or urine; headaches; and prolonged or abnormal menstrual bleeding.

Assessment

- Assess presence or absence of bleeding.
- Assess onset, duration, and severity of clinical features.
- Assess coagulation tests and additional pertinent laboratory values. Assess platelet count and risk for bleeding: less than 50,000/ mm^3 represents a moderate risk; less than 10,000 mm^3 represents a severe risk for life-threatening GI, central nervous system, or respiratory hemorrhage.

Interventions

- Administer prescribed therapies (blood or blood products, oprelvekin).
- Implement/instruct patient/caregiver regarding safety measures: use electric razor, discourage contact sports, enhance a safe environment in the home (non-skid rugs), and wear shoes and socks to protect feet.
- Minimize invasive procedures (subcutaneous or intramuscular injections, venipuncture blood sampling).
- Teach patient measures to maintain integrity of mucous membranes: blow nose gently, use water-based lubricant before having sexual intercourse, using tampons and/or using prophylactic stool softeners, and use soft toothbrush/sponge-tipped applicator for cleaning teeth.
- Teach patient to avoid having dental care (such as use of dental floss, or irrigation tools until platelet count returns to normal), avoid having sexual intercourse if platelet count is less than 50,000/mm^3, and avoid taking any medication that interferes with bleeding.
- Instruct patient/caregiver regarding signs and symptoms of thrombocytopenia and when to report certain events to the physician or nurse.

Treatment

- Review and discuss with the patient/caregiver current or over-the-counter medications that interfere/alter platelet product, and instruct him or her to discuss with the physician/nurse changes in any medication routine.

c. *Neutropenia*—A decrease in the number of circulating neutrophils in the blood evidenced by an ANC less than $1000/mm^3$. This occurs most often as a consequence of cytotoxic therapy, and commonly presents as a severe bacterial infection in patients with cancer. Neutropenia is the single most important predisposing risk factor to infection in the patient with cancer:

ANC $>1500/mm^3$ = normal risk
ANC $<1000/mm^3$ = moderate risk
ANC $<500/mm^3$ = severe risk
ANC $<100/mm^3$ = extreme risk

- The ANC is calculated as follows:
  - Total WBC, including differential count
    WBC: 1500, polys/segs: 35, bands: 25
  - Add neutrophils (*polys* [segs] and **bands**
    $35 + 25 = 60$, convert to % –60%/0.60
  - Multiply total WBC by total neutrophil
    $1500 \times 0.60 = 900$ ANC/moderate risk

Clinical Features—The clinical manifestation of neutropenia is correlated with the patient's neutropenia count (ANC $<500/mm^3$ represents a severe risk) and may not exhibit the usual signs and symptoms, such as fever and exudate at site. General signs and symptoms include fever greater than 100.5°F, tachycardia, and myalgia. Specific clinical features associated with certain sites include respiratory (cough and dyspnea on exertion), urinary tract (dysuria, frequency, hematuria, and cloudy urine), skin or mucous membrane (erythema, tenderness, hot skin, and edema), and indwelling devices (fever, erythema, pain or tenderness, edema, drainage and induration at the site).

Assessment
- Assess current/previous ANC count and correlate with treatment cycle.

- Assess presence/absence of earlier described clinical features.
- Assess nutritional status.
- Assess vital signs (blood pressure, pulse, respiratory rate, and character).

Interventions

- Obtain prescribed specimen(s) collection for culture and sensitivity tests.
- Administer prescribed therapies (hematopoietic growth factors, antimicrobials, and analgesics).
- Promote/instruct increased fluid intake and nutritionally balanced diet.
- Prevent trauma to patient's skin and mucous membranes (avoid use of catheters, enemas, rectal thermometers and suppositories, nasogastric tubes, and safety razor).
- Cleanse and protect all wounds as prescribed.
- Teach patient/caregiver signs and symptoms of infection and when to report certain events to the physician or nurse.
- Provide/educate patient/caregiver with protection measures to implement during neutropenia episodes (avoid people with cold/contagious illness, people who were recently vaccinated, and cleaning animal litter boxes/cages); instruct patients that they should NOT share food utensils, provide direct care for pets, or use tampons or enemas/rectal suppositories.
- Instruct the patient not to receive live vaccinations (polio).
- Promote/educate patient/caregiver regarding meticulous site care for vascular access device, frequent and thorough hand-washing techniques, and daily bath with mouth care before and after meals.

H. **Mucositis/Stomatitis—**
   1. *Definitions/Etiologic Factors*—Stomatitis/mucositis is an inflammatory condition of the mucosal epithelial cells, which are present on all surfaces of the GI tract from the mouth to the rectum.

Treatment

Stomatitis is mucositis in the oral cavity, esophagitis is mucositis in the esophagus, and enteritis is mucositis in the intestine. Epithelial cells in the GI tract are in a constant renewal process, and when exposed to normal influences they have the capability to repair an injury or assault. Treatment-related effects alter the integrity of the mucosal membranes and interfere with the healing and renewal process.

Chemotherapy drugs decrease this renewal rate of the basal epithelium, resulting in localized mucosal atrophy or diffuse ulceration of the mucosa and initiation of the inflammatory process. Drugs such as *5-fluorouracil, cytarabine, mercaptopurine, busulfan, melphalan, and thiotepa (with high-dose or rapid infusion); methotrexate, dactinomycin, doxorubicin, daunorubicin, etoposide, mitoxantrone,* and *procarbazine* are most noted for causing stomatitis/mucositis.

The stomatitis occurrence rate is almost 100% for patients receiving high-dose chemotherapy in preparation for peripheral blood stem cell transplantation. Secondarily, gut-related GVHD can be a consequence for the patient with an allogeneic transplantation. When the radiation treatment fields include the head and neck region, chest, abdomen, and pelvic sites, cellular changes and destruction can also occur. The greater the radiation doses and the shorter the time between doses, the greater the severity of mucositis.

Additional factors, therapies, or drugs that alter mucous membranes include oxygen therapy, dental disease or poor hygiene, ill-fitting dentures, advanced age (decreased salivary flow), anticholinergics (decreased salivary flow) and steroids (fungal overgrowth), history of alcohol or tobacco use, poor nutrition, and dehydration.

Clinical features for mucositis/stomatitis include pain, bleeding, erythema, edema of oral mucosa and tongue, mucosal ulcerations, changes in oral mucosal coloring, moisture, taste, or ability to swallow, hoarseness, and presence of white or red patches in the mouth.

2. *Assessment*
   a. Assess the patient for changes in taste, voice, pain, and ability or comfort in swallowing; examine the lips, tongue, and oral mucosa for color, moisture, shiny appearance, texture, and integrity, and examine the saliva for quantity and quality. The oral mucosal can be a "reflective picture" of changes or alterations in the remainder of the GI tract.
   b. Grades of oral mucositises/stomatitis are as follows:
      • Grade 1: Erythema of oral mucosa
      • Grade 2: Isolated small white patches and ulcerations
      • Grade 3: Confluent ulcerations covering less than 25% of oral mucosa
      • Grade 4: Hemorrhagic ulcerations
   c. Query the patient regarding GI tract–related symptoms such as burning, pain, or discharge in the rectal or vaginal areas.

3. *Interventions*
   a. *Oral Care*—Encourage frequent and consistent cleaning (after meals, at bedtime, on rising) of teeth, tongue, and mucosa; use extra-soft bristle brush or sponge swabs during neutropenia and thrombocytopenia episodes.
      • Denture care: Clean dentures daily with antimicrobial cleansing agent and soak dentures in clean water during extended hours of sleep or periods of nonuse.
      • Ensure frequent and adequate moisture; rinse mouth often (e.g., 8 ounces of water and a half teaspoon baking soda); use saliva substitute sprays or sugarless citric-flavored candy or gum.
      • Avoid using irritating and drying agents such as peroxide solutions, alcohol-based mouthwashes, and lemon-glycerine swabs and solutions.
      • Avoid use of alcohol, tobacco, and caffeine products and hot spicy foods or beverages.
      • Use mouth care products with anesthetic and coating preparations such as Moi-Stir,

Treatment

Swizzle, Ulcer Ease, Orabase, Oral Balance, Zilactin, and Hurricane.
- Maintain a diet that includes bland, moisturized food, and high-calorie/-protein foods, and use of dietary supplements, or experiment with different, healthy, nourishing foods.

b. Perineal Care
- Use perineal or sitz baths and meticulous perineal care.
- Avoid wearing tight constricting clothing or irritating (corduroy or wool) material.
- Use vaginal dryness agents (Replens) to minimize vaginal irritation.
- Avoid sexual intercourse and douching during the inflammatory stage of mucositis.
- Report signs and symptoms of infection, such as fever greater than 101°F, pain, burning, or abnormal discharge.
- Maintain fluid intake to 3000 ml per day and eat a nutritionally balanced diet.

I. **Nausea and Vomiting—**
1. *Definition/Etiologic Factors*—N&V often are the most distressing side effects of chemotherapy; they may be acute, anticipatory, delayed, or persistent. Acute N&V occur within 1 to 2 hours of treatment and last approximately 24 to 48 hours. Anticipatory N&V occur before the treatment, lasting several hours to days; N&V occurring after the initial 24 hours of treatment is referred to as delayed or persistent. The most common cause of N&V is associated with the administration of chemotherapy and biotherapy drugs and with certain radiation therapy treatments. Additional causes of N&V in the patient with cancer are metabolic disturbances, primary or metastatic tumor of the CNS, GI obstruction (delayed gastric emptying and bowel inflammation/irritation), opioid drug-related (constipation and cumulative effects of active morphine metabolites), infection, and miscellaneous (noxious odors and perfumes).

Specific chemotherapy-related risk factors for N&V include history of emesis with prior chemotherapy, poor performance status, high level of pretreatment anxiety, female gender (increased incidence of emesis), age (older age [>50 yr] experience less severe emesis), history of motion sickness, and history of pregnancy hyperemesis; patients with a history of alcohol consumption usually have a decreased incidence of emesis. When certain chemotherapy drug doses are increased or route and schedule of drug are changed, N&V usually become more severe (Table 29-1).

N&V have a significant negative impact on the patient's self-reported ability to enjoy meals and social events, maintain daily functions, and avoid personal hardships. Prompt assessments

Table 29-1   EMETOGENIC POTENTIAL OF SELECTED BIOTHERAPY AND CHEMOTHERAPY DRUGS

Low	Moderate	High/Very High
Bleomycin	Asparaginase	Amifostine
Busulfan	Daunorubicin	Carmustine
Chlorambucil	Doxorubicin	Cisplatin
Cytarabine (low dose)	5-fluorouracil	Carboplatin
Docetaxel	Gemtuzumab	Cytarabine
Epoetin alfa	Ifosfamide	Cyclophosphamide
Filgrastim	Interferons	Dacarbazine
Flutamide	Interleukin 11	Dactinomycin
Gemcitabine	Mitomycin	Etoposide
Hormones	Mitoxantrone	Interleukin-2
Hydroxyurea	Topotecan	Lomustine
Levamisole		Mechlorethamine
Paclitaxel		Methotrexate
Rituximab		Melphalan
Tamoxifen		Procarbazine
Teniposide		Semustine
Trastuzumab		Streptozocin
Vinblastine		
Vincristine		
Vinorelbine		

Treatment

with appropriate interventions are essential to help the patient maintain his or her self-esteem during this disease/treatment event.

2. *Assessment*
   a. Determine the potential causes of N&V as related to the patient (disease, therapy-related, and psychosocial).
   b. Determine the chemotherapy-related risk factors associated with N&V.
   c. Determine the patient's nutritional and hydration compromises related to the N&V.

3. *Interventions*
   a. Provide/instruct the patient to take prescribed antiemetic drugs (see Tables 25-2 and 25-3).
   b. Encourage patient to explore complementary therapies (music therapy, relaxation and distraction techniques, biofeedback, meditation, hypnotherapy, and imagery) to diminish and or cope with N&V issues.
   c. Instruct patient to take antiemetics before each treatment and on an around-the-clock schedule to prevent or diminish chemotherapy-related N&V.
   d. Dietary Interventions
      • Drink clear liquids or broths; advance diet as tolerated.
      • Avoid sweet, spicy, rich, or fatty foods or foods with noxious odors.
      • Avoid favorite foods on day of treatment and while N&V persists so that aversions to those foods do not develop.
      • Try cool foods, easily digested foods (rice, baked potato, and cooked cereal), or dry foods (crackers, toast, and dry cereal products).

J. **Pain Management—**
   1. *Definition/Etiologic Factors*—"Pain affects patients' psychological, social, and spiritual well-being and interferes with their comfort, sleep, and nutritional needs. Pain, as defined by the American Pain Society, is an unpleasant sensory and emotional experience associated with actual or potential tissue damage, or described in terms of such damage" (Ferrell 2002). Cancer pain is often

caused by direct tumor involvement (e.g., proliferation of cancer cells within the bone, nerves, viscera, and soft tissue). The site of the pain produces different sensations and intensities; also, the location of the site affects the analgesic indicated for relief. The types of pain produced by direct tumor involvement may include the following:

a. *Somatic Pain*—Results from stimulation of afferent nerves in the skin, connective tissue, muscle, joints, or bones and is described as throbbing, sharp, or aching.

b. *Visceral Pain*—Involves the organs in the thoracic or abdominal area; caused by infiltration, pressure, or distention and is described as gnawing, cramps, constant, and deep.

c. *Neuropathic Pain*—Results from peripheral or central sensory nerve trauma injury causing abnormal firing and is described as burning, shooting, lancinating, and tingling.

d. *Bone Involvement*—Involves multiple bony metastases, which cause generalized pain.

e. *Peripheral Nerves*—Most often occurs in site's chest wall and retroperitoneal space, which may produce pain in the back, abdomen, or legs.

f. *Brachial Plexus*—Usually a result of a primary lung tumor (Pancoast syndrome); aching or burning occurs in the shoulder and upper back.

g. *Epidural Spinal Cord Compression*—Patients may report pain in a specific site (e.g., a tight belt around the waist) that is constant and progressive and usually is preceded by motor or sensory deficits.

2. *Assessment*

   a. Assess **patient's self-report** of pain: *intensity* (rating best or worst scale 1 to 10, respectively), *location and radiation* (point to site[s]), *quality* (patient's description—"like hot lead"), *onset, duration, pattern variation* (start-stop, ongoing), *alleviating and aggravating factors* (what makes it better or worse), *current pain management interventions* medication(s) (doses and miscellaneous strategies [heat, cold, position]).

b. Assess patient's **pain management history:** past experience with pain, interventions, and manner of expressing pain.

c. Assess **effects of pain** on the patient's quality of life (sleep, rest, appetite, communication, concentration and mood).

d. Assess the patient's **pain goal:** comfort level rating scale 1 to 10, ability to do ADLs, and goals related to function/activities.

e. Assess **cultural, ethnic, and religious beliefs** that may have an impact on reporting or obtaining pain relief.

3. *Interventions*

a. Provide/educate patient/caregiver regarding the importance of taking analgesics on an around-the-clock schedule to provide comfort and to prevent pain.

b. Select the analgesic appropriate to the type and level of pain (see Appendix).

c. Select the easiest and most cost-effective route of administration.

d. Plan and schedule breakthrough pain medication interventions.

e. Anticipate and plan for the pain treatment–related side effects:

- Constipation: Does NOT DECREASE over time; use stool softeners
- Hallucinations, Confusion, Dizziness: Usually temporary; orient to environment
- N&V: Usually temporary and lasting about 1 week; provide antiemetics
- Pruritus: Intense itching occurs most often with intrathecal opioids; use antihistamine
- Respiratory depression: Rarely occurs
- Sedation: Usually temporary; verify that patient is alert and orientated when awake
- Urinary retention: Temporary, may require medications or catheterization

f. Instruct the patient/caregiver to explore complementary therapies (massage, music therapy, relaxation and distraction techniques, biofeedback, meditation, hypnotherapy, prayer, and imagery) to use as adjunct for pain relief.

g. Explore noninvasive pain relief techniques (heat provides comfort and relaxation; cold may produce numbness and decrease pain-causing substances) and cutaneous stimulation (transcutaneous electrical nerve stimulation unit).

h. Encourage patient/caregiver to use "pain diary" to recognize a pattern of pain occurrences, beneficial interventions, drug-related side effects, and interference with sleep, rest, appetite, or ability to do ADLs.

K. Peripheral Neuropathy—

1. *Definition/Etiologic Factors*—Peripheral neuropathy (PN) is an injury, inflammation, or degeneration of the peripheral nerve fibers. These nerve fibers can be divided into three types based on their function.

   a. *Sensory*—Modulates perception of touch, pain, temperature, position, and vibration

   b. *Motor*—Modulates voluntary movement, muscle tone, and coordination

   c. *Autonomic*—Modulates involuntary function, visceral, and vascular involvement

   Many causes of PN in patients with cancer are not directly related to chemotherapy (e.g., hereditary, vitamin or dietary deficiency, diabetes, atherosclerotic disease, and thyroid dysfunction). Chemotherapy drugs such as platinum analogs (affect perception of vibration and position), vinca alkaloids, and taxines (affect perception of pain and temperature) are associated with loss of deep tendon reflexes. With the progression, symptoms evolve up the foot and leg and develop in the fingertips and progress proximally, developing a condition known as stocking-glove syndrome. The specific chemotherapy drugs that are associated with PN include cisplatin, vincristine, vinblastine, oxaliplatin, paclitaxel, cytarabine, methotrexate, procarbazine, thalidomide, and interferon. The incidence and severity of PN are related to the drug type, drug dose, administration schedule, and cumulative dose (Almadrones 2002).

   Patients with PN commonly report symptoms of paresthesia in hands or feet, constipation, and loss of deep tendon reflexes. A sudden change in the patient's signature may indicate loss of fine-motor control and is often the symptom that gets the patient's attention, prompting him or her to report the sensory and motor changes.

2. *Assessment*
   a. *Assess*—Symmetry, lack of distal sensation, proximal extent of sensation loss, speed of onset, gait and associated symptoms of pain, bowel/bladder function, and skin changes
   b. *Motor Assessment*—Tone and reflexes (upper and lower extremities) with focus on distribution of weakness and symmetry; assess gait, balance, speech, and smoothness of muscle movement
   c. *Sensory Assessment*—Pain (pinprick), temperature (hot or cold items), position (moving digits), and vibration (tuning fork)
   d. *Autonomic Assessment*—Valsalva maneuver, intestinal motility (bowel sounds), orthostatic changes (feeling faint when suddenly sitting up/standing), and sexual function (erectile dysfunction)
   e. *Functional Assessment*—Ask the patient the following questions: Can you get up and down from the toilet, or a curb or steps? Can you dress, groom, and bathe yourself? Have you fallen or almost fallen? Do you require help to do things you previously did alone (e.g., bathe)?

3. *Interventions*
   a. *Pharmacologic Preparations*—Nonsteroidal antiinflammatory drugs, corticosteroids, antidepressants, anticonvulsants, or analgesics
   b. *Nonpharmacologic Interventions*—Physical therapy or exercise, massage, hydrotherapy, transcutaneous electrical nerve stimulation unit, diet modification, humor, or distraction
   c. Instruct patient/family regarding safety measures, for example:
      • Use protective gloves when washing dishes and use a pot holder when handling hot items.
      • Clear walkways of rugs or items that may cause falls; use non-skid shower and tub mats.

- Keep rooms and hallways well lit and without glare. Turn lights on before entering a room, hallway, or stairway.
- Keep a flashlight with you or within reach to use when lighting is not adequate.
- Wear shoes that go over the instep of the foot, gloves and warm socks in cold weather, and jewelry that you can put on without help.
- **Discuss driving skills** regarding ability to feel gas and brake pedals, ability to feel and turn steering wheel, and reaction time to driving events.

L. **Reproductive and Sexuality Issues—**
   1. *Definition/Etiologic Factors*—The systemic effects of cytotoxic therapy can affect fertility, body image, and sexual function. The impact of chemotherapy on ovarian function in premenopausal and perimenopausal women after treatment with alkylating agents is dependent on age (number of remaining ovarian follicles), type of cancer, drug dose, and duration of therapy. Destruction of the follicles by chemotherapy can cause alterations in fertility and can lead to a perimenopausal or menopausal state characterized by hot flashes, vaginal dryness, and skin changes.

   Secondary changes may occur such as temporary or permanent amenorrhea, ovarian failure or fibrosis, menstrual irregularities, difficulty becoming pregnant, decreased estradiol levels, and increased gonadotropin levels. Male patients may experience azoospermia (absence of sperm), infertility, temporary loss of libido, and spermatogenesis.

   Chemotherapy drugs that affect sexual or reproductive function include **alkylating agents** (busulfan, chlorambucil, cisplatin, cyclophosphamide, ifosfamide, melphalan, and nitrogen mustard), **antimetabolites** (5-fluorouracil, cytarabine, fludarabine, and methotrexate), **antitumor antibiotics** (dactinomycin, daunorubicin, and doxorubicin), vinca alkaloids (vinblastine and vincristine), and hormonal agents.

   Radiation therapy impacts the germ-cell function and is associated with changes such as ovarian failure (occurs with small amounts of radiation and produces symptoms associated with menopause: hot flashes, amenorrhea, decreased libido, and osteoporosis) and changes in testicular function such as erectile dysfunction and spermatogenesis, potentially resulting in permanent sterility.

2. *Assessment/Interventions*
   a. Before the cancer treatment, explore fertility options (sperm banking or in vitro fertilization) with the patient.
   b. Explore counseling consultation regarding sexual dysfunction issues.
   c. Provide information/education regarding the side effects of such therapies.
   d. Provide information/education regarding contraception to prevent pregnancy during the chemotherapy or radiation therapy treatments.

M. Skin Integrity—

1. *Definition/Etiologic Factors*—Multiple alterations in skin integrity can occur as the result of certain cancer therapies or the combination of these cancer therapies. Following is a list of alterations in skin integrity with definition, prominent clinical feature, and causal agent for these cutaneous reactions.

   a. *Acral Erythema*—A painful erythematous and edematous rash on the plantar surfaces of hands and feet; occurs as a potential chemotoxicity on the dermal vasculature
   b. *Dry Desquamation*—A skin reaction (dry, erythematous, and itching) that occurs most often from external radiation therapy
   c. *Hand and Foot Syndrome*—Acral erythema, palmar-plantar erythrodysesthesia syndrome associated with continuous infusion of 5-fluorouracil, capecitabine, and liposomal doxorubicin
   d. *Hyperpigmentation*—Increased amounts of epidermal melanin without dermal deposition in the skin, hair, nails, mucous membrane, and teeth; associated with many chemotherapy drugs (alkylating agents and antitumor antibiotics)
   e. *Inflammation of Keratoses*—Pruritus and erythema noted adjacent to previous actinic ker-

atoses (horny growth) may be the result of DNA toxicity of the keratinocytic lesions associated with chemotherapy drugs (5-fluorouracil, dacarbazine, dactinomycin, doxorubicin, and pentostatin)

f. *Nail Changes*—Includes hyperpigmentation, discoloration, nail grooving, and partial separation of nail plate from bed associated with chemotherapy drugs (bleomycin, cyclophosphamide, doxorubicin, floxuridine, procarbazine, 5-fluorouracil, and docetaxel)

g. *Pruritus*—Severe itching of skin at multiple sites; aggravated by soaps, lotions, perfumes, or medication allergy; it is associated with many biotherapy and chemotherapy drugs and external radiation therapy

h. *Radiation Enhancement*—A synergistic effect of concurrent radiation therapy and chemotherapy, related to chemotherapy drugs (doxorubicin, dactinomycin, bleomycin, hydroxyurea, 5-fluorouracil, and methotrexate) that prevent cellular repair of radiation therapy

i. *Radiation Recall*—An inflammatory reaction occurring in previously irradiated tissue; most frequently associated with doxorubicin and dactinomycin

j. *Radiation Therapy Skin Changes*—A skin reaction (dry, erythematous, itching, and moist-desquamation with peeling tissue especially in skin fold areas) that occurs most often from external radiation therapy

2. *Assessment*
   a. Perform skin assessment including nails before biotherapy, chemotherapy, and radiation therapy, and on a scheduled basis throughout the treatment noting variations from normal.
   b. Inspect palmar and plantar surfaces for sensation, color, and movement.
   c. Assess skin breakdown (location, duration, width/depth, and drainage [color, odor]).

3. *Interventions*
   a. Apply cold compresses or normal saline irrigations to affected area three to four times a day to relieve pain.

    b. Apply topical steroids, creams, or ointments **only when prescribed**.

    c. Elevate the affected areas to reduce edema.

    d. Provide analgesics or other medications to relieve pain and itching.

    e. Instruct patient to avoid wearing tight restrictive clothing such as bras or belts over the irradiated skin areas.

    f. Do not apply powders, perfumes, deodorants, or tape to irradiated skin.

    g. Avoid use of cornstarch in the axilla, groin, or gluteal folds.

    h. Use a hand-held blow dryer on a cool setting to dry the perineum and skin folds.

    i. Protect sensitive, irritated, and skin-treated area from the cold, heat, and sun.

    j. Avoid direct sun exposure, wear protective clothing, and use sunscreens with a high sun protective factor (SPF).

N. Xerostomia—

    1. Definition/Etiologic Factors—Xerostomia is an abnormal excessive dryness of the mucous membranes in the mouth that usually occurs when the radiation treatment field includes the salivary glands. As the result, the saliva changes from a thin fluid to a thick, sticky, acidic one, with the result of debris adhering more readily to the teeth and gingiva.

    The dryness in the mouth may occur 1 to 2 weeks into therapy and may result in speaking, eating, and swallowing problems requiring short- and long-term interventions.

    2. Interventions

        a. Avoid use of alcohol, tobacco, and caffeine products.

        b. Avoid use of products containing lemon or glycerine because of their irritation and drying of the mucosal membranes.

        c. Avoid use of commercial mouthwashes that contain alcohol or flavoring agents.

        d. Select a diet with bland or moist foods, add sauces and gravies in food preparation, increase fluid intake and drink fluids on a planned frequency around the clock.

e. Try nonsweetened candies or mints and use artificial saliva products.
f. Try commercially available products such as Moi-Stir, Oralbalance, and Mouth Kote provide temporary relief of xerostomia. Two to 3 ml solution is placed in the mouth and swished to coat the mucosal surfaces.
g. Use of a humidifier at bedtime helps to decrease mucosal dryness and minimize frequency of awakening to drink fluids.

CANCER RESOURCES

American Cancer Society:
www.cancer.org

Cancer Care:
www.cancercare.org

Cancer Fatigue:
www.cancerfatigue.org

I Have Cancer:
www.ihavecancer.com

National Lymphedema Network:
www.lymphnet.org

Neuropathy Association:
www.neuropathy.org

Oral Health, Cancer Care, and You:
nohic.aerie. com/campaign

Pain:
pain.com

People Living With Cancer:
www.plwc.org

Sexuality and Cancer:
www.noah-health.org/english/illness/cancer/canccer-care/library/sex/html

United Ostomy Association:
www.uoa.org

Treatment

Bibliography

Almadrones L, et al: *Chemotherapy-induced neurotoxicity, current trends in management: a multidisciplinary approach,* Philadelphia, 2002, Phillips Group Oncology Communications.

Amgen, 2002, Aranesp (darbepoetin alfa) and Neulasta (pegfilgrastim) on-line. Available at www.amgen.com/

Bender CM, Kramer PA, Miaskowoski C: *New direction in the management of cancer-related cognitive impairment, fatigue and pain,* 2002, Scientific Connexions, Ortho-Biotech Oncology.

Bender CM, McDaniel RW, Murphy-Ende K, et al: Chemotherapy-induced nausea and vomiting, *Clin J Oncol Nurs* 6(2):94, 2002.

Bodey GP: Fever in the neutropenic patient. In Abeloff MD, Armitage JO, Lichter AS, et al, editors: *Clinical oncology,* ed 2, New York, 1999, Churchill Livingstone.

Buchsel PC, Forgey A, Grape FB, et al: Granulocyte macrophage colony-stimulating factor: current practice and novel approaches, *Clin J Oncol Nurs* 6(4):198, 2002.

Buchsel PC, Murphy BJ, Newton SA: Epoetin alfa: current and future indications and nursing implications, *Clin J Oncol Nurs* 6(5):261, 2002.

Davis TC, Williams MV, Marin E: Health literacy and cancer communication, *CA Cancer J Clin* 52(3):130, 2002.

Ferrell BR, editor: *A nurses' guide to breakthrough cancer pain,* Triplei, Teterboro, NJ, 2002, Media-Media.

Gahart BL, Nazareno AR: *Intravenous medications,* ed 18, St. Louis, 2002, Mosby.

Gillespie TW: Effects of cancer-related anemia on clinical and quality-of-life outcomes, *Clin J Oncol Nurs* 6(4):206, 2002.

Given B, Given CW, McCorkle R, et al: Pain and fatigue management: results of a nursing randomized clinical trial, *Oncol Nurs Forum* 29(6):949, 2002.

Hodgson BB, Kizior RJ: *Saunders nursing drug handbook,* Philadelphia, 2003, Saunders.

Oncology Nursing Society: *Cancer chemotherapy guidelines and recommendations for practice,* Pittsburgh, Pa, 2001, Oncology Nursing Press.

Oncology Special Edition: *Annual clinical reference,* 4:2001, New York, McMahon Publishing Group, Oncologyse.com.

Otto SE, editor: *Oncology Nursing,* ed 4, St. Louis, 2001, Mosby.

Physician's desk reference, ed 57, Montvale, NJ, 2003, Medical Economics.

Rittenberg CN: A new class of antiemetic agents on the horizon, *Clin J Oncol Nurs* 6(2):103, 2002.

Segal BH, Walsh TJ, Holland SM: Infections in the cancer patient. In DeVita VT Jr, Hellman S, Rosenberg SA, editors: *Cancer principles and practice of oncology,* ed 6, Philadelphia, 2001, Lippincott Williams & Wilkins.

30

Hospice and Palliative Care

I. OVERVIEW

"The National Hospice Organization defines the hospice philosophy as: Hospice care is a specialized care for the terminally ill people with a medically directed interdisciplinary team, providing a managed program of services that focuses on the patient/family as the unit of service. The focus of care is a palliative approach rather than a curative approach with an emphasis on pain and symptom control, so that a person may live the last days of life fully, with dignity and comfort, at home or in a homelike setting" (Martinez et al 2002).

This interdisciplinary team is physician-directed with varied professionals and personnel such as social workers, chaplains, nurses, dietitians, home care staff, bereavement coordinators, pharmacists, inpatient nurses, occupational therapists, volunteers, and consultants for patient/family (funeral director). This team provides supportive and compassionate care with communication and coordination between team members and the patient/family.

II. CRITERIA FOR HOSPICE CARE

- The patient must have a primary caregiver (family member or friend) who is willing to be responsible for the patient's overall care in the home setting.
- The patient needs to reside in the geographic area of the hospice's program to receive the designated home care services.
- The patient must desire palliative, not curative, treatment.
- To receive the Medicare Hospice Benefit (MHB), two physicians must certify that the patient is terminally ill and has less than 6 months to live.

Funded through the Health Care Finance Administration, initial guidelines were developed for the MHB in 1995, which then were revised in 1996 to include non-cancer patients into hospice care. The revised guidelines added eight categories of noncancer, end-stage illness with the following comprehensive criteria: heart, pulmonary, and liver disease; dementia; and human immunodeficiency virus. This MHB covers the services of the hospice team visits in the home, medications for pain and symptom management, durable medical equipment, and supplies. Finally, the Medicare benefits cover two types of short-term inpatient admissions: admission for patients requiring pain and symptom management and admission to provide a temporary respite for caregivers who are exhausted or in a crisis (Ferrell et al 2002; Martinez et al 2001).

III. HOSPICE CARE MODELS

- Independent community-based programs providing services in the home and contracting with hospitals for inpatient care.
- Independent community-based programs providing services in the home and operating a separate setting for inpatient care.
- Hospital setting with designated acute care beds that are distributed over medical, surgical, and oncology units, where care is focused on symptom management and limitation of invasive or painful procedures. These hospital-type settings include visiting policies that are less restrictive and resources like showers and laundry services that family members can use at a low cost.
- A home health agency provides the designated home care services such as nursing, respiratory care, and occupational services, as directed by the patient's physician.

For each of these services, representatives meet with the patient and family to determine the specific patient/family needs. The type of durable equipment required for home care, team member interview or consultation, and the schedule of team members providing services in the home are arranged before patient discharge or initiation of services. A list of phone numbers is provided including the agency staff 24-hour ON-CALL phone numbers of who and when to contact for services in the event of an emergency. Finally, a specific meeting is held with the patient/family and agency nurse or social worker regarding a physician-directed "Do Not Resuscitate" order. Signed copies of such orders are kept in the home and with the agency providing the hospice services (Ferrell et al 2002; Martinez et al 2002).

IV. ETHICAL CONCERNS
A. Advance Directives—
The federal Patient Self-Determination Act, enacted in 1991, requires hospices, hospitals, and other health care agencies to provide patients, on admission, with written information about two specific areas: (1) their right to accept or refuse treatment under state law, and (2) ways to execute advance directives such as a living will and a durable power of attorney. The purpose of this legislation is to ensure that patients' wishes are carried out in the event they become mentally incapacitated or are incapable of making or communicating their decisions. Hospice team members provide whatever information is needed to assist the patient in making an informed decision, especially when it affects the patient's decision *not to have* CPR, intravenous fluids, or tube feedings (Martinez 2002).

These advanced directives may include the following:

1. *A Living Will*—This is a written document that directs treatment in accordance with a patient's wishes.
2. *A Durable Power of Attorney*—A durable power of attorney for health care (also called a medical power of attorney or health care proxy) designates a spokesperson (who may be called a health care agent, surrogate, or proxy) to represent the patient in the decision-making process. This person must base any given decision solely on the patient's known or probable wishes under the circumstances, and the decision should not be influenced by his or her own preferences.

V. CONCEPTS OF CARE
A. Palliative Care—
The focus of palliative care is to prevent, relieve, reduce, or soothe the symptoms of disease or disorder

without effecting a cure. The patient may have days, weeks, or months to live. This type of care often takes place in hospital-type settings or in the home. Diagnostic tests and invasive procedures are minimized. Palliative care provides relief from symptoms of disease but also promotes favorable outcomes by helping patients and families to reach personal goals, reconcile conflicts, and derive meaning from their life experiences.

B. **End of Life—**
Refers to the final weeks of life when death is imminent. A palliative care concept or hospice care concept at the end of life requires attention to the physical, psychological, social, and spiritual aspects of well-being of the patient and the patient's family.

C. **Hospice Care—**
Refers to a program of care (described earlier) that provides support for the patient and family throughout the dying process and for the surviving family members through bereavement.

VI. SYMPTOM MANAGEMENT AND PSYCHOSOCIAL INTERVENTIONS

Symptom management and psychosocial interventions for the patient receiving palliative or hospice care at the end of life may *include* but are not limited to the following:

A. **Pain Management—**
Pain is subjective and pain is whatever the patient says it is, existing whenever the person says it does. Pain is managed with around-the-clock coverage, with planned interventions for breakthrough pain incidents, and by using opioids, nonopioids, and other pharmacologic preparations to provide pain relief.

B. **Nutrition and Hydration—**
The goal of nutrition and hydration is to provide patient comfort and to provide adequate amounts of fluid and food.

C. **Bowel and Bladder Management—**
The goal of bowel and bladder management is to prevent or manage constipation, diarrhea, and urinary incontinence or urinary retention.

D. **Dyspnea—**
Relief of respiratory symptoms through pharmacologic preparations, positioning of the patient, or interventions to cope with changes in the respiratory status (exhale through pursed lips, taking slow deep breaths, or oxygen therapy) are the focus of dyspnea management

E. **Gastrointestinal Disorders—**
Anorexia, hiccups, dyspepsia, constipation, diarrhea, and mucositis are managed with a variety of pharmacologic preparations and interventions such as swallowing 1 teaspoon of granulated sugar, sipping ice water or crushed ice, or biting on a lemon slice for hiccups.

F. **Position of Comfort and Mobility Status—**
The patient's desire or need to communicate with family members, visitors, and home care staff guides position and mobility. Instruct family members and caregivers regarding patient positioning techniques.

G. **Skin and Hygiene Care—**
A scheduled frequency promotes rest, relaxation, and comfort.

H. **Confusion or Hallucinations—**
The patient should be reoriented to environment on a scheduled basis; provide a safe environment at the bedside or in the room, consider noise and room temperature, and speak to and touch the person with a gentle approach.

I. **Provide a "Safe Environment, Place, Trusting Relationship"—**
Allow the patient to express or share feelings or fears about the dying process, to derive meaning from life's experiences, or to "take care of unfinished business."

J. **Request for Consultation Services—**
Assist patient/family in the request for consultation services regarding funeral arrangements, financial concerns, or legal issues.

K. **Response to Facing Death—**
Assist patient/family with managing difficult responses to facing death (guilt and helplessness, anger, or depression). Help the patient and family find ways to maintain control and to express their feelings of

Treatment

sadness over dying, and give the patient/family permission to share negative feelings.

L. **Respect Patient Culture—**
   Be sensitive and incorporate strategies with respect to the patient's cultural language and spiritual needs during the dying process and at the death event.

VII. SIGNS AND SYMPTOMS OF APPROACHING DEATH

The family or caregivers providing care to the dying patient in the home or assisting with care in other settings are better prepared for the patient's day-to-day changes and at the death event when given the following information (Martinez et al 2002):

- **The patient will sleep more and may be more difficult to arouse. Hearing and vision may decrease.**
- **There may be a gradual decrease in the need for food and drink; the patient is just not hungry (doesn't have an appetite).**
- **The patient may become more confused or restless or may experience visions of people and places.**
- **The patient's hands, arms, feet, and legs may become cooler, and the skin may turn a bluish color with purplish splotches.**
- **Irregular breathing patterns may occur (space of time 10 to 30 seconds) in which there is no breathing at all (apnea). It may become difficult for the patient to cough.**

Bibliography

Bowman T: As a family ages: facing the loss of dreams, *Forum* 28(1):1, 2002.

Boyle D: Psychosocial issues: In Lin EM, editor: *Advanced practice in oncology nursing*, Philadelphia, 2001, WB Saunders.

Burke C, editor: *Psychosocial dimensions of oncology nursing care*, Pittsburgh, Pa, 1998, Oncology Nursing Press.

Demaree AC, Thornton G, Zanich ML: Bereavement Support Group: challenges in a Rural Hospice, *Forum* 26(5):1, 2000.

DeSpelder LA, Strickland AL: *The last dance*, ed 4, Mountain View, Calif, 1996, Mayfield Publishing.

Ferrell BR, Coyle N: An overview of palliative nursing care, *Am J Nurs* 102(5):26, 2002.

Halstead MT, Roscoe ST: Restoring the spirit at the end of life: music as an intervention for oncology nurses, *Clin J Oncol Nurs* 6(6):332, 2002

Harrold JK: Palliative care: helping patients and families cope with the ambiguity of dying, *Forum* 28(4):1, 2002.

Henry M: Descending into delirium, *Am J Nurs* 102(3):49, 2002.

Herman CP: Spiritual needs of dying patients: a qualitative study, *Oncol Nurs Forum* 28(1):67, 2001.

Luggen AS, Meiner SE, editors: *Handbook for the care of the older adult with cancer,* Pittsburgh, Pa, 2000, Oncology Nursing Press.

Martinez J, Wagner S: Hospice care. In Thompson JM, McFarland GK, Hirsch JE, et al, editors: *Mosby's clinical nursing,* ed 5, St. Louis, 2002, Mosby.

Nail LM: I'm coping as fast as I can: psychological adjustment to cancer and cancer treatment, *Oncol Nurs Forum* 28(6):967, 2001.

Paice JA: Managing psychological conditions in palliative care, *Am J Nurs* 102(11):36, 2002.

Pessagno RA: Differentiating between grief and depression, *Clin J Oncol Nurs* 3(1):31, 1999.

Scanlon C: Ethical concerns in end-of-life care, *Am J Nurs* 103(1):48, 2003.

Sinna A: Art of healing, *Cure Cancer Updates, Research and Education* 1(3):46, 2002.

Stanley KJ: The healing power of presence: respite from the fear of abandonment, *Oncol Nurs Forum* 29(6):935, 2002.

Tobin DR, Lindsey K: *Peaceful dying,* Cambridge, 1999, Perseus Books.

Waller A, Caroline NL: *Handbook of palliative care in cancer,* ed 2, Boston, 2000, Butterworth Heinemann.

Treatment

31 Grief and Bereavement Issues

I. OVERVIEW

Grief and bereavement issues, such as the circumstances of the death event, resources available to the bereaved person, and life experiences of the bereaved person, have many determinants that impact the grief and mourning process for a person who has experienced a significant loss. J. William Worden, a noted authority in grief and bereavement, defines grief, mourning, and bereavement and describes the four steps of mourning that the individual needs to accomplish for reconciliation in the grieving process as follows:

A. Grief—

The thoughts and feelings that are experienced within oneself with the loss or death of someone or something one loved. Grieving is a normal reaction to loss with a wide variety of emotional expressions such as sadness, crying, anger, guilt and self-reproach, anxiety, helplessness, shock, relief, and numbness. Physical symptoms or sensations experienced include feeling a hollowness in the stomach, tightness in the chest and throat, feeling short of breath, having a dry mouth, nausea, feeling very weak or not having energy to complete certain tasks, and the sensation of things occurring without their control.

B. Mourning—

The ability to take the internal experience of grief and express it outside of oneself, such as the following:
1. *To accept the reality* of the loss/death
2. *To work through the pain* of grief
3. *To adjust to an environment* in which the deceased loved one or thing is missing

4. To emotionally relocate the deceased loved one/ something loved and replace it with another relationship or to move on in life

The mourning process may have many variables regarding the person's ability or permission to express grief, such as the circumstances of the death event regarding whether the death was sudden and unexpected with a sense that it did not happen versus an anticipatory process that occurs with an extended illness with the bereaved persons involved in the care components for the deceased and being in attendance and communicating feelings on an ongoing basis, saying good-byes, and having a sense of closure facilitates the bereaved person's tasks of mourning. Mourning is an ongoing process and evolves over time as the person experiences episodes of great sadness to periods of happiness with less sadness. The sadness changes over time to a peaceful kind of sadness that is incorporated into the person's changed life.

C. **Bereavement—**
   The period of mourning does not have a certain time frame for resolution. Cultural, religious, and past experiences are some of the influences that impact the person's bereavement process. Role expectations regarding returning to work or school, participation in religious or community activities, and the length of an acceptable bereavement period have many different meanings to different people. For those recently experiencing a loss, "their world" has changed, and to those not affected by the loss, time quickly passes on to new expectations. The person who died and the nature of that relationship with regard to the newly bereaved being able to emotionally relocate their loved one and move on to a different life are a day-to-day evolving process. There is a sense in which mourning can be finished, that is, when people regain an interest in life, feel more hopeful, experience gratification again, and adapt to new roles. There is also a sense in which mourning is never finished.

II. DETERMINANTS OF GRIEF
Individual experiences regarding the grief process may be described by some as a very intense experience,

whereas others may describe their experience as less intense, and others have many episodes of highs and lows. Some important determinants of grief are related to the bereaved person's developmental level and conflict issues regarding the deceased person. Following are additional issues that affect individual grief experiences:

A. **Who the Person Was Who Died—**

Who is affected by the death of this person? Who was in this person's daily life? Was he or she a close or extended family member?

B. **Nature of the Attachment or Relationship—**

The security of the attachment to or the intensity of the love for the person who died affects the bereaved person's ability to cope and meet the new challenges of a changed life.

C. **Mode of Death—**

Was the death "anticipated" or was it "a sudden unexpected event"?

D. **Social Variables—**

What family, friends, and financial resources are available to the newly bereaved? The degree of perceived emotional and social support from others, both inside and outside the family, is significant during the bereavement process.

E. **Concurrent Stresses—**

Other factors that affect the bereavement process are the concurrent changes and crises that may follow a death event, such as depletion of finances, loss of job or home, and the need to geographically relocate, thereby losing friends and other extended relationships.

III. BEREAVEMENT SUPPORT

Bereavement support is a significant component of a hospice and palliative care program and is required under Medicare regulations. The goal of bereavement support is to facilitate the survivor's progression through the grief, mourning, and bereavement phases and to help the survivor have a sense of resolution regarding his or her loss. Hospice program personnel usually follow up with the survivors for at least 1 year after the death event. Bereavement interventions can be an initial assessment of the survivors with the chaplain or social worker to determine significant circumstances or issues that may affect the grieving process. The hospice program staff can determine at this time or at the scheduled follow-up contacts whether professional counseling is necessary for abnormal grief reactions or complications regarding the grief process.

In addition, contact with the survivors can include regularly scheduled phone calls to assess survivors' needs or to offer other services such as participation in grief support groups. The usual participants in these groups have similar experiences, are of similar ages or circumstances, and allow the "survivor" to be himself or herself, share as desired, and listen to the group's comments. Competent and skilled personnel will provide additional information on the grieving process through specific topics and will lead the grief support groups. These groups meet at designated times, and sessions usually last from 1 to 2 hours over an 8- to 12-week period. Friendships and support systems develop within the group that often develop into temporary or lasting friendships, thereby providing the bereaved person with new social outlets. Finally, hospice programs offer and conduct on a scheduled frequency "memorial services" and invite all previous survivors to attend these special services to facilitate resolution of the grief process.

Bibliography

Bowman T: As a family ages: facing the loss of dreams, *Forum* 28(1):1, 2002.

Burke C, editor: *Psychosocial dimensions of oncology nursing care,* Pittsburgh, Pa, 1998, Oncology Nursing Press.

Demaree AC, Thornton G, Zanich ML: Bereavement Support Group: challenges in a rural hospice, *Forum* 26(5):1, 2000.

DeSpelder LA, Strickland AL: *The last dance,* ed 4, Mountain View, Calif, 1996, Mayfield Publishing.

Doaka KJ, Davidson JD, editors: *Living with grief, who we how we grieve,* Philadelphia, 1998, Brunner/Mazel.

Hofsess R: Grief and loss in the workplace, *Forum* 28(2):1, 2002.

Kubler-Ross E: *The wheel of life,* New York, 1997, Touchstone Edition, Simon & Schuster.

Pessagno RA: Differentiating between grief and depression, *Clin J Oncol Nurs* 3(1):31,1999.

Wolfelt AD: *Understanding grief, helping yourself heal,* Muncie, 1992, Accelerated Development.

Worden JW: *Grief counseling & grief therapy,* ed 2, New York, 1991, Springer Publishing.

Treatment

UNIT IV

ONCOLOGIC EMERGENCIES

I. OVERVIEW

Oncologic emergencies occur frequently in patients with cancer and are usually the direct result of the disease process or the cancer treatment. The onset of the symptoms and progressive changes vary with each patient's underlying disease, functional status, and presence or absence of other complications or conditions such as compromised cardiac, hepatic, hematologic, neurologic, respiratory, or renal systems. Prompt recognition of the clinical features with appropriate intervention(s) is the critical factor that contributes to improved patient quality-of-life outcomes.

II. ANAPHYLAXIS, HYPERSENSITIVITY REACTIONS—

Severe reactions or anaphylaxis that occur from a life-threatening immunologic response to a foreign substance or antigen. Chemotherapeutic agents like other drugs or products may be recognized by the body's immune system as "not self." This process may initiate a type I reaction characterized by the release of histamines and other inflammatory mediators that induce the

Oncologic Emergencies

symptoms of anaphylaxis such as respiratory distress
and cardiovascular failure.

A. **Pathophysiology—**

Anaphylactic and hypersensitivity reactions occur in
three phases. The *sensitization phase* occurs when a
patient is exposed to a foreign substance, thus causing formation of specific antibodies (IgE) that attach
to the receptors on basophils and mast cells.

The second exposure to the antigen is called the *activation phase*, where the antigen attaches to the IgE molecules on the mast cell surface resulting in release of
preformed chemical mediators such as histamine,
heparin, and chemotactins into the surrounding tissue
and serum. This mediated response releases prostaglandins, leukotrienes, and histamines that stimulate H1 and H2 receptors located in the myocardium,
vessel walls, smooth muscle lining of the lung, ureters,
bladder, and the gastrointestinal tract.

The last phase is the *effector phase.* This process
involves the immediate neuromuscular and vascular
responses evidenced in the organs (skin, vasculature,
connective tissue, and gastrointestinal tract) targeted
by the chemical mediators.

B. **Patient Population at Risk—**

An increased incidence occurs with type, administration route, and the immunologic characteristics of
certain drugs. Chemotherapeutic drugs with high-
risk potential include L-asparaginase, bleomycin,
docetaxel, paclitaxel, procarbazine, teniposide, rituximab, and trastuzumab. Patient age, sex, genetic
make-up, nutritional status, stress level, and hormonal factors are also contributing factors.

C. **Clinical Features—**

The reactions may occur within minutes or may take
hours depending on the drug metabolism. The most
common presenting *initial* symptoms include dyspnea, agitation, hypotension, chest or back pain,
urticaria, feeling of tightness in throat and chest,
wheezing, and a feeling of intense warmth; secondary symptoms include headache, nausea, vomiting,
diarrhea, and abdominal cramping.

D. **Medical and Nursing Management—**

1. *Primary prevention* is key to diminishing hypersensitivity and anaphylaxis events. Prior to any

drug administration, obtain an accurate assessment of the patient's allergy history, type of reaction(s) experienced, and what interventions were needed to treat the reaction(s). Knowledge of the potential side effects of a drug is imperative so that the necessary precautions can be taken for patients at high risk for anaphylaxis who are scheduled to receive the drug. Follow the drug product administration guidelines for premedication regimens to diminish the potential side effects (Table 32-1).

2. Before and during drug/product administration, *monitor the patient for signs of anaphylaxis or hypersensitivity reactions*, including monitoring of blood pressure, pulse, and oxygen saturation. Emergency equipment, supplies, and medications must be readily available (Table 32-2).

3. *In the event of an anaphylaxis or hypersensitivity occurrence:*
   - STOP the drug/solution infusion.
   - CALL for assistance.
   - REMAIN with the patient.
   - ASSESS airway patency.
   - PREPARE for ventilation assistance and cardiopulmonary resuscitation.
   - ADMINISTER medications as prescribed by protocol such as epinephrine, diphenhydramine, Solu-Medrol.
   - MAINTAIN intravenous (IV) access with isotonic solutions (0.9% normal saline solution [NS]) to maintain blood pressure.
   - PREPARE for administration of secondary medications/solutions such as vasopressors, bronchodilators, diuretics, or previously prescribed medications the patient may be currently taking on a scheduled frequency.

4. Outcomes related to anaphylaxis and hypersensitivity reactions depend on *prompt recognition and treatment of such events*. The patient should be monitored until all symptoms have resolved. Instructions to the patient and family should include scheduled physician follow-up visits to monitor long-term effects.

Oncologic Emergencies

Table 32-1   CHEMOTHERAPY DRUGS: POTENTIAL FOR ANAPHYLAXIS NURSING MANAGEMENT

Drugs	Signs and Symptoms	Precautions
Asparaginase (Elspar)	Respiratory distress, increased pulse and respirations, hypotension, facial edema, anxiety, flushed appearance, hives itching*	Test dose prior to initial IV/IM dosing. MONITOR Q 30 min/IV 60 min/IM post-drug adm. KEEP vein open IV-N/S before, during, and 30–60 minutes post IV drug infusion. INITIATE IV drug infusion slowly (mg/m^2-titrate rate). CODE CART, O_2, suction supplies, and emergent drugs at/near patient bedside.

Test dose procedure: Prepare 10,000 IU asparaginase with 5 ml NS: Inject 0.1 ml of this solution (200 IU) into 9.9 ml NS; inject *intradermally* 0.1 ml of this concentration (2 IU) to make a wheal in the inner aspect of the forearm; observe wheal 60 min for erythema, swelling, or itching before initiating the drug infusion.

Bleomycin (Blenoxane)	Dyspnea, hypotension, rash, increased pulse, respirations	Test dose before initial IV dosing; initiate drug infusion slowly (10–20 ml/15 min). Monitor VS and auscultate breath sounds during the infusion and on scheduled frequency.

Test dose procedure: Inject 2 U bleomycin *intradermally* to make a wheal in the inner aspect of the forearm; observe wheal (60 min) for erythema, itching, or edema *prior to the initial 2 doses of the bleomycin infusion.*

Paclitaxel (Taxol) Docetaxel (Taxotere)	Increased/decreased blood pressure, increased temperature and pulse, restlessness, dyspnea, hives, bronchospasm, facial flush. *If any of these symptoms occur, STOP THE DRUG INFUSION AND NOTIFY PHYSICIAN IMMEDIATELY.*	Premedicate with the following PRIOR to Taxol/Taxotere infusion: Dexamethasone 10–20 mg PO/IV 12 and 6 hr; Benadryl 10–20 mg PO/IV 12 and 6 hr; Benadryl 50 mg IVP 30–60 min; cimetidine 300 mg IV over 30 min. Infuse Taxol/Taxotere in a glass bottle with non-PVC tubing and a 0.22-micron filter. Obtain baseline VS: then every 15 min for an hour, for 4 hours during the infusion. ***Ensure emergent medications:*** Benadryl 50 mg; hydrocortisone 100 mg; adrenalin 1:1000 (Epinephrine) all IV BOLUS; oxygen, suction, equipment assembled and ready for use.

Continued

Table 32-1   CHEMOTHERAPY DRUGS: POTENTIAL FOR ANAPHYLAXIS NURSING MANAGEMENT—cont'd

Drugs	Signs and Symptoms	Precautions
Etoposide (VePesid)	Hypotension, chest pain, chills, bronchospasm, facial flush, fever, diaphoresis, increased pulse and respirations	Initiate drug infusion slowly (10–20 ml/15 min). Infuse total volume over at least 1 hour. MONITOR VS every 15 min for at least 60 min.
Teniposide (Vumon)	SEVERE hypotension, anxiety, fever, increased pulse and respirations	Initiate drug infusion slowly (10–20 ml *slowly* over 30 min). Total infusion time is 1 to 2 hours. MONITOR VS every 15 min 4 times, then every 30 min twice during infusion.

Source: Modified from Otto SE: Chemotherapy. In Otto SE, editor: *Oncology nursing,* ed 4, St. Louis, 2001, Mosby.
IM, intramuscular; *IV,* intravenous; *IVP,* intravenous push; *NS,* normal saline solution; *PO,* per os (by mouth); *VS,* vital signs.
*****Risk** for anaphylaxis increases with each dose.

Table 32-2   DRUGS AND SUPPLIES USED IN MANAGEMENT OF HYPERSENSITIVITY AND ANAPHYLAXIS

Drug	Concentration	Usage
Epinephrine (Adrenalin)	1:10,000 solution IVP	Administer 0.1–0.5mg IVP no less than 3 to 5 min
Diphenhydramine hydrochloride (Benadryl)	50 mg IVP	Administer IV to block further antigen/antibody reaction
Corticosteroids		
Methyl prednisolone (Solu Medrol)	30–60 mg IVP	Administer IV to ease bronchoconstriction cardiac dysfunction.
Hydrocortisone (Solu Cortef)	100–500 mg IVP	
Dexamethasone (Decadron)	10–20 mg IVP	
Aminophylline	5 mg/kg IV infusion	Administer IV infusion over 3C min to enhance bronchodilation.
Dopamine (Intropin)	2 mcg/kg/min IV Infusion	Administer IV to increase perfusion.
Histamine H$_2$ Antagonist		
Cimetidine (Tagamet)	300 mg IV over 30 min	Diminishes aspiration potential and laryngeal edema
Famotidine (Pepcid)	20 mg IV over 10 min	Diminishes aspiration potential and laryngeal edema
Ranitidine (Zantac)	50 mg IV over 15–30 min	Diminishes aspiration potential and laryngeal edema

IV, intravenously; IVP, intravenous push.
Drug doses are for adults only. Supplies include oxygen, cardiac monitor with defibrillator, incubation supplies, intravenous tubing, solutions, venous access and blood sampling supplies, syringes, needles, and medication/solution diluent.

Oncologic Emergencies

III. CARDIAC TAMPONADE—

A compression of the heart muscle caused by pathologic fluid accumulation within the pericardial sac. This increase in intrapericardiac pressure may occur because of fluid accumulation in the pericardial sac, direct or metastatic tumor invasion to the pericardial sac, and fibrosis of the pericardial sac related to radiation therapy. Compression of the myocardium interferes with dilation of the heart chambers, which prevents adequate cardiac filling during diastole. As this intrapericardiac pressure *increases, left* ventricular filling *decreases;* the ability of the heart to pump *decreases,* thus resulting in decreased cardiac output.

A. **Patient Population at Risk—**
   Patients with lung cancer, breast cancer, leukemia, and non–Hodgkin's lymphoma (80%); sarcoma, gastrointestinal tract cancer, or melanoma cancer; and patients receiving more than 400 Gy of radiation to a field in which the heart is located are at risk for cardiac tamponade. Approximately 90% of these cases occur within 1 year after radiation treatment. Nonmalignant conditions that may cause cardiac tamponade include heart surgery, chest trauma, aneurysm, rupture of a great vessel, cardiac procedures (e.g., angiography, insertion/removal of pacemaker wires), and infectious pericarditis.

B. **Clinical Features—**
   EARLY symptoms include retrosternal chest pain (*relieved* by leaning forward and *intensified* when lying supine), dyspnea, cough, orthopnea, muffled or distant heart sounds, weak/absent apical pulse, anxiety, agitation, and hiccups. **LATE symptoms** include tachycardia, tachypnea, *decreased* systolic pressure and *increasing* diastolic pressure *(narrowing pulse pressure)*, peripheral edema, altered levels of consciousness, pulse paradox greater than 10 mm Hg, increased central venous pressure, and oliguria.

C. **Medical and Nursing Management**
   1. *Diagnostic tests*—Chest radiograph; two-dimensional, transesophageal, stress, and intraarterial echocardiography; computed tomography (CT) scan; or magnetic resonance imaging (MRI)

to detect pleural effusion/pericardial thickening; and electrocardiogram (ECG) to detect electrical alterations (e.g., premature atrial contractions [PACs] premature ventricular contractions [PVC]). Cardiac catheterization can confirm the diagnosis of tamponade and also determine the size and location of the pericardial fluid.

2. *The initial goal of treatment is to drain the peri-cardial fluid* (pericardiocentesis with cytology of fluid). Additional procedures may include total pericardectomy, pericardial sclerosis (sclerotherapy, e.g., bleomycin; instill drug when there is no drainage for 24 hours), and radiation therapy or chemotherapy to treat primary tumor.

3. *Pharmacologic therapy:* corticosteroids (prednisone 40 to 60 mg/day), diuretics (furosemide 40 mg/day), non-steroidal anti-inflammatory drugs, vasoactive drugs (dopamine, dobutamine), IV fluids, blood products, and analgesics.

4. *Initiate oxygen therapy.*

5. *Assess and monitor clinical features* (level of consciousness [LOC], vital signs, respirations) for narrowing pulse pressure, paradoxical pulse, peripheral edema, and progression of symptoms.

6. *Elevate head of bed* to position of comfort and provide measures to relieve pain.

7. *Monitor cardiac output, intake and output, laboratory values, and test results.*

IV. CAROTID ARTERY RUPTURE—

Carotid artery rupture or "blowout" and hemorrhage is an oncologic emergency in patients with head and neck cancer that has a potentially life-threatening outcome. Both the patient and the staff witnessing this clinical event are often terrified and unprepared for this unfolding emergency and its consequences. Carotid artery rupture, similar to many other oncologic emergencies, arises from the ability of the cancer to spread by contiguous invasion of adjacent structures or by the metastatic process to other sites resulting in hemorrhage, obstruction of vessels, or an abnormal infiltration of serous membranes with effusion.

Oncologic Emergencies

A. **Patient Population at Risk—**

Patients with head and neck cancer with tumor growth invasion, fistula formation, postsurgical infection, poor wound healing, exposure of artery at surgery, or previous radiation therapy are at risk for carotid artery rupture.

B. **Clinical Features—**

This sudden clinical event can occur without warning, with an eruption of a massive artery spurting blood several feet into the air. Initially, the patient is hemodynamically stable and conscious. Depending on the **immediate interventions for the hemorrhage**, the patient can quickly exsanguinate, become severely hypotensive and hypoxic, and lose consciousness.

C. **Medical and Nursing Management**

1. *The most important therapeutic intervention is to control the bleeding with a firm thumb pressure over the ruptured site of the vessel.* Firm digital pressure usually controls bleeding and must be maintained continuously until the patient arrives in the surgical suite for immediate ligation of the carotid vessel.

2. *Use a gauze pad under the thumb rather* than a bulky external dressing, which is not effective to maintain pressure and to stop the bleeding.

3. *Initiate immediate oxygen therapy, IV fluids, and blood products* to correct the hypotension and the significant blood loss.

4. *The most common surgical procedure will be a double ligation of the artery excised through a new clean surgical field.* Secondarily, a debridement of the necrotic tissue is done to diminish further infection, hemorrhage potential, or both.

5. *Monitor postoperative signs and symptoms of hemorrhage* such as continuous oozing of blood around the surgical site, drains, tracheotomy, and laryngectomy, which are unrelated to manipulation of suctioning or other procedures.

6. *Monitor postoperative signs and symptoms of arterial erosion/rupture* such as evidence of arterial erosion, incision site color (red, pallor, black), vascularity (evidence of bleeding and bruising, pulsations, arterial exposure), incision skin tem-

perature changes (warm, cool, unilateral), edema (present or absence), and skin turgor (taut, mobile).

7. *Monitor postoperative signs and symptoms of infection* such as drainage or odor at or near the surgical site, change in vital signs (elevated temperature), and erythema or edema at the surgical incision area.

V. DISSEMINATED INTRAVASCULAR COAGULATION (DIC)—

The inappropriate, accelerated, or systematic activation of the coagulation cascade, resulting in thrombosis and subsequently hemorrhage.

A. Pathophysiology—

Homeostasis is maintained through a balanced system of **thrombosis** and **fibrinolysis**. The *thrombosis process* is initiated through a disruption of the endothelial membrane, which activates a cascade of clotting factors in the intrinsic pathway (coagulation factors 8 to 12), resulting in coagulation, tissue injury, or both. This insult/injury initiates the release of tissue thromboplastin into the circulation and the activation of the extrinsic pathway (tissue thromboplastin), resulting in coagulation. *Fibrinolysis* is the process of reactions that occur when **clotting** is **inhibited**, developed clots are destroyed, or the formation of fibrin clots is initiated. Fibrin-degradation products or fibrin-split products are released into the circulation and **NOW function as** *anticoagulants.*

In the presence of an underlying condition (e.g., bacterial sepsis infection, malignancy, or trauma) the intrinsic and/or extrinsic pathway of the clotting cascade is triggered; thrombosis is accelerated, and fibrin clots are formed and deposited into the microcirculation; the **consumption** of coagulation factors is **greater** than the ability of the body for replacement, and consequently coagulation is inhibited; and fibrinolysis is initiated—fibrin-degradation products are not effectively removed from the circulation and an accumulation of the anticoagulant substances occurs.

B. Patient Population at Risk—

Patients with cancer diseases such as leukemia (acute promyelocytic leukemia) or breast, prostate, colon, or lung cancer, with a history of cancer treatment—chemotherapy, surgery, blood/stem cell transplantation, radiation therapy—or with an overwhelming viral or bacterial infection/sepsis are at risk for DIC. Nonmalignant conditions such as trauma, burns, shock, pregnancy or obstetric complications, liver disease, recent blood transfusions, or hemolytic transfusion reaction may also be a contributing factor to DIC.

C. **Clinical Features**—
   Tachycardia, diminished peripheral pulses, tachypnea, dyspnea, hypotension, hemolysis, hemoptysis, hematuria, decreased urinary output, joint pain, abdominal distention, positive guaiac stool test, petechiae, ecchymosis, purpura, acral cyanosis (blue/gray coloration), lethargy, restlessness, or alterations in mental status are clinical features of DIC. Changes, abnormalities, or both in DIC screening tests are also indicative of DIC (Box 32-1).

D. **Medical and Nursing Management**—
   1. **The goal is to treat the underlying condition** (e.g., chemotherapy for chemotherapy, antimicro-

---

Box 32-1
DISSEMINATED INTRAVASCULAR COAGULATION SCREEN

D-Dimer assay	>0.5 µg/ml
Fibrin degradation products	>10 µg/ml
Fibrin split products	>4 µg/ml
Prothrombin time	>25 seconds
Partial thrombo-plastin time	>45 seconds
Thrombin time (TT)	>20 seconds
Fibrinogen level	<160 mg/dl
Hematocrit	<37%
Hemoglobin	<10 g/dl
Platelet count	<150,000 mm³
Protamine sulfate	positive
Antithrombin level	<85 decreased

bials for sepsis). *Replacement of coagulation factors* and platelets with cryoprecipitate (provides fibrinogen and factor VIII), platelet concentrate, fresh-frozen plasma (provides plasma and fibrinogen to increase the clotting factors), and packed red blood cells is one treatment method.

2. ***Inhibition of coagulation or fibrinolysis process***— Plasmapheresis and heparin interfere with thrombin production (goal: maintain partial thromboplastin time at 1½ to 2 times normal level— primary effect is bleeding); ε-aminocaproic acid inhibits fibrinolysis—primary effect is clotting; antithrombin III inhibits procoagulants and fibrinolytic process. Heparin infusion to inactivate thrombin and inhibit clotting; platelet transfusion and fresh frozen plasma [FFP]; Amicar IV to inhibit fibrinolysis.

3. ***Provide interventions to maximize safety;*** decrease severity of symptoms, for example, direct pressure to sites of active bleeding.

4. **Monitor clinical features** for progressive DIC (e.g., hypotension, anuria, LOC), interventions in response to treatment (e.g., weigh dressings, count peripads, measure blood drainage), changes in laboratory levels, and symptoms of fluid overload.

5. **Assess tissue perfusion parameters** (e.g., color, temperature, peripheral pulses, and respiratory and cardiovascular status).

VI. HYPERCALCEMIA—

A serum calcium level greater than 14 mg/dl (8.5 to 10.5 mg/dl) is most often associated with malignant tumors **bone metastasis**, resulting from a disturbance of the hormonal mechanisms that maintain calcium homeostasis in the body. *Hypercalcemia is the most common oncologic complication.* Bone metastasis is the movement of cancer cells from one part of the body to another or a *change in location of disease.* This disease process may spread through the lymphatic circulation, the blood stream, or cerebrospinal fluid.

A. **Pathophysiology**—

Normal levels of calcium are regulated by the action of the parathyroid gland (production of parathyroid hormone), gastrointestinal tract (absorption of vitamin D), and the kidneys (excretion). When calcium levels decrease to below normal, the parathyroid gland is stimulated to produce parathyroid hormone, which acts on the bone (a reservoir for calcium) and causes an increase in the amount of calcium released from the bone (resorption) into the circulation and ultimately the extracellular fluid. When the calcium levels increase above normal, the kidney increases excretion of calcium to return the level to normal.

Bone remodeling is a constant process as minor imperfections are removed and new bone is formed. This remodeling process maintains a balance between two types of cells: *osteoclasts* break down or resorb bone and *osteoblasts* reconstruct new bone. During bone destruction, as in bone metastasis, the *osteoclast activity predominates and bone is steadily resorbed*, resulting in a fragile bone structure and pathologic bone fractures. In addition, the malignant cells secrete a multitude of factors (prostaglandin E, growth factors, cytokines e.g., lymphotoxin, IL-1, IL-6, tumor necrosis factor, transforming growth factor, parathyroid hormone–related peptides) to recruit osteoclast precursors and stimulate osteoclast activity or stimulate production of the cytokines (Figure 32-1).

B. **Patient Population at Risk—**
The potential causes of hypercalcemia among persons with cancer include an increased bone resorption secondary to an increased osteoclast activity; direct tumor invasion of the bone and prostaglandin secretion by the tumor (e.g., 30% to 40% for breast cancer, 20% to 40% for multiple myeloma, 12% to 32% for squamous cell lung cancer, 25% for head and neck cancer), lymphoma, leukemia, and renal cancers. Bone metastasis occurs most often in the following anatomic sites: vertebrae (70%), pelvis (41%), long bones/femur (25%), and the skull (14%).

C. **Clinical Features—**
The symptoms, severity, and onset of hypercalcemia vary among patients (age, performance status, sites of bone metastasis, and renal or hepatic failure). Varied clinical features include: serum calcium concentration **greater than 14 mg/dl** (9 to 11 ml/dl),

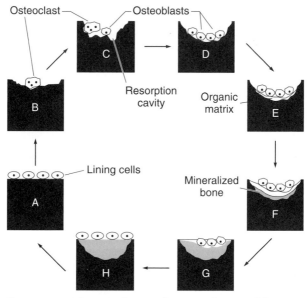

Figure 32-1 Schematic diagram illustrating the normal bone (**A**) Remodeling cycle. Osteoclasts attract to a site of fatigued bone to create an erosion cavity (**B-C**). Osteoblasts are attracted and synthesize the organic matrix, which will fill the resorption cavity (**D-F**). The new bone is then remineralized to complete the remodeling process (**G-H**). (From Abeloff MD, Armitage JO, Lichter AS, et al, editors: *Clinical oncology*, ed 2, New York, 2000, Churchill Livingstone.)

thirst-polydipsia, polyuria, nocturia, pruritus, nausea/vomiting, anorexia, constipation, LOC changes, lethargy, profound muscle weakness and fatigue, hypertension, bradycardia, and multiple changes in ECG rhythm strip (prolonged PR interval [PRI], shortened QT interval [QTI], and widened Q wave), renal calculi, or renal failure. **Bone pain** is the most common symptom in bone metastasis and usually is the symptom that motivates the patient to seek medical attention. The pain becomes progressively worse over weeks or months accompanied by inability to move or discomfort in mobility.

D. **Medical and Nursing Management**
   1. *Diagnostic Tests*—Hypercalcemias: serum calcium (8.5 to 10.5 mg/dl) and urine calcium, serum

potassium, sodium, phosphorus, blood urea nitrogen, creatinine, and an ECG.

Approximately one half of the circulating calcium is bound by albumin and the remaining unbound ionized calcium (normal range 4.5 to 5. 1 mg/dl) is responsible for biologic effects. In patients with hypoalbuminemia, the ionized calcium may be greater and the effective total calcium should be calculated.

Corrected Calcium (mg/dl) = measured Calcium (mg/dl) – albumin (g/dl) + 4

Additional diagnostic tests for bone metastasis include bone scans, x-ray of affected area, CT scans, MRI, myelogram, and bone density studies.

2. *Nonpharmacologic interventions:* Hydration with saline diuresis (5 to 8 L NS intravenously during initial 24 hours, then approximately 1 L every 8 hours); maintain mobility status; potential for dialysis to provide rapid, temporary relief.

3. *Bone metastasis management* is aimed at patient comfort, bone stabilization, spinal stabilization, preventing spinal cord compression, and providing prophylactic fixation of fracture with surgery. The primary cancer diagnosis determines the additional choice and type of therapy (e.g., Does the primary metastatic tumor respond to radiation therapy or chemotherapy? What is the best drug?).

4. *Pharmacologic Interventions:* Hypercalcemia IV bisphosphonates to inhibit osteoclast activity. The serum calcium will usually normalize in 3 to 4 days after administration. Furosemide: blocks calcium reabsorption and inhibits sodium absorption (e.g., Lasix 80 to 100 mg IV). Prednisone: inhibits bone resorption; the dose varies with severity of disease process.

5. *Bisphosphonate therapy options* include:
   a. Calcitonin—Inhibits bone resorption: administer 4 IU sub-Q/intramuscularly every 12 hours, if ineffective increase to 8 IU.
   b. Etidronate (Didronel)—Inhibits bone resorption, limits calcium absorption from gut, promotes soft-tissue and skeletal calcification; administer 7.5 mg/kg per day IV fluid/250 ml

NS for approximately 2 hours for 4 to 5 days or 20 mg/kg per day PO (by mouth).

c. Gallium nitrate—Inhibits bone resorption; administer 200 mg/m^2 per day IV for 24 hours for 4 to 5 days.

d. Pamidronate disodium (Aredia)—Inhibits bone resorption, limits calcium absorption from gut, promotes soft-tissue and skeletal calcification in cancer diseases that metastasize to bone; administer 90 mg in 100 ml NS/D5W and infuse over 1 to 2 hours.

e. Zoledronic acid (Zometa)—this drug is third generation of pamidronate, is approximately 100 to 1000 times more potent, and provides the same benefit; administer 4 mg in 30 ml IV-NS solution over 15 minutes.

f. Prophylactic bisphosphonate therapy recommendations—Breast and prostate cancer: administer Pamidronate 90 mg in 100 ml over 1 to 2 hours IV infusion every 3 to 4 weeks; multiple myeloma: 90 mg in 500 ml over 2 to 4 hours IV infusion every month. This treatment approach reduces the rate of skeletal complications and bone pain.

6. Promote/maintain activity and mobility; *restrict activity if fracture exists.*

7. *Provide measures/analgesia to control pain.*

8. *Maintain strict intake and output and obtain daily weights.*

VII. INCREASED INTRACRANIAL PRESSURE (ICP)—

An increase in the ICP can result when the volume of any (brain tissue, vascular tissue, or cerebrospinal fluid) of these three compartments increases through displacement of brain tissue (primary/metastatic tumors), edema of brain tissue, obstruction of cerebrospinal fluid flow, or increased vascularity associated with tumor growth. Brain metastasis occurs in approximately 20% to 40% of patients with cancer and is the most common cause of ICP.

A. **Patient Population at Risk**—

Patients with primary tumors of brain (e.g., neuroblastoma); spinal cord, lung, breast, testicular, thyroid,

stomach, or kidney cancer; leukemia; or melanoma
are at risk for ICP.

B. **Clinical Features—**

EARLY symptoms include: headaches (early morning,
bilateral, located in occipital or frontal areas);
headaches initiated or aggravated by Valsalva maneuver, coughing, or bending over; loss of appetite, nau-
sea/occasional vomiting; blurred vision or decreased
vision. *LATE symptoms* include: bradycardia, *widened*
pulse pressure; tachypnea; slow, shallow, or Cheyne-
Stokes respirations; *decreased* ability to concentrate
and level of consciousness; hemiplegia, hemiparesis,
seizures, and pupillary and personality changes.

C. **Medical and Nursing Management—**

The goal is to have a *rapid reduction of cerebral edema
and a decompression of ICP* to minimize harm to the
brain.

1. *Diagnostic tests:* MRI, cerebral angiography, CT
   scan, CT-guided biopsy, and myelography.

2. *The treatment(s)* may include surgical procedure
   with a complete resection of primary tumor or
   single brains metastasis or a shunt placement.
   Radiation therapy as a primary or palliative
   approach, depending on the radiosensitivity of
   tumor (e.g., stereotactic radiosurgery with gamma
   knife). Chemotherapy is administered through
   intraarterial, intrathecal, or intratumor routes.

3. *Pharmacologic therapy* corticosteroids to decrease
   peritumoral edema; anticonvulsants to lessen potential seizure events; osmotic diuretics (e.g., mannitol)
   to decrease cerebral edema by increasing plasma
   osmolarity, thus drawing extracellular fluid back
   into the plasma where it can be excreted by the kidneys; and loop diuretics to enhance the excretion of
   sodium and water from the brain. Diuretics may
   also be combined with fluid restrictions.

4. *Assess and monitor clinical features* (baseline neurologic status, LOC, vital signs, respiratory status, pulse pressure) or progression of
   symptoms.

5. *Maintain bedrest;* elevate head of bed 30 to
   45 degrees to promote venous drainage.

6. *Monitor serum electrolytes, osmolarity, and creatinine.*

7. *Implement measures to decrease stress* (calm environment, minimal external noise/light).

VIII. MALIGNANT PLEURAL EFFUSIONS (MPE)—

The presence of abnormal amounts (>5 to 15 ml) of fluid in the pleural space. MPE has malignant cells present in this fluid, in the pleural cavity, or in both.

A. **Pathophysiology**—

Benign pleural effusion may be caused by increased hydrostatic pressure (CHF), increased permeability in the microvascular circulation (infection, trauma), increased negative pressure in the pleural space (atelectasis), or decreased oncotic pressure in the microvascular areas (e.g., nephrotic syndrome, cirrhosis, hypoalbuminemia). MPE may be caused by direct extension of primary lung tumor to the pleura or mediastinum, impaired lymphatic drainage from the pleural space (obstruction caused by tumor), increased permeability caused by inflammation, or altered mucosal lung or mediastinal tissue (e.g., radiation therapy restricts the lung's ability to expand) (Figure 32-2).

B. **Patient Population at Risk**—

MPE develops in approximately 50% of patients with cancer, with more than 100,000 cases annually. Lung and breast cancers account for 75% of cases; 12% have an unknown primary cause. Lymphoma or hematopoietic system and *prior* pleural effusions also can lead to MPE. Additional causes include radiation therapy to chest, thorax, or abdomen and the surgical modification of venous or lymphatic vessels.

C. **Clinical Features**—

Tachypnea, restricted chest wall expansion, dullness to percussion, diminished or absent breath sounds, egophony (nasal type sound heard in chest auscultation on affected side), dyspnea, dry nonproductive cough (the most common symptom), pleural friction rub, compression atelectasis, and fever.

D. **Medical and Nursing Management**—

1. *Diagnostic tests:* chest radiograph, thoracentesis (25 to 50 ml for cytology testing and culture), and pleural biopsy. *Therapeutic thoracentesis* (not to exceed 1500 ml at one time) to improve comfort

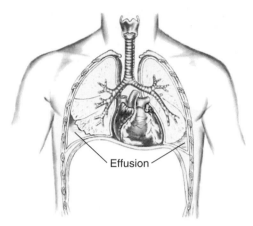

Effusion

Figure 32-2 Pleural effusion. (From Wilson SF, Thompson JM: *Mosby's clinical nursing series: respiratory disorder,* St. Louis, 1990, Mosby.)

and relieve dyspnea (reaccumulation of fluid) is common; however, there is potential for hypoproteinemia, pneumothorax, and empyema.

2. *Complete drainage through chest tube:* promotes adherence of the visceral and parietal pleural surfaces by removal of accumulated fluid.

3. *Sclerotherapy:* instillation of sclerosing agents intrapleurally to produce mesothelial fibrosis (tetracycline, nitrogen mustard, bleomycin [used 60% to 80%], talc, and **lidocaine** added to the sclerosing agent decreases discomfort).

4. *Parietal pleurectomy:* open or videothorascopic pleurectomy; insertion of pleuroperitoneal shunt; chemotherapy, radiation therapy, or both to the mediastinal area to decrease the tumor burden.

5. *Implement safety and comfort measures* (position, analgesia, using assistive devices for mobility).

6. *Report critical changes* (chest pain, fever, and character of respiratory status) immediately to the physician.

7. *Monitor respiratory status/comfort status and effectiveness of interventions.* Keep head of bed raised more than 30 to 45 degrees to improve respiratory process.

IX. SEPTIC SHOCK (SS)—

Comprises a group of diverse life-threatening syndromes that result from different pathologic circumstances (e.g., decreased cardiac function, hemorrhage, trauma, antigen/antibody reaction, or sepsis). The three major classifications of shock are: *hypovolemic* (decreased intravascular volume), *cardiogenic* (impaired ability of the heart to adequately pump blood), and *vasogenic* or distributive (an abnormality [e.g., anaphylaxis, neurogenic event] in the vascular or neurologic systems). The incidence of SS has increased steadily in the past 20 years, and the mortality rates range from 10% to 90%.

A. **Pathophysiology—**
   SS is a complex interaction of hemodynamic (vasoconstriction/vasodilation), humoral, cellular, and metabolic (metabolic acidosis) abnormalities. SS can be caused by bacterial, fungal, viral, and protozoa organisms. When released, a proliferate gram-negative bacterium activates the coagulation complement and kinin systems, thus causing a toxin-induced reaction. This reactive process activates the humoral cellular and immunologic defense mechanisms leading to a generalized inflammatory response. Evidence of this response is the production of the varied chemical mediators such as prostaglandins, endorphins, and kinins that modulate the different multisystem alterations in SS.

B. **Patient Population at Risk—**
   Immunosuppressed patients with cancer receiving marrow ablative therapies (blood stem cell transplantation) and/or combination therapies (chemotherapy and radiation therapy) are most at risk of SS; patients with leukemia, Hodgkin's disease, lymphoma, and multiple myeloma are also at risk.

C. **Clinical Features—**
   Initial phase: normal, above, or below normal temperature; tachycardia; tachypnea; rales; hyperglycemia;

peripheral cyanosis; altered mental status; restlessness; irritability; disorientation; and normal or slightly elevated blood pressure with a widening pulse pressure. **Intermediate phase:** complaints of thirst; peripheral edema; increasing tachycardia; decreasing and shallow respirations; decreased urine output; pale, cool, and clammy skin; decreased blood pressure with a narrow pulse pressure; abdominal distention; and presence of hemorrhagic lesions. **Late (refractory shock) phase:** decreased cardiac output, cold and cyanotic skin, subnormal temperature, tachycardia, weak or absent pulses, hypotension, decreased respirations, hypoglycemia, diminished or no urine output, altered mental status (coma-like state), and presence of hemorrhagic lesions.

D. **Medical and Nursing Management—**
The specific phase of SS will dictate the appropriate and timely interventions. The primary goal is to determine the cause of SS and immediately provide the appropriate interventions such as maintaining blood pressure and tissue perfusion while treating the underlying pathogen.

1. *Diagnostic tests:* complete blood count; coagulation studies, blood and anatomic site(s) (nose, throat, sputum, and urine) specimen(s) for culture and sensitivity studies, serum electrolytes and creatinine levels, and CT scans or radiograph of chest, abdomen, and pelvis.

2. *Pharmacologic therapy:* appropriate antimicrobial interventions specific to the causal organism, fluid replacement with crystalloids or colloids to correct hypovolemia, vasopressors to maintain perfusion to vital organs, and correction of electrolyte imbalances.

3. *Nonpharmacologic therapy:* hemodynamic monitoring, blood products if patient is bleeding, glucose monitoring with interventions for hypoglycemia or hyperglycemia, oxygen or ventilatory assistance to maintain oxygenation, and parenteral nutritional support.

4. *Prevent disease transmission and cross-contamination* by careful nurse/patient assignments.

5. *Monitor clinical features for progressive SS:* change in vital signs, urine output, skin integrity and color, mental status, or presence of hemorrhagic lesions.
6. *Obtain blood, urine, and sputum cultures in a timely manner.*
7. *Assess tissue perfusion parameters* (e.g., color, temperature, peripheral pulses, and respiratory and cardiovascular status).

X. SPINAL CORD COMPRESSION—

A compression of the spinal cord that may occur as the result of tumor invasion of the vertebrae and subsequent collapse on the spinal cord or tumor invasion of the spinal cord that results in increased pressure, primary tumors of the spinal cord, or both.

A. Pathophysiology—
The spinal cord is a cylindrical body of nervous tissue that occupies the upper two thirds of the vertebral canal. It contains the motor, sensory, and autonomic functions for the body. Compression of the spinal cord can result in minor changes in motor, sensory, and autonomic function to complete paralysis. Spinal cord compression occurs at cervical (10%), lumbar (20%), and thoracic (70%) sites (Figure 32-3).

B. Patient Population at Risk—
Patients with primary cancers of the spinal cord (ependymoma, astrocytoma, and glioma), cancers that metastasize to the spinal cord (lymphoma, seminoma, and neuroblastoma), and cancers that metastasized to the bone (breast, lung, prostate [50% to 60%], renal, and myeloma) are at risk for spinal cord compression. The patient's *pertinent history* (e.g., time since onset of symptoms, level and degree of compression) is the best predictor for patient's motor/sensory functional outcome.

C. Clinical Features—
The *presenting signs and symptoms vary with the location and severity of the compression:* neck or **back pain** (initial symptom in **96%** and most common symptom in **95%** of patients) that may be local, constant, or dull and aching and is usually progressive; radicular pain that may be constant or initiated with movement; pain that is usually worse when sitting up;

Oncologic Emergencies

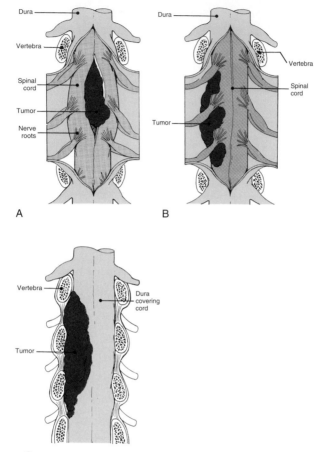

A

B

C

Figure 32-3 Spinal cord tumors. **A,** Intramedullary tumors. **B,** Intradural/extramedullary tumor. **C,** Extramedullary tumors. (From Thompson JM, McFarland GK, Hirsch JE, et al: *Mosby's clinical nursing,* ed 5, St. Louis, 2002, Mosby.)

pain exacerbated by straining, coughing, or flexion of neck; **motor weakness** or dysfunction followed by **sensory loss** for deep pressure and position; incontinence or retention of urine or stool; paralysis;

muscle atrophy; tenderness over spinal cord compression site; hyperactive deep tendon reflexes and Babinski response.

D. **Medical and Nursing Management—**

1. *Diagnostic tests:* spinal radiograph (shows bone abnormalities or soft tissue masses); bone scan (identifies metastases to vertebral bodies); **MRI** (more sensitive than myelography, which identifies extradural, intradural, and extramedullary lesions; compression; and bone destruction); CT scan; myelogram (with or without CT scan when the MRI is nondiagnostic). CSF protein increases to greater than 100 mg/ml are noted in most patients with spinal cord compression.

2. *Nonpharmacologic interventions:* immediate intervention with *radiation therapy* to start as soon as the clinical diagnosis is confirmed and to continue for 2 to 4 weeks (300 to 400 Gy). *Surgery* is chosen if the tumor is not responsive to radiation therapy (decompression by laminectomy or resection of a vertebral body), or after radiation therapy. High-dose ketoconazole (400 mg PO every 8 hours) rapidly reduces testosterone levels into the castration range and should be considered in patients with spinal cord compression known or suspected to be caused by prostate cancer. In addition, replacement doses of corticosteroids (prednisone 5 mg PO every morning and 2.5 mg PO every evening) are necessary because ketoconazole may cause adrenal insufficiency.

3. *Pharmacologic interventions:* corticosteroids to reduce spinal cord edema and pain and chemotherapy agents used as an adjuvant treatment to radiation therapy, surgery, or both. With tumors responsive to drugs (e.g., lymphoma, germ cell) or with neuroblastoma, corticosteroids are used as the preferred treatment for children and infants because radiation therapy to the spinal column can inhibit growth projection. Analgesics for pain management are administered as needed.

4. *Assess and monitor clinical features, and progression.*

5. *Implement safety and mobility measures regarding findings of stable or unstable spine.*

Oncologic Emergencies

6. *Monitor bowel and bladder elimination patterns and effectiveness.*
7. *Initiate a consultation with a physical therapist for assessment of motor and sensory functions* (muscle strength, coordination of hands and feet, *mobility,* sensory perception) and consult with sex therapist to address changes in sexual function.

XI. SUPERIOR VENA CAVA SYNDROME (SVCS)—

The compression or obstruction of the superior vena cava resulting in impaired venous return *to the heart* from the head, neck, thorax, and upper extremities, thereby causing *increased* **venous pressure** and *decreased* **cardiac output** (Figure 32-4).

A. **Pathophysiology—**
   The superior vena cava is a thin-walled major vessel that returns blood to the right atrium of the heart from the head, neck, upper thorax, and upper extremities. It is located in the mediastinum and is surrounded by the rigid structures of the sternum, trachea, vertebrae, aorta, right bronchus, lymph nodes, and the pulmonary artery. This low-pressure vessel is easily compressed by direct tumor invasion, enlarged lymph nodes, or a thrombus within the vessel.

B. **Patient Population at Risk—**
   The following are risk factors for SVCS: presence of lymphoma (15% to 20%) involving the mediastinum, germ cell tumors, or breast and small-cell lung cancers; Kaposi's sarcoma; presence of central venous catheters and pacemakers; previous radiation therapy to the mediastinum; and associated conditions such as histoplasmosis, benign tumors, and aortic aneurysm.

C. **Clinical Features—**
   Clinical features include facial swelling on arising in the morning; periorbital edema; swelling of the upper extremities (neck and neck veins, arms, hands [rings tight]); **dyspnea** (the most common symptom); hoarseness; nonproductive cough; cyanosis of upper torso; stridor; headache; irritability; visual disturbances; dizziness; and changes in mental status.

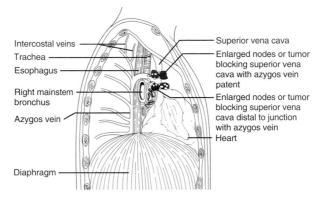

Figure 32-4 Lateral view of the thorax with superior vena cava syndrome. (From Abeloff MD, Armitage JO, Lichter AS, et al, editors. *Clinical oncology,* ed 2, New York, 2000, Churchill Livingstone.

D. Medical and Nursing Management—

1. *Diagnostic tests:* chest radiograph (abnormal 80%; findings include mass, pleural effusion, and superior mediastinal widening); CT imaging of the chest; bronchoscopy; mediastinoscopy; thoracentesis; sputum specimen; biopsy of palpable nodes; and bone marrow biopsy.

2. *Nonpharmacologic interventions:* radiation therapy is the primary treatment for SVCS if the patient has non–small-cell lung cancer or a histologic diagnosis *cannot* be made. Other interventions include removal of the central venous catheter if cause is catheter-induced SVCS; insertion of expendable wire stents to open and maintain patency of superior vena cava; *percutaneous transluminal angioplasty* using balloon technique; and oxygen therapy.

3. *Pharmacologic interventions:* chemotherapy (platinum-based, small-cell lung cancer) for patients who have had previous mediastinal radiation therapy; chemotherapy + radiation therapy; corticosteroids, diuretics, or thrombolytic therapy.

4. *Avoid/minimize procedures in upper extremities* (e.g., venipunctures, IV fluid administration, or

obtaining blood pressure); remove rings and restrictive clothing.

5. *Evaluate laboratory studies* (arterial blood gases, electrolytes, complete blood count, coagulation studies).
6. *Implement measures to decrease severity of symptoms* (e.g., elevate head of bed).
7. *Monitor the sequelae of SVCS or treatment: increased* respiratory rate; stridor; anxiety; confusion; adventitious breath sounds; swelling in face, arms, or neck; venous distention of the neck or thorax; *decreased* blood pressure; *decreased* or absent peripheral pulses; pale or cyanotic skin of the face, extremities, or nail beds.

XII. SYNDROME OF INAPPROPRIATE ANTIDIURETIC HORMONE SECRETION (SIADH)—

An endocrine paraneoplastic syndrome that causes a disorder of water balance, characterized by elevated serum blood levels of antidiuretic hormone, hyponatremia, and excessive water retention.

A. Pathophysiology—
   Antidiuretic hormone (ADH) is released normally from the posterior pituitary in response to *increased* plasma osmolarity and *decreased* plasma volume. The *ADH* acts on the distal renal tubules and collecting ducts to increase permeability and thus *increase water reabsorption*. **Excess production of ADH** from tumors or inappropriate stimulation of the posterior pituitary gland results in **excessive water retention** and dilutional hyponatremia.

B. Patient Population at Risk—
   Approximately two thirds of patients with SIADH have a neoplasm; small-cell lung, pancreas, duodenum, prostate, brain, head and neck, or Hodgkin's disease; pulmonary infection (e.g., pneumonia, tuberculosis); history of trauma, infection, or lesions of the central nervous system; previous cancer therapy (e.g., chemotherapy, cisplatin, cyclophosfamide, vincristine); history of medication use (e.g., thiazide diuretics, morphine, antidepressants); concurrent cardiac, renal, or hepatic disease.

C. **Clinical Features—**

Clinical features include (central nervous system) confusion, irritability, headache, lethargy, change in LOC; thirst, nausea/vomiting, diarrhea, anorexia, decreased urinary output, weight gain, muscle cramping, weakness, anorexia and generalized weakness, hyponatremia, hypokalemia, hypocalcemia, decreased serum osmolarity; increased urine osmolarity; increased urinary excretion of sodium.

D. **Medical and Nursing Management—**

1. *Diagnostic tests:* serum sodium <130 mEq/L (135 to 145 mEq/L: normal level); serum osmolality <280 mOsm/kg of body weight (280 to 300); urine sodium >20 mEq/L; urinary osmolality >1400 mOsm/L (100 to 1000 mOsm/kg); blood urea nitrogen >20 (10 to 20); creatinine level >0.7 to 1.4 mg/dl; uric acid serum <2.2 mg/dl (3.2 to 8 mg/dl); urine-specific gravity <1.003 (1.015 to 1.025).

2. *Nonpharmacologic interventions:*

   a. Moderate hyponatremia: initiate fluid restriction 800 to 1000 ml/24 hours—**corrects** decreased sodium level over 7 to 10 days; NOT recommended for chronic SIADH and acute symptoms.

   b. Severe hyponatremia: *initiate hypertonic* saline solution (3% to 5%) infused IV through pump over 2 to 3 hours. Furosemide (Lasix) usually is given concurrently to increase fluid excretion.

3. *Pharmacologic interventions:* treat the underlying condition (cancer/therapy, infection/antimicrobials); *discontinue* drugs contributing to SIADH (e.g., morphine, diuretics, antidepressants); administer medications to treat SIADH (e.g., demeclocycline) (interferes with ADH action), lithium (interferes with ADH action), urea (causes osmotic diuresis).

4. *Assess central nervous system* function or changes and provide interventions to maximize safety.

5. *Restrict fluids* (divide amount of fluids over 24 hours).

6. *Maintain strict intake and output.*

XIII. TUMOR LYSIS SYNDROME (TLS)—

A metabolic imbalance that occurs with the rapid release of intracellular potassium, phosphorus, and nucleic acid into the blood as a result of tumor cell death (rapid lysis of cancer cells) from chemotherapy or radiation therapy treatments.

A. **Pathophysiology—**

Hyperuricemia results from the conversion of nucleic acid to uric acid. TLS also includes hyperkalemia, hyperphosphatemia, and hypocalcemia (results from the increased phosphorus binding to calcium to form calcium phosphate salts). The potential harmful effects include renal failure of the kidneys (the primary route of elimination for phosphorus, uric acid, and potassium) and cardiac arrhythmia.

B. **Patient Population at Risk—**

Patients at risk for TLS are those with cancer diseases with a high growth fraction or elevated lactate dehydrogenase; acute lymphoblastic leukemia, Hodgkin's lymphoma; testicular or small-cell lung cancer; recent chemotherapy or radiation therapy treatment for cancer; concurrent renal or cardiac disease.

C. **Clinical Features—**

Clinical features of TLS include cardiac arrhythmias, bradycardia, muscle weakness, paresthesia, oliguria, flank pain, hematuria, edema, weight gain, lethargy, fatigue, tetany, confusion, seizures, acute renal failure, cardiac arrhythmias, and cardiopulmonary arrest. The patient will have abnormalities in the serum electrolytes with evidence of hyperkalemia, hypocalcemia, hyperphosphatemia, and hyperuricemia.

D. **Medical and Nursing Management—**

1. *Diagnostic tests:* blood urea nitrogen, lactate dehydrogenase, potassium, phosphorus and uric acid (**elevated levels indicative of TLS**), serum calcium and creatinine clearance (**decreased levels indicative of TLS**), and ECG.

2. *Nonpharmacologic interventions:* hydration (oral/IV 6 to 8 L fluid in 24 hours) **before and after cancer treatment,** hemapheresis, dialysis, and potassium and phosphorus restrictions.

3. **Prevention measures** can be initiated before and during initial treatment. All patients should have volume repletion with isotonic fluids infused at 200 to 300 ml/hr to achieve a brisk diuresis during the first 2 to 3 days of chemotherapy. The goal of hydration is to preserve renal function and to eliminate cellular breakdown products as they are released. Allopurinol (PO/IV at 600 mg/day starting 24 to 48 hours before chemotherapy) blocks purine metabolism by preventing the conversion of xanthine to uric acid, thereby decreasing uric acid production.
4. **Report critical changes** (anuria, cardiac arrhythmia) **immediately** to the physician.
5. **Maintain an accurate intake and output.**

Bibliography

Almadrones L, et al: *Chemotherapy-induced neurotoxicity: current trends in management—a multidisciplinary approach*, Philadelphia, 2002, Phillips Group Oncology Communications.

Armitage JO, Mauch PM, Harris NL, et al: Non-Hodgkin's lymphoma. In DeVita VT Jr, Hellman S, Rosenberg SA, editors: *Cancer principles and practice of oncology*, ed 6, Philadelphia, 2001, JB Lippincott.

Bosl GJ, et al: Cancer of the testes. In DeVita VT Jr, Hellman S, Rosenberg S, editors: *Cancer principles and practice of oncology*, ed 5, Philadelphia, 1997, Lippincott-Raven.

Boyle D: Psychosocial issues. In Lin EM, editor: *Advanced practice in oncology nursing*, Philadelphia, 2001, WB Saunders.

Brown HK, Healey JH: Metastatic cancer to the bone. In DeVita VT Jr, Hellman S, Rosenberg SA, editors: *Cancer principles and practice of oncology*, ed 6, Philadelphia, 2001, JB Lippincott.

Camp-Sorrell D: Surviving the cancer, surviving the treatment: acute cardiac and pulmonary toxicity, *Oncol Nurs Forum* 26(6):983, 1999.

Chu E, DeVita VT Jr: Principles of cancer management: chemotherapy. In DeVita VT Jr, Hellman S, Rosenberg SA, editors: *Cancer principles and practice of oncology*, ed 6, Philadelphia, 2001, JB Lippincott.

Diehl V, Mauch PM, Harris NL: Hodgkin's disease. In DeVita VT Jr, Hellman S, Rosenberg SA, editors: *Cancer principles and practice of oncology*, ed 6, Philadelphia, 2001, JB Lippincott.

Flounders JA, Ott BB: Oncology emergency modules: spinal cord compression, http://www.ons.org, 2003.

Oncologic Emergencies

Ginsberg RJ, Vokes EE, Rosenzweig K: Non-small-cell lung cancer. In DeVita VT Jr, Hellman S, Rosenberg SA, editors: *Cancer principles and practice of oncology,* ed 6, Philadelphia, 2001, JB Lippincott.

Hawkins R: Mastering the intricate maze of metastasis, *Oncol Nurs Forum* 28(6):959, 2001.

Henry JB, editor: *Clinical diagnosis and management by laboratory methods,* ed 20, Philadelphia, 2001, WB Saunders.

Henry M: Descending into delirium, *Am J Nurs* 102(3):49, 2002.

Hodgson BB, Kizior RJ: *Saunders nursing drug handbook 2003,* Philadelphia, 2003, WB Saunders.

King CR, Hinds PS: *Quality of life: from nursing and patient perspectives,* Boston, 1998, Jones and Bartlett.

Lin EM: Laboratory value assessment. In Lin EM, editor: *Advanced practice in oncology nursing,* Philadelphia, 2001, WB Saunders.

Morris JC, Holland JF: Oncologic emergencies. In Holland JF, Frei E III, Bast RC Jr, et al, editors: *Cancer medicine,* ed 5, American Cancer Society, Hamilton, London, 2000, BC Decker.

Murren J, Glatstein E, Pass HI: Small-cell lung cancer. In DeVita VT Jr, Hellman S, Rosenberg SA, editors: *Cancer principles and practice of oncology,* ed 6, Philadelphia, 2001, JB Lippincott.

Myers JS: Oncologic complications. In Otto SE, editor: *Oncology nursing,* ed 4, St. Louis, 2001, Mosby.

Novartis: Bisphosphonate use in metastatic prostate cancer: emerging treatment options, Strategic Institute for Continuing Health Care Education, February 2002, East Hanover, NJ.

Oncology Nursing Society: *Cancer chemotherapy guidelines and recommendations for practice,* Pittsburgh, 2001, Oncology Nursing Press.

Read W, Denes A: Oncologic emergencies. In Govindan R, Arquette MA, editors: *The Washington manual of oncology,* Philadelphia, 2002, Lippincott Williams & Wilkins.

Redner A: Central nervous system malignancies. In Lanzkowsky P, editor: *Manual of pediatric hematology and oncology,* ed 3, San Diego, 2000, Academic Press.

Rosenberg SA: Principles of cancer management: surgical oncology. In DeVita VT Jr, Hellman S, Rosenberg SA, editors: *Cancer principles and practice of oncology,* ed 6, Philadelphia, 2001, JB Lippincott.

Schrump DS, Nguyen DM: Malignant pleural and pericardial effusions. In DeVita VT Jr, Hellman S, Rosenberg SA, editors: *Cancer principles and practice of oncology,* ed 6, Philadelphia, 2001, JB Lippincott.

Segal BH, Walsh TJ, Holland SM: Infections in the cancer patient. In DeVita VT Jr, Hellman S, Rosenberg SA, editors:

Cancer principles and practice of oncology, ed 6, Philadelphia, 2001, JB Lippincott.

Wickham R: Dyspnea: recognizing and managing an invisible problem, *Oncol Nurs Forum* 29(6):925, 2002.

RESOURCES

33

Cancer Resources

I. NURSING ORGANIZATIONS WEBSITES

American Nurses Association:
   www.ana.org
American Radiological Nurses Association:
   www.arna.net
American Society of Pain Management Nurses:
   www.aspmn.org
Association of Nurses in AIDS Care:
   www.anacnet.org
Association of Pediatric Oncology Nurses:
   www. apon.org
Association of Rehabilitation Nurses:
   www. rehabnurse.org
Case Management Society of America:
   www. cmsa.org
Home Healthcare Nurses Association:
   www. nahc.org/hhna
Hospice and Palliative Nurses Association:
   www.hpna.org
International Transplant Nurses Society:
   www.itns.org
Intravenous Nurses Society:
   www.ins1.org
National Association of Nurse Massage Therapists:
   www.nanmt.org
National Council of State Boards of Nursing:
   www.ncsbn.org

Resources

National Gerontological Nursing Association:
   www.ngna.org
National League for Nursing:
   www.nln.org
Oncology Nursing Society:
   www.ons.org
Society for Vascular Nursing:
   www.svnnet.org
Wound, Ostomy and Continence Nurses Society:
   www.wocn.org

II. PROFESSIONAL ORGANIZATION WEBSITES

Alternative Medicine Foundation:
   www.AM Foundation.org
American Academy of Family Physicians:
   www. aafp.org
American Alliance of Cancer Pain Initiatives:
   www.aacpi.org
American Association of Blood Banks:
   www.aabb.org
American Cancer Society:
   www.cancer.org
American Cancer Society Complementary & Alternative Methods:
   www.cancer.org/docroot/ETO/ ETO_5.asp?sitearea
   =ETO
American Geriatrics Society:
   www.americangeriatrics.org
American Health Decisions:
   www.ahd.org
American Hospital Association:
   www.aha.org
American Medical Association:
   www.ama-assn.org
Americans for Better Care of the Dying:
   www.abcd-caring.com
American Red Cross:
   www.redcross.org
American Society for Bioethics and Humanities:
   www.asbh.org
American Society for Enteral and Parenteral Nutrition:
   www.clinnutr.org
American Society of Clinical Oncology (ASCO):
   www.asco.org

American Pain Society:
  www.ampainsoc.org
Cancer Centers Program:
  http://cancer.gov/cancercenters
Cancer Hope Network:
  www.cancerhopenetwork.org
Cancer Research Institute:
  www.cancerresearch. org
Clinical Trials Listings:
  www.cancer.gov/clinicaltrials
Candlelighters Childhood Cancer Foundation:
  www.candlclighters.org
Choice in Dying: Partnership for Caring:
  www. choices.org
Hospice Association of America:
  www.hospice-america.org
International Myeloma Foundation:
  www. myeloma.org
Joint Commission on Accreditation of Healthcare
Organizations:
  www.jcaho.org
Last Acts:
  www.lastacts.org
Leukemia and Lymphoma Society:
  www. leukemia-lymphoma.org
Look Good . . . Feel Better:
  www.lookgoodfeelbetter.org
Make-A-Wish Foundation:
  www.wish.org
National Alliance of Breast Cancer Organizations:
  www.nabco.org
National Association for Home Care and
Hospice:
  www.nahc.org
National Brain Tumor Foundation:
  www.braintumor.org
National Cancer Survivors Day (NCSD):
  www. NCSDF.org
National Coalition for Cancer Survivorship:
  www.canceradvocacy.org
National Family Caregivers Association:
  www. nfcacares.org
National Foundation for Cancer Research:
  www.nfcr.org

Resources

National Hospice and Palliative Care Organization:
www.nho.org
National Lymphedema Network:
www.lymphnet.org
National Marrow Donor Program (NMDP):
www.marrow.org
Neuropathy Association:
www.neuropathy.org
Susan G. Komen Breast Cancer Foundation:
www.komen.org
Y-Me National Breast Cancer Organization:
www.y-me.org

III. GOVERNMENT AND REGULATORY WEBSITES

Agency for Healthcare Research and Quality (AHRQ);
formerly the Agency for Health Care Policy and
Research (AHCPR):
www.ahcpr.gov
Centers for Disease Control and Prevention (CDC):
www.cdc.gov
Food and Drug Administration:
www.fda.gov
FDA MedWatch Program:
www.fda.gov/medwatch
National Institutes of Health:
www.nih.gov
National Center for Complementary and Alternative
Medicine:
nccam.nih.gov
Occupational Safety and Health Administration (OSHA):
www.osha.gov
Office of Minority Health Resource Center (OMH-RC):
www.omhrc.gov/omhrc
PDQ Cancer:
www.nci.nih.gov/cancerinfo/pdq
World Health Organization (WHO):
www. who.int

IV. PHARMACEUTICAL AND INFUSION THERAPY PRODUCTS AND SOURCES WEBSITES

3M Health Care:
www.3M.com/us/healthcare

Abbott Laboratories:
  www.abbotthosp.com
ALARIS Medical System:
  www.alaris.com
Alpha Therapeutic Corporation:
  www.alphather. com
Amgen Inc.:
  www.amgen.com
Arrow International:
  www.arrowintl.com
AstraZeneca:
  astraZeneca.com
Aventis:
  www.aventis.com
Axcan Scandipharm:
  www.axcanscandipharm. com
B. Braun:
  www.bbraunusa.com
Bard Access Systems:
  www.bardaccess.com
Bayer Corporation:
  www.bayer.com
Baxter Healthcare Corporation:
  www.baxter.com
BD (Becton, Dickinson, and Company):
  www.bd. com
Berlex Laboratories:
  www.berlex.com
Best Glove Manufacturing Company:
  www.bestglove.com
Bio-Plexis:
  www.bio-plexis.com
Bioject:
  www.bioject.com
Braintree Laboratories:
  www.braintreelabs.com
Bristol-Myers Squibb:
  www.bms.com
Cathflow:
  www.cathflow.com
Celgene:
  www.celgene.com
Cell Therapeutics:
  www.cticseattle.com

Centocor:
  www.centocor.com
Cephalon:
  www.cephalon.com
Chiron:
  www.chiron.com
ConMed Corporation:
  www.conmed.com
Cook Incorporated:
  www.cookgroup.com
Deltec:
  www.deltec.com
Diagnostic Ultrasound:
  www.dxu.com
Eli Lilly and Company:
  www.lilly.com
Genentech BioOncology:
  www.gene.com
GlaxoSmithKline:
  www.gsk.com
HMP:
  www.hmpvascular.com
ICU Medical:
  www.icumed.com
IDEC Pharmaceuticals Corporation:
  www.idecpharm.com
Imclone Systems:
  www.imclone.com
Immunex (acquired by Amgen on July 15, 2002):
  www.immunex.com
IMPAC Medical Systems:
  www.impac.com
Infusystem:
  www.infusystem.com
Ivax Pharmaceuticals:
  www.ivaxpharmaceuticals.com
Kendall:
  www.kendallhq.com
Ladies First:
  www.wvi.com/~ladies1/
Ligand Pharmaceuticals Incorporated:
  www.ligand.com
Maxim Pharmaceuticals:
  www.maxim.com

Mead Johnson Nutritionals:
www.meadjohnson. com
Med-Derm Pharmaceuticals:
www.delrayderm. com/medderm.asp
Medi-Flex Hospital Products:
www.medi-flex. com
MedImmune:
www.medimmune.com
Medix Pharmaceuticals America:
www.biafine. com
Medtronic:
www.medtronic.com
Merck Human Health:
www.merck.com
Myriad Genetic Laboratories:
www.myriad.com
Nabi Biopharmaceuticals:
www.nabi.com
Navion Biomedical:
www.navionbiomedical.com
Novartis Pharmaceutical Corporation:
www. pharma.us.novartis.com
Now Medical:
www.now-med.com
Pall Corporation:
www.pall.com/industry/health/asp
Pall Medical:
www.pall.com/applicant/bio-pharm/
Oncology Supply:
www.oncologysupply.com
Ortho Biotech Oncology:
www.orthobiotech. com
Pharmacia Oncology:
www.pharmaciaoncology. com
Priority Healthcare Corporation:
www.priorityhealthcare.com
Purdue Pharma, LP:
www.partnersagainstpain. com
Roche Laboratories:
www.roche.com
Ross Products Division:
www.ross.com
Roxane Laboratories:
www.roxane.com

Scale-Tronix:
  www.scale-tronix.com
Schering-Plough Corporation:
  www.sch-plough. com
Solvay Pharmaceuticals:
  www.solvay.com
SuperGen:
  www.supergen.com
Tap Pharmaceuticals:
  www.tap.com
Tyco Healthcare/Kendall-LTP:
  www.kendall-ltp. com
US Labs:
  www.uslabs.net
US Oncology:
  www.usoncology.com
Vata:
  www.vatainc.com
Wyeth Pharmaceuticals:
  www.wyeth.com
Zefron International:
Zila Pharmaceuticals:
  www.zila.com

V. DRESSINGS, TAPES, AND SKIN CARE PRODUCTS RESOURCES
3M Health Care, 800-228-3957
Alba Health Products, 800-262-2404
Aloe Life International, 800-414-2563
Amerx Health Care, 800-448-9599
Bard Medical Division, 800-526-4455
Beiersdorf-Jbbst, 800-537-1063
B. Braun/McGaw, 800-227-2862
Brennen Medical, 800-328-9105
Brown Medical Industries, 800-843-4395
Care-Tech Laboratories, 800-325-9681
Carrington Laboratories, 800-358-5205
Centurion Specialty Care, 800-248-4058
Coloplast Corporation, 800-533-0464
ConvaTec, 800-422-8811
Derma Sciences, 800-825-4325
DeRoyal, 800-337-6925
Ferris Manufacturing Corporation, 800-765-9636
FNC Medical Corporation, 800-440-2888

Genelogic, 800-976-9090
Glenwood, 800-542-0772
GOJO Industries, 800-321-9647
Hollister, 800-323-4060
Hyperion Medical, 800-743-8111
Johnson & Johnson, 800-255-2500
Kendall Healthcare Products, 800-962-9888
Lantiseptic Division Summit Industries, 800-241-6996
Medicom, 800-361-2862
Mohmlcke Health Care, 800-992-9939
Nu-Hope Laboratories, 800-899-5017
Orion Medical Products, 800-669-5079
Rynel, 800-945-4992
Sage Products, 800-323-2220
SiliPOs, 800-229-4404
Smith & Nephew, 800-876-1261
Ulmer Pharmacal Company, 800-848-5637
Winfield Laboratories, 800-527-4616

VI. SUPPORT SURFACES RESOURCES

AirCare Therapy, 800-942-7678
AliMed, 800-225-2610
Anatomic Concepts, 800-874-7237
B.G. Industries, 800-822-8288
Blue Chip Medical Products, 800-795-6115
Comfortex, 800-445-4007
Creative Bedding Technologies, 800-526-2158
Crown Therapeutics, 800-851-3449
EROB, 800-966-3462
FloCare, 800-356-2337
Gaymar Industries, 800-828-7341
Grant Airmass Corporation, 800-243-5237
Heelbo, 800-323-5444
Hermell Products, 800-233-2342
Hill-Rom, 800-638-2546
Huntleigh Healthcare, 800-223-1218
Invacare Corporation, 800-333-6900
James Consolidated, 800-884-3317
KCI (Kinetic Concepts Inc.), 800-531-5346
Lunax Corporation, 800-264-4144
Marcon Group, 800-547-5021
Mason Medical Products, 800-233-4454
Mastex Industries, 800-343-7444
Mediq FST, 800-490-4744

Resources

Medline Industries, 800-633-5463
Neuropedic, 800-327-6759
Next Generation Company, 800-598-4303
Pegasus Airwave, 800-443-4325
Plexus/Medical, 800-690-6113
Precision Dynamics Corporation, 800-847-0670
Regency Products International, 800-845-7931
Restorative Care of America, 800-627-1595
SenTech Medical Systems, 800-474-4225
Sleepnet Corporation, 800-742-3646
Span-America Medical Systems, 800-888-6752
Standard Textile Company, 800-999-0400
Sunrise Medical Inc. Bio Clinic, 800-333-4000
Tempur-Medical, 800-878-8889
Tetra Medical Supply Corporation, 800-621-4041
Turnsoft, 800-944-8876

Appendix
Commonly Used Medications

All drug information for this appendix is borrowed with permission from Hodgson B, Kizior R: *Saunders Nursing Drug Handbook 2004*, St. Louis, 2004, Saunders.

Medications

Antacids

USES

Relief of symptoms associated with hyperacidity (e.g., heartburn, acid indigestion, sour stomach), hyperacidity associated with gastric/duodenal ulcers, treatment of pathologic gastric hypersecretion associated with Zollinger-Ellison syndrome, symptomatic treatment of gastroesophageal reflux disease (GERD), prevention and treatment of upper gastrointestinal stress-induced ulceration and bleeding (especially in intensive care unit).

ACTION

Act primarily in the stomach to neutralize gastric acid (increase pH). Antacids do not have a direct effect on acid output. The ability to increase pH depends on the dose, dosage form used, presence or absence of food in the stomach, and acid-neutralizing capacity (ANC). ANC is the number of mEq of hydrochloric acid that can be neutralized by a particular weight or volume of antacid.

ANTACIDS

Antacid	Brand Names	Availability	Dosage Range	Side Effects
Aluminum Carbonate	Basaljel	**T, C:** 608 mg **S:** 400 mg/5 ml	**2 T** or **C** or 10 ml **S** up to 12 times/day	Chalky taste, mild constipation, stomach cramps *Long-term use:* Neurotoxicity in dialysis patients, hypercalcemia, osteoporosis *Large doses:* Fecal impaction, swelling of feet/legs
Aluminum Hydroxide	Amphojel, Alu-Tab, Dialume	**T:** 300 mg, 500 mg, 600 mg **C:** 500 mg	500–1500 mg 3–6 times/day	Same as aluminum carbonate

Calcium

Carbonate	Tums, Maalox, Antacid	**T (chewable):** 500 mg, 750 mg, 1000 mg	500–1500 mg as needed	Chalky taste *Large doses:* Fecal impaction, swelling of feet/legs, metabolic alkalosis *Long-term use:* Difficult/painful urination

Magnesium

Hydroxide	Milk of Magnesia	**T (chewable):** 311 mg **L:** 400 mg/5 ml, 800 mg/5 ml	**T:** 622–1244 mg up to 4 times/day **L:** 2.5–7.5 ml up to 4 times/day	Chalky taste, diarrhea, laxative effect, electrolyte imbalance (dizziness, irregular heartbeat, fatigue)
Magnesium Oxide	Mag-Ox 400, Maox 420	**T:** 400, 420, 500 mg	400–800 mg/day	Same as magnesium hydroxide

C, Capsules; *L,* liquid; *S,* suspension; *T,* tablets.

Antianxiety Agents

USES

Treatment of anxiety. In addition, some benzodiazepines are used as hypnotics, anticonvulsants to prevent delirium tremors during alcohol withdrawal and as adjunctive therapy for relaxation of skeletal muscle spasms.

ACTION

Benzodiazepines are the largest and most frequently prescribed group of antianxiety agents. The exact mechanism is unknown.

Medications

BENZODIAZEPINE ANTIANXIETY AGENTS

Name	Availability	Uses	Dosage Range (per day)	Side Effects
Alprazolam (Xanax)	**T:** 0.25 mg, 0.5 mg, 1 mg, 2 mg **S:** 0.5 mg/5 ml, 1 mg/ml	Anxiety, panic disorder	0.75–10 mg	Drowsiness, weakness or fatigue, ataxia, slurred speech, confusion, lack of coordination, impaired memory, paradoxical agitation, dizziness, nausea
Chlordiazepoxide (Librium, Libritabs)	**C:** 5 mg, 10 mg, 25 mg **T:** 10 mg, 25 mg	Anxiety, alcohol withdrawal	5–300 mg	Same as alprazolam
Clorazepate (Tranxene)	**C:** 3.75 mg, 7.5 mg, 15 mg **SD:** 11.25 mg, 22.5 mg	Anxiety, alcohol withdrawal, anticonvulsant	7.5–90 mg	Same as alprazolam
Diazepam (Valium)	**T:** 2.5 mg, 5 mg, 10 mg **S:** 5 mg/5 ml, 5 mg/ml **I:** 5 mg/ml	Anxiety, alcohol withdrawal, anticonvulsant, muscle relaxant	2–40 mg	Same as alprazolam
Lorazepam (Ativan)	**T:** 0.5 mg, 1 mg, 2 mg **S:** 2 mg/ml **I:** 2 mg/ml, 4 mg/ml	Anxiety	0.5–10 mg	Same as alprazolam
Oxazepam (Serax)	**C:** 10 mg, 15 mg, 30 mg **T:** 15 mg	Anxiety, alcohol withdrawal	30–120 mg	Same as alprazolam

Nonbenzodiazepine Antianxiety Agents

Buspirone (BuSpar)	**T:** 5 mg, 10 mg, 15 mg, 30 mg	Anxiety	7.5–60 mg	Dizziness, lightheadedness, headache, nausea, restlessness
Hydroxyzine (Atarax, Vistaril)	**T:** 10 mg, 25 mg, 50 mg, 100 mg	Anxiety, rhinitis, pruritus, urticaria, nausea or vomiting	100–400 mg	Drowsiness; dry mouth, nose, and throat
Paroxetine (Paxil)	**S:** 10 mg/5 ml **T:** 10 mg, 20 mg, 30 mg, 40 mg **T(EC):** 12.5 mg, 25 mg, 37.5 mg	Anxiety, depression, obsessive-compulsive disorder, panic disorder	10–50 mg	Drowsiness; dry mouth, nose, and throat; dizziness; diarrhea; increased sweating; constipation; vomiting; tremors
Trazodone (Desyrel)	**T:** 50 mg, 100 mg, 150 mg, 300 mg	Anxiety, depression	100–400 mg	Drowsiness, dizziness, headache, dry mouth, nausea, vomiting, unpleasant taste
Venlafaxine (Effexor)	**C:** 37.5 mg, 75 mg, 150 mg	Anxiety, depression	37.5–225 mg	Drowsiness, nausea, headache, dry mouth

C, Capsules; *I*, injection; *S*, solution; *SD*, single dose; *T*, tablets.

Medications

Antibiotics

USES

Treatment of wide range of gram-positive or gram-negative bacterial infections; suppression of intestinal flora before surgery; control of acne; prophylactically to prevent rheumatic fever; prophylactically in high-risk situations (e.g., some surgical procedures or medical states) to prevent bacterial infection.

ACTION

Antibiotics (antimicrobial agents) are natural or synthetic compounds that have the ability to kill or suppress the growth of microorganisms.

SELECTION OF ANTIMICROBIAL AGENTS

The goal of therapy is to produce a favorable therapeutic result by achieving antimicrobial action at the site of infection sufficient to inhibit the growth of the microorganism. The agent selected should be the most active against the most likely infecting organism, least likely to cause toxicity or allergic reaction. Factors to consider in selection of an antimicrobial agent include the following:

- Sensitivity pattern of the infecting microorganism
- Location and severity of infection (may determine route of administration)
- Patient's ability to eliminate the drug (status of renal and liver functions)
- Patient's defense mechanisms (includes both cellular and humoral immunity)
- Patient's age, whether pregnant, genetic factors, allergies, central nervous system disorder, preexisting medical problems

CATEGORIZATION OF ORGANISMS BY GRAM STAINING

Gram-Positive Cocci	Gram-Negative Cocci	Gram-Positive Bacilli	Gram-Negative Bacilli
Aerobic	**Aerobic**	**Aerobic**	**Aerobic**
Staphylococcus aureus	*Neisseria gonorrhoeae*	*Listeria monocytogenes*	*E. coli*
Staphylococcus epidermidis	*Neisseria meningitidis*	*Bacillus antrocis*	*Klebsiella pneumoniae*
Streptococcus pneumoniae	*Moraxella catarrhalis*	*Corynebacterium diphtheriae*	*Proteus mirabilis*
Streptococcus pyogenes		**Anaerobic**	*Serratia marcescens*
Viridans streptococci		*Clostridium difficile*	*Pseudomonas aeruginosa*
Enterococcus faecalis		*Clostridium perfringens*	*Enterobacter spp.*
Enterococcus faecium		*Clostridium tetani*	*Haemophilus influenzae*
Anaerobic		*Actinomyces spp.*	*Legionella pneumophila*
Peptostreptococcus spp.			**Anaerobic**
Peptococcus spp.			*Bacteroides fragilis*
			Fusobacterium spp.

Antibiotics: Aminoglycosides

USES

Treatment of serious infections when other, less toxic agents are not effective, are contraindicated, or require adjunctive therapy (e.g., with penicillins or cephalosporins). Used primarily in the treatment of infections caused by gram-negative microorganisms, such as those caused by *Proteus, Klebsiella, Pseudomonas, Escherichia coli, Serratia, and Enterobacter.*

ACTION

Bactericidal. Transported across bacterial cell membrane; irreversibly binds to specific receptor proteins of bacterial ribosomes. Interfere with protein synthesis, preventing cell reproduction, and eventually causing cell death.

Medications

ANTIBIOTICS: AMINOGLYCOSIDES

Name	Availability	Dosage Range	Side Effects
Amikacin (Amikin)	**I:** 250 mg/ml, 50 mg/ml	**A:** 15 mg/kg/day **C:** 15 mg/kg/day	Nephrotoxicity, neurotoxicity, ototoxicity (both auditory and vestibular), hypersensitivity (skin itching, redness, rash, swelling)
Gentamicin (Garamycin)	**I:** 40 mg/ml, 10 mg/ml	**A:** 3–5 mg/kg/day **C:** 6–7.5 mg/kg/day	Same as amikacin
Neomycin	**T:** 500 mg	**A:** 1 g for 3 doses as preop	Nausea, vomiting, diarrhea
Netilmicin (Netromycin)	**I:** 100 mg/ml	**A:** 3–6.5 mg/kg/day **C:** 5.5–8 mg/kg/day	Same as amikacin
Streptomycin	**I:** 1 g	**A:** 15 mg/kg/day **C:** 20–40 mg/kg/day **Max:** 1 g	Same as amikacin Peripheral neuritis (numbness), optic neuritis (any vision loss)
Tobramycin (Nebcin)	**I:** 40 mg/ml, 10 mg/ml	**A:** 3–5 mg/kg/day **C:** 6–7.5 mg/kg/day	Same as amikacin

A, Adults; *C*, children; *I*, injection; *T*, tablets.

Antibiotics: Cephalosporins

USES

Broad-spectrum antibiotics, which, like penicillins, may be used in a number of diseases, including respiratory diseases, skin and soft tissue infection, bone/joint infections, gastric ulcer infections, prophylactically in some surgical procedures.

First-generation cephalosporins have good activity against gram-positive organisms and moderate activity against gram-negative organisms.

Second-generation cephalosporins have increased activity against gram-negative organisms.

Third-generation cephalosporins are less active against gram-positive organisms but more active against the Enterobacteriaceae with some activity against *Pseudomonas aeruginosa.*

Fourth-generation cephalosporins have good activity against gram-positive organisms and gram-negative organisms.

ACTION

Cephalosporins inhibit cell wall synthesis or activate enzymes that disrupt cell wall, causing a weakening in the cell wall, cell lysis, and cell death. May be bacteriostatic or bactericidal. Most effective against rapidly dividing cells.

ANTIBIOTIC: CEPHALOSPORINS

Name	Availability	Dosage Range	Side Effects
First-Generation			
Cefadroxil (Duricef)	**C:** 500 mg **T:** 1 g **S:** 125 mg/5 ml, 250 mg/5 ml, 500 mg/5 ml	**A:** 1–2 g/day **C:** 30 mg/kg/day	Abdominal or stomach cramps/pain, fever, nausea, vomiting, diarrhea, headaches, oral/vaginal candidiasis

(Continued)

Medications

ANTIBIOTIC: CEPHALOSPORINS—cont'd

Name	Availability	Dosage Range	Side Effects
First-Generation—cont'd			
Cefazolin (Ancef, Kefzol)	**I:** 500 mg, 1 g, 2 g	**A:** 0.75–6 g/day **C:** 25–100 mg/kg/day	Same as cefadroxil
Cephalexin (Keftab)	**C:** 250 mg, 500 mg **T:** 250 mg, 500 mg, 1 g	**A:** 1–4 g/day **C:** 25–100 mg/kg/day	Same as cefadroxil
Second-Generation			
Cefaclor (Ceclor)	**C:** 250 mg, 500 mg **T (ER):** 375 mg, 500 mg **S:** 125 mg/5 ml, 187 mg/5 ml, 250 mg/5 ml, 375 mg/5 ml	**A:** 250–500 mg q8h **C:** 20–40 mg/kg/day	Same as cefadroxil May have serum sickness–like reaction
Cefmetazole (Zefazone)	**I:** 1 g, 2 g	**A:** 4–8 g/day	Same as cefadroxil
Cefotetan (Cefotan)	**I:** 1 g, 2 g	**A:** 1–6 g/day	Same as cefadroxil May cause unusual bleeding/bruising
Cefoxitin (Mefoxin)	**I:** 1 g, 2 g	**A:** 3–12 g/day	Same as cefadroxil
Cefpodoxime (Vantin)	**T:** 100 mg, 200 mg **S:** 50 mg/5 ml, 100 mg/5 ml	**A:** 200–800 mg/day **C:** 10 mg/kg/day	Same as cefadroxil
Cefprozil (Cefzil)	**T:** 250 mg, 500 mg **S:** 125 mg/5 ml, 250 mg/5 ml	**A:** 0.5–1 g/day **C:** 30 mg/kg/day	Same as cefadroxil

Cefuroxime (Ceftin, Kefurox, Zinacef)	**T:** 125 mg, 250 mg, 500 mg **S:** 125 mg/5 ml, 250 mg/5 ml **I:** 750 mg, 1.5 g	**A (PO):** 0.25–1 g/day; **(IM/IV):** 2.25–9 g/day **C (PO):** 250–500 mg/day; **(IM/IV):** 50–100 mg/kg/day	Same as cefadroxil
Loracarbef (Lorabid)	**C:** 200 mg, 400 mg **S:** 100 mg/5 ml, 200 mg/5 ml	**A:** 200–800 mg/day **C:** 15–30 mg/kg/day	Same as cefadroxil
Third-Generation			
Cefdinir (Omnicef)	**C:** 300 mg **S:** 125 mg/5 ml	**A:** 600 mg/day **C:** 14 mg/kg/day	Same as cefadroxil
Cefditoren (Spectracef)	**T:** 200 mg	**A:** 400–800 mg/day	Same as cefadroxil
Cefotaxime (Claforan)	**I:** 500 mg, 1 g, 2 g	**A:** 2–12 g/day **C:** 100–200 mg/kg/day	Same as cefadroxil
Ceftazidime (Fortaz, Tazicef, Tazidime)	**I:** 500 mg, 1 g, 2 g	**A:** 0.5–6 g/day **C:** 90–150 mg/kg/day	Same as cefadroxil
Ceftibuten (Cedax)	**C:** 400 mg **S:** 90 mg/5 ml, 180 mg/5 ml	**A:** 400 mg/day **C:** 9 mg/kg/day	Same as cefadroxil
Ceftizoxime (Cefizox)	**I:** 500 mg, 1 g, 2 g	**A:** 1–12 g/day **C:** 150–200 mg/kg/day	Same as cefadroxil
Ceftriaxone (Rocephin)	**I:** 250 mg, 500 mg, 1 g, 2 g	**A:** 1–4 g/day **C:** 50–100 mg/kg/day	Same as cefadroxil
Fourth-Generation			
Cefepime (Maxipime)	**I:** 500 mg, 1 g, 2 g	**A:** 1–6 g/day	Same as cefadroxil

A, Adults; *C,* capsules; *C* (dosage), children; *I,* injection; *IM,* intramuscularly; *IV,* intravenously; *PO,* by mouth; *S,* suspension; *T,* tablets.

Medications

Antibiotics: Fluoroquinolones

USES

Fluoroquinolones act against a wide range of gram-negative and gram-positive organisms. They are used primarily in the treatment of lower respiratory infections, skin/skin structure infection, urinary tract infections, and sexually transmitted diseases.

ACTION

Bactericidal. Inhibit DNA gyrase in susceptible microorganisms, interfering with bacterial DNA replication and repair.

ANTIBIOTICS: FLUOROQUINOLONES

Name	Availability	Dosage Range	Side Effects
Ciprofloxacin (Cipro)	**T:** 250 mg, 500 mg, 750 mg **S:** 5 g/100 ml **I:** 200 mg, 400 mg	**A (PO):** 250–750 mg q12h; **(IV):** 200–400 mg q12h	Dizziness, headaches, nervousness, drowsiness, insomnia, abdominal pain, nausea, diarrhea, vomiting, phlebitis (parenteral)
Enoxacin (Penetrex)	**T:** 200 mg, 400 mg	**A:** 200–400 mg q12h	Same as ciprofloxacin
Gatifloxacin (Tequin)	**T:** 200 mg, 400 mg **I:** 200 mg, 400 mg	**A:** 200–400 mg q12h	Same as ciprofloxacin
Levofloxacin (Levaquin)	**T:** 250 mg, 500 mg, 750 mg **I:** 250 mg, 500 mg, 750 mg	**A (PO/IV):** 250–750 mg/day as single dose	Same as ciprofloxacin
Lomefloxacin (Maxaquin)	**T:** 400 mg	**A:** 400 mg/day	Same as ciprofloxacin

Moxifloxacin (Avelox)	**T:** 400 mg **I:** 400 mg	**A:** 400 mg/day	Same as ciprofloxacin; may prolong QT interval
Norfloxacin (Noroxin)	**T:** 400 mg	**A:** 400 mg q12h	Same as ciprofloxacin
Ofloxacin (Floxin)	**T:** 200 mg, 300 mg, 400 mg	**A:** 200–400 mg q12h	Same as ciprofloxacin
Sparfloxacin (Zagam)	**T:** 200 mg	**A:** 400 mg once, then 200 mg/day	Same as ciprofloxacin; photosensitivity, QT prolongation, vaginitis

A, Adults; *I,* injection; *IV,* intravenously; *PO,* by mouth; *S,* suspension; *T,* tablets.

Antibiotics: Macrolides

USES	ACTION
Macrolides act primarily against gram-positive microorganisms and gram-negative cocci. Macrolides are used in the treatment of pharyngitis/tonsillitis, sinusitis, chronic bronchitis, pneumonia, uncomplicated skin/skin structure infections.	Bacteriostatic or bactericidal. Reversibly bind to the P site of the 50S ribosomal subunit of susceptible organisms, inhibiting RNA-dependent protein synthesis.

Medications

ANTIBIOTICS: MACROLIDES

Name	Availability	Dosage Range	Side Effects
Azithromycin (Zithromax)	**T:** 250 mg, 600 mg **S:** 100 mg/5 ml, 200 mg/5 ml, 1 g packet **I:** 500 mg	**A (PO):** 500 mg once, then 250 mg days 2–5; **(IV):** 500 mg/day **C (PO):** 10 mg/kg once, then 5 mg/kg/day on days 2–5	**PO:** Nausea, diarrhea, vomiting, abdominal pain **IV:** Pain, redness, swelling at injection site
Clarithromycin (Biaxin)	**T:** 250 mg, 500 mg **T (XL):** 500 mg **S:** 125 mg/5 ml	**A:** 250–500 mg q12h **C:** 7.5 mg/kg q12h	Headaches, loss of taste, nausea, vomiting, diarrhea, abdominal pain/discomfort
Dirithromycin (Dynabec)	**T:** 250 mg	**A, C (>12 yrs):** 500 mg/day as a single daily dose	Dizziness, nausea, vomiting, diarrhea, abdominal pain, headaches, weakness
Erythromycin (Erytab, PCE. Eryc. EES, Eryped, Erythrocin)	**T:** 200 mg, 250 mg, 333 mg, 400 mg, 500 mg **C:** 250 mg **S:** 125 mg/5 ml, 200 mg/5 ml, 250 mg/5 ml, 400 mg/5 ml, 100 mg/2.5 ml	**A (PO):** 250–500 mg q6h **C (PO):** 30–50 mg/kg/day **A, C (IV):** 15–20 mg/kg/day **Max:** 4 g/day	**PO:** Nausea, vomiting, diarrhea, abdominal pain **IV:** Inflammation, phlebitis at injection site

A, Adults; *C,* capsules; *C* (dosage), children; *I,* injection; *IV,* intravenously; *PO,* by mouth; *S,* suspension; *T,* tablets; *XL,* long acting.

Antibiotics: Penicillins

USES

Penicillins may be used to treat a large number of infections, including pneumonia and other respiratory diseases, urinary tract infections, septicemia, meningitis, intraabdominal infections, gonorrhea and syphilis, bone/joint infection.

Penicillins are classified based on an antimicrobial spectrum:

Natural penicillins are very active against gram-positive cocci but ineffective against most strains of *Staphylococcus aureus* (inactivated by enzyme penicillinase).

Penicillinase-resistant penicillins are effective against penicillinase-producing *Staphylococcus aureus* but are less effective against gram-positive cocci than the natural penicillins.

Broad-spectrum penicillins are effective against gram-positive cocci and some gram-negative bacteria (e.g., *Haemophilus influenzae, Escherichia coli, Proteus mirabilis*).

Extended-spectrum penicillins are effective against *Pseudomonas aeruginosa, Enterobacter, Proteus species, Klebsiella*, and some other gram-negative microorganisms.

ACTION

Penicillins inhibit cell wall synthesis or activate enzymes, which disrupt bacterial cell wall, causing a weakening in the cell wall, cell lysis, and cell death.

May be bacteriostatic or bactericidal. Most effective against bacteria undergoing active growth and division.

Medications

ANTIBIOTICS: PENICILLINS

Name	Availability	Dosage Range	Side Effects
Natural			
Penicillin G benzathine (Bicillin)	**I:** 600,000 U, 1.2 million U, 2.4 million U	**A:** 1.2 million U/day **C:** 0.3–1.2 million U/day	Mild diarrhea, nausea, vomiting, headaches, sore mouth/tongue, vaginal itching/discharge, allergic reaction (including anaphylaxis, skin rash, hives, itching)
Penicillin G potassium (Pfizerpen)	**I:** 1, 2, 3, 5 million U vials	**A:** 2–24 million U/day **C:** 100–250,000 U/kg/day	Same as penicillin G benzathine
Penicillin G procaine (Wycillin)	**I:** 600,000 U, 1.2 million U, 2.4 million U	**A, C:** 0.6–1.2 million U/day	Same as penicillin G benzathine; increased risk of mental disturbances
Penicillin V (Pen-Vee K, V-Cillin-K)	**T:** 250 mg, 500 mg **S:** 125 mg/5 ml, 250 mg/5 ml	**A:** 0.5–2 g/day **C:** 25–50 mg/kg/day	Same as penicillin G benzathine
Penicillinase-Resistant			
Cloxacillin (Tegopen)	**C:** 250 mg, 500 mg **S:** 125 mg/5 ml	**A:** 1–2 g/day **C:** 50–100 mg/kg/day	Same as penicillin G benzathine; increased risk of liver toxicity
Dicloxacillin (Dynapen, Pathocil)	**C:** 125 mg, 250 mg, 500 mg **S:** 62.5 mg/5 ml	**A:** 1–2 g/day **C:** 12.5–25 mg/kg/day	Same as penicillin G benzathine Increased risk of liver toxicity
Nafcillin (Nafcil, Unipen)	**C:** 250 mg **I:** 500 mg, 1 g, 2 g	**A (PO):** 1–6 g/day; **(IV):** 2–6 g/day **C (PO):** 25–50 mg/kg/day; **(IV):** 50 mg/kg/day	Same as penicillin G benzathine; increased risk of interstitial nephritis

Oxacillin (Bactocill)	**C:** 250 mg, 500 mg **S:** 250 mg/5 ml **I:** 250 mg, 500 mg, 1 g, 2 g	**A (PO/IV):** 2–6 g/day **C (PO/IV):** 50–100 mg/kg/day	Same as penicillin G benzathine; increased risk of liver toxicity, interstitial nephritis
Broad-Spectrum			
Amoxicillin (Amoxil, Polymox, Trimox)	**T:** 125 mg, 250 mg, 500 mg, 875 mg **C:** 250 mg, 500 mg **S:** 50 mg/ml, 125 mg/5 ml, 250 mg/5 ml	**A:** 0.75–1.5 g/day **C:** 20–40 mg/kg/day	Same as penicillin G benzathine
Amoxicillin/clavulanate (Augmentin)	**T:** 250 mg, 500 mg, 875 mg **T (chewable):** 125 mg, 200 mg, 250 mg, 400 mg **S:** 125 mg/5 ml, 200 mg/5 ml, 250 mg/5 ml, 400 mg/5 ml	**A:** 0.75–1.5 g/day **C:** 20–40 mg/kg/day	Same as penicillin G benzathine
Ampicillin (Omnipen, Polycillin, Principen)	**C:** 250 mg, 500 mg **S:** 125 mg/5 ml, 250 mg/5 ml **I:** 125 mg, 250 mg, 500 mg, 1 g, 2 g	**A:** 1–12 g/day **C:** 50–200 mg/kg/day	Same as penicillin G benzathine
Ampicillin/sulbactam (Unasyn)	**I:** 1.5 g, 3 g	**A:** 6–12 g/day **C:** 100–200 mg/kg/day	Same as penicillin G benzathine
Bacampicillin (Spectrobid)	**T:** 400 mg	**A:** 800–1,600 mg/day **C:** 25–50 mg/kg/day	Same as penicillin G benzathine

(Continued)

Medications

ANTIBIOTICS: PENICILLINS—cont'd

Name	Availability	Dosage Range	Side Effects
Extended-Spectrum			
Carbenicillin (Geocillin)	**T:** 382 mg	**A:** 382–764 mg 4 times/day	Same as penicillin G benzathine
Piperacillin/tazobactam (Zosyn)	**I:** 2.25 g, 3.375 g, 4.5 g	**A:** 2.25–4.5 g q6–8h **C:** 200–400 mg/kg/day	Same as penicillin G benzathine
Ticarcillin/clavulanate (Timentin)	**I:** 3.1 g	**A:** 3.1 g q4–6h **C:** 200–300 mg/kg/day	Same as penicillin G benzathine

A, Adults; *C,* capsules; *C* (dosage), children; *I,* injection; *S,* suspension; *T,* tablets.

Anticoagulants/Antiplatelets/Thrombolytics

USES

Treatment and prevention of venous thromboembolism, acute MI, acute cerebral embolism; reduce risk of acute MI; occlusion of saphenous grafts following open heart surgery; embolism in select patients with atrial fibrillation, prosthetic heart valves, valvular heart disease, cardiomyopathy. Heparin also used for acute/chronic consumption coagulopathies (disseminated intravascular coagulation).

ACTION

Anticoagulants: Inhibit blood coagulation by preventing the formation of new clots and extension of existing ones. *Do not dissolve formed clots.* Anticoagulants are subdivided into two common classes: *Heparin:* Indirectly interferes with blood coagulation by blocking the conversion of prothrombin to thrombin and fibrinogen to fibrin. *Coumarin:* Acts indirectly to prevent synthesis in the liver of vitamin K-dependent clotting factors.

Antiplatelets: Interfere with platelet aggregation. Effects are irreversible for life of platelet. Medications in this group act by different mechanisms and are used in combinations to provide desired effect.

Thrombolytics: Act directly or indirectly on fibrinolytic system to dissolve clots (converting plasminogen to plasmin, an enzyme that digests fibrin clot).

ANTICOAGULANTS/ANTIPLATELETS/THROMBOLYTICS

Name	Availability	Uses	Dosage Range	Side Effects
Anticoagulants				
Dalteparin (Fragmin)	**I:** 2500 IU, 5000 IU	DVT prophylaxis, unstable angina	**DVT:** 2500–5000 IU/day **Angina:** 120 IU/kg q12h	Hematoma at injection site, bleeding
Danaparoid (Orgaran)	**I:** 750 units	DVT prophylaxis	750 U q12h	Pain at injection site, bleeding
Enoxaparin (Lovenox)	**I:** 30 mg, 40 mg, 60 mg, 80 mg, 100 mg	DVT treatment/ prophylaxis, DVT, unstable angina	**DVT prophylaxis:** 40 mg/ day or 30 mg q12h **DVT, angina:** 1 mg/kg q12h	Same as dalteparin
Heparin	**I:** 5000 U, 10,000 U, 20,000 U	DVT prophylaxis, thrombosis, embolism, coagulopathies	**DVT prophylaxis:** 5000 U q8–12h **DVT, embolism:** IV bolus, then IV infusion of 20,000–40,000 U/day	Bleeding
Tinzaparin (Innohep)	**I:** 20,000 IU/ml	DVT treatment	175 IU/kg once daily	Same as danaparoid
Warfarin (Coumadin)	**T:** 1 mg, 2 mg, 2.5 mg, 3 mg, 4 mg, 5 mg, 6 mg, 7.5 mg, 10 mg	Thromboembolic complications with AF, PE, DVT	Initially, 5–10 mg, then 2–10 mg/day	Same as heparin
Antiplatelets				
Abciximab (ReoPro)	**I:** 2 m/ml	ACS	IV bolus of 0.25 mg/kg, then 10 µg/min	Bleeding, hypotension

(Continued)

Medications

ANTICOAGULANTS/ANTIPLATELETS/THROMBOLYTICS—cont'd

Name	Availability	Uses	Dosage Range	Side Effects
Antiplatelets—cont'd				
Anagrelide (Agrylin)	**C:** 0.5 mg, 1 mg	Thrombocythemia	2–10 mg/day	Abdominal pain, weakness, dizziness, shortness of breath
Aspirin	**T:** 80 mg, 160 mg, 325 mg	Atherosclerotic events	81–325 mg/day	GI irritation
Clopidogrel (Plavix)	**T:** 75 mg	Atherosclerotic events	75 mg/day	Pain, dizziness, heartburn, headaches, flulike symptoms
Dipyridamole (Persantine)	**T:** 25 mg, 50 mg, 75 mg	Thromboembolic complications	75–100 mg 4 times/day	Abdominal discomfort, diarrhea, dizziness, headaches
Eptifibatide (Integrilin)	**I:** 0.75 mg/ml, 2 mg/ml	ACS	IV bolus of 180 µg/kg, then 2 µg/kg/min	Same as abciximab
Ticlopidine (Ticlid)	**T:** 250 mg	Stroke	250 mg 2 times/day	Skin rash, abdominal pain, diarrhea, nausea, indigestion
Tirofiban (Aggrastat)	**I:** 50 µg/ml, 250 µg/ml	ACS	IV bolus of 0.4 µg/kg/min, then 0.1 µg/kg/min	Same as abciximab
Thrombolytics				
Alteplase (Activase)	**I:** 50 mg, 100 mg	AMI, acute ischemic stroke, PE	**IV:** 100 mg over 3 hrs (PE over 2 hrs)	Same as abciximab
Anistreplase (Eminase)	**I:** 30 U	AMI	**IV:** 30 U over 2–5 min	Same as abciximab

Reteplase (Retavase)	*I:* 10 U		IV: 10 U q30 min 2 times	Same as abciximab
Streptokinase	*I:* 250,000 U, 500,000 U, 1.5 million U	AMI, PE, arterial thrombus	**AMI:** 1.5 million U over 60 min **PE, arterial thrombus:** 250,000 U bolus, then 100,000 U/hr	Same as abciximab
Tenecteplase (TNKase)	*I:* 50 mg	AMI	Based on patient weight **Max:** 50 mg	Same as abciximab

ACS, Acute coronary syndrome; *AF,* atrial fibrillation; *AMI,* acute myocardial infarction; *C,* capsules; *DVT,* deep vein thrombosis; *GI,* gastrointestinal; *I,* injection; *IV,* intravenously; *MI,* myocardial infarction; *PE,* pulmonary embolism; *T,* tablets.

Anticonvulsants

USES

Anticonvulsants are used to treat seizures. Seizures can be divided into two broad categories: partial seizures and generalized seizures. Partial seizures begin focally in the cerebral cortex, undergoing limited spread. Simple partial seizures do not involve loss of consciousness but may evolve secondarily into generalized seizures. Complex partial seizures involve impairment of consciousness.

ACTION

Anticonvulsants can prevent or reduce excessive discharge of neurons with seizure foci or decrease the spread of excitation from seizure foci to normal neurons. The exact mechanism is unknown but may be caused by (1) suppressing sodium influx; (2) suppressing calcium influx; or (3) increasing the action of GABA, which inhibits neurotransmitters throughout the brain.

Medications

ANTICONVULSANTS

Name	Availability	Uses	Dosage Range	Side Effects
Barbiturates				
Phenobarbital	**T:** 30 mg, 60 mg, 100 mg, **I:** 65 mg, 130 mg	Tonic-clonic, partial, status epilepticus	**A (PO):** 100–300 mg/day; **(IM/IV):** 200–600 mg; **C (PO):** 3–5 mg/kg/day; **(IM/IV):** 100–400 mg	CNS depression, sedation, paradoxical excitement and hyperactivity, rash
Primidone (Mysoline)	**T:** 50 mg, 250 mg **S:** 250 mg/5 ml	Complex, partial, akinetic, tonic-clonic	**A:** 750–2000 mg/day **C:** 10–25 mg/kg/day	CNS depression, sedation, paradoxical excitement and hyperactivity, rash, dizziness, ataxia
Benzodiazepines				
Clonazepam (Klonopin)	**T:** 0.5 mg, 1 mg, 2 mg	Petit mal, akinetic, myoclonic, absence seizure	**A:** 1.5–20 mg/day	CNS depression, sedation, ataxia, confusion, depression
Diazepam (Valium)	**T:** 2 mg, 5 mg, 10 mg **I:** 5 mg/ml **R:** 2.5 mg, 5 mg, 10 mg, 20 mg	Adjunctive therapy status epilepticus	**A (PO):** 4–40 mg/day; **(IM/IV):** 5–30 mg **C (PO):** 3–10 mg/day; **(IM/IV):** 1–10 mg	CNS depression, sedation, confusion, depression, respiratory suppression
Hydantoins				
Fosphenytoin (Cerebyx)	**I:** 50 mg PE/ml	Status epilepticus, seizures occurring during neurosurgery	**A:** 15–20 mg PE/kg bolus, then 4–6 mg PE/kg/day maintenance	Burning, itching, paresthesia, nystagmus, ataxia

			A (PO): 300–600 mg/day; IV): 150–250 mg/day; C (PO): 4–8 mg/kg/day; IV): 10–15 mg/kg	Nystagmus, ataxia, hypertrichosis, gingival hyperplasia, rash, osteomalacia, lymphadenopathy
Phenytoin (Dilantin)	C: 100 mg T (chewable): 50 mg S: 125 mg/5 ml I: 50 mg/ml	Tonic-clonic psychomotor seizures		
Miscellaneous				
Carbamazepine (Tegretol)	S: 100 mg/5 ml T (chewable): 100 mg T: 200 mg T (ER): 100 mg, 200 mg, 400 mg C (ER): 200 mg, 300 mg	Complex partial, tonic-clonic, mixed seizures, trigeminal neuralgia	A: 800–1200 mg/day C: 400–800 mg/day	Dizziness, diplopia, leukopenia
Gabapentin (Neurontin)	C: 100 mg, 300 mg, 400 mg	Partial seizures with and without secondary generalization	A: 900–1800 mg/day	CNS depression, fatigue, somnolence, dizziness, ataxia
Lamotrigine (Lamictal)	T: 25 mg, 100 mg, 150 mg, 200 mg	Partial seizures	A: 100–500 mg/day	Dizziness, ataxia, somnolence, diplopia, nausea, rash
Levetiracetam (Keppra)	T: 250 mg, 500 mg, 750 mg	Partial-onset seizures	A: 1000–3000 mg/day	Asthenia, dizziness, flulike symptoms, headache, rhinitis, somnolence
Oxcarbazepine (Trileptal)	T: 150 mg, 300 mg, 600 mg	Partial seizures	A: 900–1800 mg/day	Drowsiness, dizziness, blurred vision
Tiagabine (Gabitril)	T: 4 mg, 12 mg, 16 mg, 20 mg	Partial seizures	A: Initially, 4 mg up to 56 mg C: Initially, 4 mg up to 32 mg	Dizziness, asthenia, nervousness, tremors, abdominal pain

(Continued)

Medications

ANTICONVULSANTS—cont'd

Name	Availability	Uses	Dosage Range	Side Effects
Miscellaneous—cont'd				
Topiramate (Topamax)	**T:** 25 mg, 100 mg, 200 mg	Partial seizures	**A:** 25–400 mg/day **C:** 1–9 mg/kg/day	Difficulty concentrating, speech problems, fatigue
Valproic acid (Depakene, Depakote)	**C:** 250 mg **S:** 250 mg/5 ml **Sprinkles:** 125 mg **T:** 125 mg, 250 mg, 500 mg **T (ER):** 500 mg **I:** 100 mg/ml	Complex partial seizures, absence seizures	**A, C:** 15–60 mg/kg/day	Nausea, vomiting, tremors, thrombocytopenia, hair loss, liver dysfunction
Zonisamide (Zonegran)	**C:** 100 mg	Partial seizures	**A:** 500 mg/day	Somnolence, dizziness, anorexia, headaches, nausea

A, Adults; *C,* (dosage), children; *CNS,* central nervous system; *ER,* extended-release; *I,* injection; *PE,* pulmonary embolism; *R,* rectal; *S,* suspension; *T,* tablets.

Antidepressants

USES

Used primarily for the treatment of depression. Imipramine is also used for childhood enuresis. Clomipramine is used only for obsessive-compulsive disorder (OCD). Monoamine oxidase (MAO) inhibitors are rarely used as initial therapy except for patients unresponsive to other therapy or when other therapy is contraindicated.

ACTION

Antidepressants are classified as tricyclic, MAO inhibitors, or second-generation antidepressants (further subdivided into selective serotonin reuptake inhibitors [SSRIs] and atypical antidepressants). Antidepressants block metabolism, increase amount/effects of monoamine neurotransmitters, and act at receptor sites.

ANTIDEPRESSANTS

Name	Availability	Uses	Dosage Range (per day)	Side Effects
Tricyclics				
Amitriptyline (Elavil)	**T:** 10 mg, 25 mg, 50 mg, 75 mg, 100 mg, 150 mg	Depression	40–300 mg	Drowsiness, blurred vision, constipation, confusion, postural hypotension, conduction defects, weight gain, seizure tendency
Clomipramine (Anafranil)	**C:** 25 mg, 50 mg, 75 mg	OCD	25–250 mg	Same as amitriptyline
Desipramine (Norpramin, Pertofrane)	**T:** 10 mg, 25 mg, 50 mg, 75 mg, 100 mg, 150 mg	Depression	25–100 mg	Same as amitriptyline
Doxepin (Sinequan)	**C:** 10 mg, 25 mg, 50 mg, 75 mg, 100 mg, 150 mg **OC:** 10 mg/ml	Depression	25–300 mg	Same as amitriptyline
Imipramine (Janimine, Tofranil)	**T:** 10 mg, 25 mg, 50 mg **C:** 75 mg, 100 mg, 125 mg, 150 mg	Depression, enuresis	30–300 mg	Same as amitriptyline
Nortriptyline (Aventyl, Pamelor)	**C:** 10 mg, 25 mg, 50 mg, 75 mg **S:** 10 mg/5 ml	Depression	25–100 mg	Same as amitriptyline
Protriptyline (Vivactil)	**T:** 5 mg, 10 mg	Depression	15–60 mg	Same as amitriptyline

(Continued)

Medications

ANTIDEPRESSANTS—cont'd

Name	Availability	Uses	Dosage Range (per day)	Side Effects
Monoamine Oxidase Inhibitors (MAOIs)				
Phenelzine (Nardil)	**T:** 15 mg	Depression	15-90 mg	Sedation, hypertensive crisis, weight gain, orthostatic hypotension
Tranylcypromine (Parnate)	**T:** 10 mg	Depression	30-60 mg	Same as amitriptyline
Selective Serotonin Reuptake Inhibitors (SSRIs)				
Citalopram (Celexa)	**T:** 20 mg, 40 mg **S:** 10 mg/5 ml	Depression	25-60 mg	Insomnia or sedation, nausea, agitation, headaches
Escitalopram (Lexapro)	**T:** 5 mg, 10 mg, 20 mg	Depression	10-20 mg	Insomnia or sedation, nausea, agitation, headaches
Fluoxetine (Prozac)	**C:** 10 mg, 20 mg, 40 mg **T:** 10 mg **S:** 20 mg/5 ml	Depression, OCD, bulimia	10-80 mg	Akathisia, sexual dysfunction, skin rash, hives, itching, decreased appetite, asthenia, diarrhea, drowsiness, headache, increased sweating, insomnia, nausea, tremors
Fluvoxamine (Luvox)	**T:** 25 mg, 50 mg, 100 mg	OCD	100-300 mg	Sexual dysfunction, fatigue, constipation, dizziness, drowsiness, headache, insomnia, nausea, vomiting
Paroxetine (Paxil)	**T:** 10 mg, 20 mg, 30 mg, 40 mg **S:** 10 mg/5 ml	Depression, OCD, panic attack, social anxiety disorder	20-50 mg	Asthenia, constipation, diarrhea, sweating, insomnia, nausea, sexual dysfunction, tremor, vomiting, urinary frequency or retention

Sertraline (Zoloft)	**T:** 25 mg, 50 mg, 100 mg **S:** 20 mg/ml	Depression, OCD, panic attack	50–200 mg	Sexual dysfunction, dizziness, drowsiness, anorexia, diarrhea, nausea, dry mouth, stomach cramps, decreased weight, headache, increased sweating, tremor, insomnia
Atypical				
Bupropion (Wellbutrin)	**T:** 75 mg, 100 mg **SR:** 100 mg, 150 mg	Depression	150–450 mg	Insomnia, irritability, seizures
Mirtazapine (Remeron)	**T:** 15 mg, 30 mg, 45 mg	Depression	15–45 mg	Sedation, dry mouth, weight gain, agranulocytosis, liver toxicity
Nefazodone (Serzone)	**T:** 50 mg, 100 mg, 150 mg, 200 mg, 250 mg	Depression	200–600 mg	Sedation, orthostatic hypotension, nausea
Trazodone (Desyrel)	**T:** 50 mg, 100 mg, 150 mg, 300 mg	Depression	50–600 mg	Sedation, orthostatic hypotension, priapism
Venlafaxine (Effexor)	**T:** 25 mg, 37.5 mg, 50 mg, 75 mg, 100 mg **T (ER):** 37.5 mg, 75 mg, 150 mg	Depression, anxiety	75–375 mg	Increased blood pressure, agitation, sedation, insomnia, nausea

C, Capsules; *ER,* extended-release; *OC,* oral concentrate; *OCD,* obsessive-compulsive disorder; *S,* suspension; *SR,* sustained-release; *T,* tablets.

Antidiarrheals

USES

Acute diarrhea, chronic diarrhea of inflammatory bowel disease, reduction of fluid from ileostomies.

ACTION

Systemic agents: Disrupt peristaltic movements, decrease gastrointestinal motility, increase transit time of intestinal contents.

Local agents: Adsorb toxic substances and fluids to large surface areas of particles in the preparation.

Medications

ANTIDIARRHEALS

Name	Availability	Type	Dosage Range
Bismuth subsalicylate (Pepto-Bismol)	**T:** 262 mg **C:** 262 mg **L:** 130 mg/15 ml, 262 262 mg/15 ml, 524 mg/15 ml	Local	**A:** 2 T or 30 ml **C (9–12 yrs):** 1 T or 15 ml **C (6–9 yrs):** ⅔ T or 10 ml **C (3–6 yrs):** ⅓ T or 5 ml
Diphenoxylate (with atropine) (Lomotil)	**T:** 2.5 mg **L:** 2.5 mg/5 ml	Systemic	**A:** 5 mg 4 times/day **C:** 0.3–0.4 mg/kg/day in 4 divided doses **(L)**
Kaolin (with pectin) (Kaopectate)	**Suspension**	Local	**A:** 60–120 ml after each bowel movement **C (6–12 yrs):** 30–60 ml **C (3–6 yrs):** 15–30 ml
Loperamide (Imodium)	**C:** 2 mg **T:** 2 mg **L:** 1 mg/5 ml, 1 mg/ml	Systemic	**A:** Initially, 4 mg; 16 mg/day maximum **C (8–12 yrs):** 2 mg 3 times/day **(5–8 yrs):** 2 mg 2 times/day **(2–5 yrs):** 1 mg 3 times/day (L)

A, Adults; *C*, capsules; *C* (dosage), children; *L*, liquid; *T*, tablets.

Antihistamines

USES

Symptomatic relief of upper respiratory allergic disorders. Allergic reactions associated with other drugs respond to antihistamines, as do blood transfusion reactions. Used as a second-choice drug in treatment of angioneurotic edema. Effective in treatment of acute urticaria and other dermatologic conditions.

ACTION

Antihistamines (H_1 antagonists) inhibit vasoconstrictor effects and vasodilator effects on endothelial cells of histamine. They block increased capillary permeability, formation of edema/wheal caused by histamine. Many antihistamines can bind to receptors in central nervous system, causing primarily depression but also stimulation.

ANTIHISTAMINES

Name	Availability	Dosage Range	Side Effects
Chlorpheniramine (Chlor-Trimeton)	**T:** 4 mg **T (chewable):** 2 mg **T (SR):** 8 mg, 12 mg **S:** 2 mg/5 ml	**A:** 2–4 mg q4–6h or **SR:** 8–12 mg q12–24 h **C:** 0.35 mg/kg/day	Dry mouth, urinary retention, blurred vision
Brompheniramine (Dimetane)	**T:** 4 mg **T (SR):** 4 mg, 6 mg **S:** 2 mg/5 ml	**A:** 4–8 mg q4–6h or **T (SR):** 8–12 mg q12–24 h **C:** 0.5 mg/kg/day	Same as chlorpheniramine
Dexchlorpheniramine (Polaramine)	**T:** 2 mg **S:** 2 mg/5 ml	**A:** 2 mg q4–6h **C:** 0.5–1 mg q4–6h	Same as chlorpheniramine
Diphenhydramine (Benadryl)	**T:** 25 mg, 50 mg **C:** 25 mg, 50 mg **L:** 6.25 mg/5 ml, 12.5 mg/5 ml	**A:** 25–50 mg q6–8h **C (6–11 yrs):** 12.5–25 mg q4–6h; **(2–5 yrs):** 6.25 mg q4–6h	Dry mouth, urinary retention, blurred vision, sedation, dizziness, paradoxical excitement
Clemastine (Tavist)	**T:** 1.34 mg, 2.68 mg **S:** 0.67 mg/5 ml	**A:** 1.34–2.68 mg q8–12h **C (6–12 yrs):** 0.67–1.34 mg q8–12h	Same as diphenhydramine
Promethazine (Phenergan)	**T:** 12.5 mg, 25 mg, 50 mg **S:** 6.25 mg/5 ml, 25 mg/5 ml	**A:** 25 mg at bedtime or 12.5 mg q8h **C:** 0.5 mg/kg at bedtime or 0.1 mg/kg q6–8h	Same as diphenhydramine
Cyproheptadine (Periactin)	**T:** 4 mg **S:** 2 mg/5 ml	**A:** 4 mg q8h **C:** 0.25 mg/kg/day	Same as diphenhydramine

(Continued)

Medications

ANTIHISTAMINES—cont'd

Name	Availability	Dosage Range	Side Effects
Azatadine (Optimine)	**T:** 1 mg	**A:** 1–2 mg q12h **C:** 0.05 mg/kg/day	Same as diphenhydramine
Hydroxyzine (Atarax, Vistaril)	**T:** 10 mg, 25 mg, 50 mg, 100 mg **C:** 25 mg, 50 mg, 100 mg **S:** 10 mg/5 ml, 25 mg/5 ml	**A:** 25 mg q6–8h **C:** 2 mg/kg/day	Same as diphenhydramine
Cetirizine (Zyrtec)	**T:** 5 mg, 10 mg **S:** 5 mg/5 ml	**A:** 5–10 mg/day **C (6–12 yrs):** 5–10 mg/day; **(2–5 yrs):** 2.5–5 mg/day	Minimal CNS, anticholinergic side effects
Fexofenadine (Allegra)	**T:** 30 mg, 60 mg, 180 mg	**A:** 60 mg q12h or 180 mg/day; **C (6–11 yrs):** 30 mg q12h	Same as cetirizine
Loratadine (Claritin)	**T:** 10 mg **S:** 1 mg/ml	**A:** 10 mg/day **C (6–12 yrs):** 10 mg/day	Same as cetirizine

A, Adults; *C,* capsules; *C* (dosage), children; *L,* liquid; *S,* syrup; *SR,* sustained-release; *T,* tablets.

Antivirals

USES

Treatment of HIV infection. Treatment of CMV retinitis in patients with AIDS, acute herpes zoster (shingles), genital herpes (recurrent), mucosal and cutaneous herpes simplex virus, chickenpox, and influenza A viral illness.

ACTION

Possible mechanisms of action of antivirals used for non-HIV infection may include interference with viral DNA synthesis and viral replication, inactivation of viral DNA polymerases, incorporation and termination of the growing viral DNA chain, prevention of release of viral nucleic acid into the host cell, or interference with viral penetration into cells.

ANTIVIRALS

Name	Availability	Uses	Side Effects
Abacavir (Ziagen)	**T:** 300 mg **OS:** 20 mg/ml	HIV infection	Nausea, vomiting, loss of appetite, diarrhea, headaches, fatigue
Acyclovir (Zovirax)	**T:** 400 mg, 800 mg **C:** 200 mg **I:** 50 mg/ml	Mucosal/cutaneous HSV-1 and HSV-2, varicella-zoster (shingles), genital herpes, herpes simplex, encephalitis, chickenpox	Malaise, anorexia, nausea, vomiting, light-headedness
Amantadine (Symmetrel)	**C:** 100 mg **S:** 50 mg/5 ml	Influenza A	Anxiety, dizziness, lightheadedness, headaches, nausea, loss of appetite
Amprenavir (Agenerase)	**C:** 50 mg, 150 mg **OS:** 15 mg/ml	HIV infection	Hyperglycemia, rash, abdominal pain, nausea, vomiting, diarrhea

(Continued)

Medications

ANTIVIRALS—cont'd

Name	Availability	Uses	Side Effects
Atazanavir (Reyataz)	N/A	HIV infection	Increased liver function tests, jaundice, scleral icterus
Cidofovir (Vistide)	**I:** 75 mg/ml	CMV retinitis	Decreased urination, fever, chills, diarrhea, nausea, vomiting, headaches, loss of appetite
Delavirdine (Rescriptor)	**T:** 100 mg, 200 mg	HIV infection	Diarrhea, fatigue, rash, headaches, nausea
Didanosine (Videx)	**T:** 25 mg, 50 mg, 100 mg, 150 mg, 200 mg **C:** 125 mg, 200 mg **Powder for suspension:** 100 mg, 167 mg, 250 mg	HIV infection	Peripheral neuropathy, anxiety, headaches, rash, nausea, diarrhea, dry mouth
Efavirenz (Sustiva)	**C:** 50 mg, 100 mg, 200 mg	HIV infection	Diarrhea, dizziness, headaches, insomnia, nausea, vomiting, drowsiness
Entricitabine (Emtriva, FTC)	N/A	HIV infection	Hyperpigmentation of palms, soles
Famciclovir (Famvir)	**T:** 125 mg, 250 mg, 500 mg	Herpes zoster, genital herpes	Headaches
Foscarnet (Foscavir)	**I:** 24 mg/ml	CMV retinitis, HSV infections	Decreased urination, abdominal pain, nausea, vomiting, dizziness, fatigue, headaches
Ganciclovir (Cytovene)	**C:** 250 mg, 500 mg **I:** 500 mg	CMV retinitis, CMV disease	Sore throat, fever, unusual bleeding/bruising

Indinavir (Crixivan)	**C:** 200 mg, 400 mg	HIV infection	Blood in urine, weakness, nausea, vomiting, diarrhea, headaches, insomnia, altered taste
Lamivudine (Epivir)	**T:** 100 mg, 150 mg **OS:** 5 mg/ml, 10 mg/ml	HIV infection	Nausea, vomiting, stomach pain, tingling, numbness
Lopinavir/ritonavir (Kaletra)	**C:** 133/33 mg **OS:** 80/20 mg	HIV infection	Diarrhea, nausea
Nelfinavir (Viracept)	**T:** 250 mg **Powder:** 50 mg/g	HIV infection	Diarrhea
Oseltamivir (Tamiflu)	**C:** 75 mg **S:** 12 mg/ml	Influenza	Diarrhea, nausea, vomiting
Ribavirin (Virazole)	**Aerosol:** 6 g	Lowers respiratory infections in infants, children due to respiratory syncytial virus (RSV)	Anemia
Ritonavir (Norvir)	**C:** 100 mg **OS:** 80 mg/ml	HIV infection	Weakness, diarrhea, nausea, decreased appetite, vomiting, altered taste
Saquinavir (Invirase)	**C:** 200 mg	HIV infection	Weakness, diarrhea, nausea, mouth ulcers, abdominal pain
Stavudine (Zerit)	**C:** 15 mg, 20 mg, 30 mg, 40 mg **OS:** 1 mg/ml	HIV infection	Numbness in hands/feet, decreased appetite, chills, fever, rash
Tenofovir (Viread)	**T:** 300 mg	HIV infection	Diarrhea, nausea, pharyngitis, headaches

(Continued)

Medications

ANTIVIRALS—cont'd

Name	Availability	Uses	Side Effects
Valacyclovir (Valtrex)	**T:** 500 mg	Herpes zoster, genital herpes	Headaches, nausea
Valganciclovir (Valcyte)	**T:** 450 mg	CMV retinitis	Anemia, abdominal pain, diarrhea, headaches, nausea, vomiting, numbness in hands/feet
Zalcitabine (Hivid)	**T:** 0.375 mg, 0.75 mg	HIV infection	Numbness in arms/feet/legs, joint pain, rash, nausea, vomiting
Zanamivir (Relenza)	**Inhalation:** 5 mg	Influenza	Cough, diarrhea, dizziness, headaches, nausea, vomiting
Zidovudine (Retrovir)	**T:** 300 mg **C:** 100 mg **S:** 50 mg/5 ml	HIV infection	Unusual tiredness, fever, chills, headaches, nausea, muscle pain

AIDS, Acquired immune deficiency syndrome; *C,* capsules; *CMV,* cytomegalovirus; *HIV,* human immunodeficiency virus; *HSV-1,* herpes simplex virus type 1; *HSV-2,* herpes simplex virus type 2; *I,* injection; *OS,* oral solution; *S,* syrup; *T,* tablets.

Cancer Chemotherapeutic Agents

USES

Treatment of a variety of cancers; may be palliative or curative. Treatment of choice in hematologic cancers. Frequently used as adjunctive therapy (e.g., with surgery or

ACTION

Most antineoplastics inhibit cell replication by interfering with the supply of nutrients or genetic components of the cell (DNA or RNA). Some antineoplastics,

irradiation); most effective when tumor mass has been removed or reduced by radiation. Frequently used in combinations to increase therapeutic results, decrease toxic effects. Certain agents may be used in nonmalignant conditions; polycythemia vera, psoriasis, rheumatoid arthritis, or immunosuppression in organ transplantation.

referred to as *cell cycle-specific* (CCS), are particularly effective during a specific phase of cell reproduction (e.g., antimetabolites and plant alkaloids). Other antineoplastics, referred to as *cell cycle-nonspecific*, act independently of a specific phase of cell division (e.g., alkylating agents and antibiotics). Some hormones are also classified as antineoplastics.

CANCER CHEMOTHERAPEUTIC AGENTS

Name	Availability	Side Effects
Aldesleukin (Proleukin)	I: 22 million U Powder	Hypotension, sinus tachycardia, nausea, vomiting, diarrhea, renal impairment, anemia, rash fatigue, agitation, pulmonary congestion, dyspnea, fever, chills, oliguria, weight gain, dizziness
Alemtuzumab (Campath)	I: 30 mg/3 ml	Rigors, fever, fatigue, hypotension, neutropenia, anemia, sepsis, dyspnea, bronchitis, pneumonia, urticaria
Alitretinoin (Panretin)	Gel: 0.1%	Burning, pain, edema, dermatitis, rash, skin disorders
Altretamine (Hexalen)	C: 50 mg	Nausea, vomiting, myelosuppression, peripheral neuropathy, altered mood, ataxia, dizziness, nervousness, vertigo
Aminoglutethimide (Cytadren)	T: 250 mg	Orthostatic hypotension, hypothyroidism, vomiting, anorexia, rash, drowsiness, headaches, fever, myalgia
Anastrozole (Arimidex)	T: 1 mg	Peripheral edema, chest pain, nausea, vomiting, diarrhea, constipation, abdominal pain, anorexia, pharyngitis, vaginal hemorrhage, anemia, leukopenia, rash, weight gain, sweating, increased appetite, pain, headaches, dizziness, depression, paresthesias, hot flashes, increased cough, dry mouth, asthenia, dyspnea, phlebitis

(Continued)

Medications

CANCER CHEMOTHERAPEUTIC AGENTS—cont'd

Name	Availability	Side Effects
Arsenic trioxide (Trisenox)	**I:** 10 mg/ml	Atrioventricular block, GI hemorrhage, hypertension, hypoglycemia, hypokalemia, hypomagnesemia, neutropenia, oliguria, prolonged QT interval, seizures, sepsis, thrombocytopenia
Asparaginase (Elspar)	**I:** 10,000 U	Anorexia, nausea, vomiting, liver toxicity, pancreatitis, nephrotoxicity, clotting factor abnormalities, malaise, confusion, lethargy, EEG changes, respiratory distress, fever, hyperglycemia, depression, stomatitis, allergic reactions, drowsiness
BCG (Tice BCG, TheraCys)	**I:** 50 mg, 81 mg	Nausea, vomiting, anorexia, diarrhea, dysuria, hematuria, cystitis, urinary urgency, anemia, malaise, fever, chills
Bexarotene (Targretin)	**C:** 75 mg **Gel:** 1%	Anemia, dermatitis, fever, hypercholesterolemia, infection, leukopenia, peripheral edema
Bicalutamide (Casodex)	**T:** 50 mg	Gynecomastia, hot flashes, breast pain, nausea, diarrhea, constipation, nocturia, impotence, pain, muscle pain, asthenia, abdominal pain
Bleomycin (Blenoxane)	**I:** 15 U, 30 U	Nausea, vomiting, anorexia, stomatitis, hyperpigmentation, nail changes, alopecia, pruritus, hyperkeratosis, urticaria, pneumonitis progression to fibrosis, decreased weight, rash
Busulfan (Myleran)	**T:** 2 mg	Nausea, vomiting, hyperuricemia, myelosuppression, skin hyperpigmentation, alopecia, anorexia, decreased weight, diarrhea, stomatitis
Capecitabine (Xeloda)	**T:** 150 mg, 300 mg	Nausea, vomiting, diarrhea, stomatitis, bone marrow depression, hand-and-foot syndrome, dermatitis, fatigue, anorexia
Carboplatin (Paraplatin)	**I:** 50 mg, 150 mg, 450 mg	Nausea, vomiting, nephrotoxicity, bone marrow suppression, alopecia, peripheral neuropathy, hypersensitivity, ototoxicity, asthenia, diarrhea, constipation

Carmustine (BiCNU)	**I:** 100 mg	Anorexia, nausea, vomiting, bone marrow depression, pulmonary fibrosis, pain at injection site, diarrhea, skin discoloration
Chlorambucil (Leukeran)	**T:** 2 mg	Bone marrow suppression, dermatitis, nausea, vomiting, liver toxicity, anorexia, diarrhea, abdominal discomfort, rash
Cisplatin (Platinol)	**I:** 50 mg, 100 mg	Nausea, vomiting, nephrotoxicity, bone marrow depression, neuropathies, ototoxicity, anaphylactic-like reactions, hyperuricemia, hypomagnesemia, hypophosphatemia, hypokalemia, hypocalcemia, pain at injection site
Cladribine (Leustatin)	**I:** 1 mg/ml	Nausea, vomiting, diarrhea, bone marrow depression, chills, fatigue, rash, fever, headaches, anorexia, diaphoresis
Cyclophosphamide (Cytoxan)	**I:** 100 mg, 200 mg, 500 mg, 1 g, 2 g **T:** 25 mg, 50 mg	Nausea, vomiting, hemorrhagic cystitis, bone marrow depression, alopecia, interstitial pulmonary fibrosis, amenorrhea, azoospermia, diarrhea, darkening skin/fingernails, headaches, diaphoresis
Cytarabine (Cytosar, Ara-C)	**I:** 100 mg, 500 mg, 1 g, 2 g	Anorexia, nausea, vomiting, stomatitis, esophagitis, diarrhea, bone marrow depression, alopecia, rash, fever, neuropathies, abdominal pain
Dacarbazine (DTIC)	**I:** 200 mg	Nausea, vomiting, anorexia, liver necrosis, bone marrow depression, alopecia, rash, facial flushing, photosensitivity, flulike syndrome, confusion, blurred vision
Dactinomycin (Cosmegen)	**I:** 0.5 mg vial	Nausea, vomiting, stomatitis, esophagitis, pharyngitis, GI ulceration, proctitis, diarrhea, bone marrow depression, alopecia, erythema, acne, skin eruptions, hypocalcemia, fever, fatigue, myalgia, anorexia
Daunorubicin (Cerubidine)	**I:** 20 mg	CHF, nausea, vomiting, stomatitis, mucositis, diarrhea, red urine, bone marrow depression, alopecia, fever, chills, abdominal pain

(Continued)

Medications

CANCER CHEMOTHERAPEUTIC AGENTS—cont'd

Name	Availability	Side Effects
Daunorubicin (DaunoXome)	**I:** 50 mg	Nausea, diarrhea, abdominal pain, anorexia, vomiting, stomatitis, myelosuppression, rigors, back pain, headaches, neuropathy, depression, dyspnea, fatigue, fever, cough, allergic reactions, sweating
Denileukin (Ontak)	**I:** 300 µg/2 ml	Hypersensitivity reaction, back pain, dyspnea, rash, chest pain, tachycardia, asthenia, flulike syndrome, chills, nausea, vomiting, infection
Docetaxel (Taxotere)	**I:** 20 mg, 80 mg	Hypotension, nausea, vomiting, diarrhea, mucositis, bone marrow suppression, rash, paresthesia, hypersensitivity, fluid retention, alopecia, asthenia, stomatitis, fever
Doxorubicin (Adriamycin)	**I:** 10 mg, 20 mg, 50 mg, 75 mg, 150 mg, 200 mg	Cardiotoxicity; including; CHF; arrhythmias; nausea; vomiting; stomatitis; esophagitis; GI ulceration; diarrhea; anorexia; red urine; bone marrow depression; alopecia; hyperpigmentation of nail beds and skin; local inflammation at injection site; rash; fever; chills; urticaria; lacrimation; conjunctivitis
Doxorubicin (Doxil)	**I:** 20 mg, 50 mg	Neutropenia, palmoplantar erythrodysesthesia syndrome, cardiomyopathy, CHF
Epirubicin (Ellence)	**I:** 2 mg/ml	Anemia, leukopenia, neutropenia, infection, mucositis
Estramustine (Emcyt)	**C:** 140 mg	Increased risk of thrombosis, gynecomastia, nausea, vomiting, diarrhea, thrombocytopenia, peripheral edema
Etoposide (VePesid)	**I:** 20 mg/ml **C:** 50 mg	Nausea, vomiting, anorexia, bone marrow depression, alopecia, diarrhea, somnolence, peripheral neuropathies
Exemestane (Aromasin)	**T:** 25 mg	Dyspnea, edema, hypertension, mental depression
Floxuridine (FUDR)	**I:** 500-mg vial	Aphthous, stomatitis, enteritis

Fludarabine (Fludara)	**I:** 50 mg	Nausea, diarrhea, stomatitis, bleeding, anemia, bone marrow depression, skin rash, weakness, confusion, visual disturbances, peripheral neuropathy, coma, pneumonia, peripheral edema, anorexia
Fluorouracil	**I:** 50 mg/ml **Cream:** 1%, 5% **Solution:** 1%, 2%, 5%	Nausea, vomiting, stomatitis, GI ulceration, diarrhea, anorexia, bone marrow depression, alopecia, skin hyperpigmentation, nail changes, headaches, drowsiness, blurred vision, fever
Flutamide (Eulexin)	**C:** 125 mg	Hot flashes, nausea, vomiting, diarrhea, hepatitis, impotence, decreased libido, rash, anorexia
Fulvestrant (Faslodex)	**I:** 250 mg/5 ml, 125 mg/ 2.5 ml syringes	Asthenia, pain, headache, injection site pain, flulike symptoms, fever, nausea, vomiting, constipation, anorexia, diarrhea, peripheral edema, dizziness, depression, anxiety, rash, increased cough, UTI
Gemcitabine (Gemzar)	**I:** 200 mg, 1 g	Increased LFTs, nausea, vomiting, diarrhea, stomatitis, hematuria, myelosuppression, rash, mild paresthesias, dyspnea, fever, edema, flulike symptoms, constipation
Gemtuzumab (Mylotarg)	**I:** 5 mg/20 ml	Anemia, hematuria, liver toxicity, pneumonia, herpes simplex, nausea, vomiting, dyspnea, headaches, hypotension, hypoxia, mucositis, myelosuppression, peripheral edema, tachycardia, thrombocytopenia
Goserelin (Zoladex)	**I:** 3.6 mg, 10.8 mg	Hot flashes, sexual dysfunction, decreased erections, gynecomastia, breast swelling, lethargy, pain, lower urinary tract symptoms, headaches, nausea, depression, sweating
Hydroxyurea (Hydrea)	**C:** 500 mg	Anorexia, nausea, vomiting, stomatitis, diarrhea, constipation, bone marrow depression, fever, chills, malaise
Ibritumomab (Zevalin)	Injection kit	Neutropenia, thrombocytopenia, anemia, infection, asthenia, abdominal pain, fever, pain, headache, nausea, peripheral edema, allergic reaction, GI hemorrhage, apnea

(Continued)

Medications

CANCER CHEMOTHERAPEUTIC AGENTS—cont'd

Name	Availability	Side Effects
Idarubicin (Idamycin)	**I:** 5 mg, 10 mg, 20 mg	CHF, arrhythmias, nausea, vomiting, stomatitis, bone marrow depression, alopecia, rash, urticaria, hyperuricemia, abdominal pain, diarrhea, esophagitis, anorexia
Ifosfamide (Ifex)	**I:** 1 g, 3 g	Nausea, vomiting, hemorrhagic cystitis, bone marrow depression, alopecia, lethargy, somnolence, confusion, hallucinations, hematuria
Imatinib (Gleevec)	**C:** 100 mg	Nausea, fluid retention, hemorrhage, musculoskeletal pain, arthralgia, weight gain, pyrexia, abdominal pain, dyspnea, pneumonia
Interferon alfa 2a (Roferon-A)	**I:** 3 million U, 6 million U, 9 million U, 18 million U	Anorexia, nausea, diarrhea, bone marrow depression, pruritus, myalgia, dizziness, headaches, paresthesias, numbness, fatigue, fever, chills, dyspnea, flulike symptoms, vomiting, coughing, altered taste
Interferon alfa 2b (Intron-A)	**I:** 3 million U, 5 million U, 10 million U, 18 million U, 25 million U, 50 million U	Mild hypotension, hypertension, tachycardia with high fever, nausea, diarrhea, altered taste, weight loss, thrombocytopenia, bone marrow depression, rash, pruritus, myalgia, arthralgia associated with flulike syndromes
Irinotecan (Camptosar)	**I:** 40 mg, 100 mg	Diarrhea, nausea, vomiting, abdominal cramping, anorexia, stomatitis, increased SGOT (AST), severe myelosuppression, alopecia, sweating, rash, decreased weight, dehydration, increased alkaline phosphatase, headaches, insomnia, dizziness, dyspnea, cough, asthenia, rhinitis, fever, pain, back pain, chills
Letrozole (Femara)	**T:** 2.5 mg	Hypertension, nausea, vomiting, constipation, diarrhea, abdominal pain, anorexia, rash, pruritus, musculoskeletal pain, back pain, arm/leg pain, arthralgia, fatigue, headaches, dyspnea, coughing, hot flashes

Leuprolide (Lupron)	**I:** 3.75 mg, 5 mg, 7.5 mg, 11.25 mg, 15 mg, 22.5 mg,30 mg	Hot flashes, gynecomastia, nausea, vomiting, constipation, anorexia, dizziness, headaches, insomnia, paresthesias, bone pain
Lomustine (CeeNU)	**C:** 10 mg, 40 mg, 100 mg	Anorexia, nausea, vomiting, stomatitis, liver toxicity, nephrotoxicity, bone marrow depression, alopecia, confusion, slurred speech
Mechlorethamine (Mustargen)	**I:** 10 mg/ml	Severe nausea and vomiting, metallic taste, diarrhea, bone marrow depression, alopecia, phlebitis, vertigo, tinnitus, hyperuricemia, infertility, azoospermia, anorexia, headaches, drowsiness, fever
Megestrol (Megace)	**T:** 20 mg, 40 mg **Suspension:** 40 mg/ml	Deep vein thrombosis, Cushing-like syndrome, alopecia, carpal tunnel syndrome, weight gain, nausea
Melphalan (Alkeran)	**T:** 2 mg	Anorexia, nausea, vomiting, bone marrow depression, diarrhea, stomatitis
Mercaptopurine (Purinethol)	**T:** 50 mg	Anorexia, nausea, vomiting, stomatitis, liver toxicity, bone marrow depression, hyperuricemia, diarrhea, rash
Methotrexate	**T:** 2.5 mg, 5 mg, 7.5 mg, 10 mg,15 mg **I:** 5 mg, 50 mg, 100 mg, 200 mg, 250 mg	Nausea, vomiting, stomatitis, GI ulceration, diarrhea, liver toxicity, renal failure, cystitis, bone marrow suppression, alopecia, urticaria, acne, photosensitivity, interstitial pneumonitis, fever, malaise, chills, anorexia
Mitomycin-C (Mutamycin)	**I:** 20 mg, 40 mg	Anorexia, nausea, vomiting, stomatitis, diarrhea, renal toxicity, bone marrow depression, alopecia, pruritus, fever, hemolytic uremic syndrome, weakness
Mitotane (Lysodren)	**T:** 500 mg	Anorexia, nausea, vomiting, diarrhea, skin rashes, depression, lethargy, somnolence, dizziness, adrenal insufficiency, blurred vision, decreased hearing

(Continued)

Medications

CANCER CHEMOTHERAPEUTIC AGENTS—cont'd

Name	Availability	Side Effects
Mitoxantrone (Novantrone)	I: 20 mg, 25 mg, 30 mg	CHF, tachycardia, ECG changes, chest pain, nausea, vomiting, stomatitis, mucositis, myelosuppression, rash, alopecia, urine color change to bluish green, phlebitis, diarrhea, cough, headaches, fever
Nilutamide (Nilandron)	T: 50 mg	Hypertension, angina, hot flashes, nausea, anorexia, increased liver enzymes, dizziness, dyspnea, visual disturbances, impaired adaptation to dark, constipation, loss of libido
Oxaliplatin (Eloxatin)	I: 50 mg, 100 mg	Fatigue, neuropathy, abdominal pain, dyspnea, diarrhea, nausea, vomiting, anorexia, fever, edema, chest pain, anemia, thrombocytopenia, thromboembolism, altered LFTs
Paclitaxel (Taxol)	I: 30 mg, 100 mg	Hypertension, bradycardia, ECG changes, nausea, vomiting, diarrhea, mucositis, bone marrow depression, alopecia, peripheral neuropathies, hypersensitivity reaction, arthralgia, myalgia
Pegasparase (Oncaspar)	I: 750 IU/ml	Hypotension, anorexia, nausea, vomiting, liver toxicity, pancreatitis, depression of clotting factors, malaise, confusion, lethargy, EEG changes, respiratory distress, hypersensitivity reaction, fever, hyperglycemia, stomatitis
Pentostatin (Nipent)	I: 10 mg	Nausea, vomiting, liver disorder, elevated LFTs, leukopenia, anemia, thrombocytopenia, rash, fever, upper respiratory infection, fatigue, hematuria, headaches, myalgia, arthralgia, diarrhea, anorexia
Plicamycin (Mithracin)	I: 2.5 mg	Anorexia, nausea, vomiting, stomatitis, diarrhea, clotting factor disorders, facial flushing, mental depression, confusion, fever, hypocalcemia, hypophosphatemia, hypokalemia, headaches, dizziness, rash

Procarbazine (Matulane)	**C:** 50 mg	Nausea, vomiting, stomatitis, diarrhea, constipation, bone marrow depression, pruritus, hyperpigmentation, alopecia, myalgia, paresthesias, confusion, lethargy, mental depression, fever, liver toxicity, arthralgia, respiratory disorders
Rituximab (Rituxan)	**I:** 100 mg, 500 mg	Hypotension, arrhythmias, peripheral edema, nausea, vomiting, abdominal pain, leukopenia, thrombocytopenia, neutropenia, rash, pruritus, urticaria, angioedema, myalgia, headaches, dizziness, throat irritation, rhinitis, bronchospasm, hypersensitivity reaction
Streptozocin (Zanosar)	**I:** 1 g	May lead to insulin-dependent diabetes, nausea, vomiting, nephrotoxicity, renal tubular acidosis, bone marrow depression, lethargy, diarrhea, confusion, depression
Tamoxifen (Nolvadex)	**T:** 10 mg, 20 mg	Skin rash, nausea, vomiting, anorexia, menstrual irregularities, hot flashes, pruritus, vaginal discharge or bleeding, bone marrow depression, headaches, tumor or bone pain, ophthalmic changes, weight gain, confusion
Temozolomide (Temodar)	**C:** 5 mg, 20 mg, 100 mg, 250 mg	Amnesia, fever, infection, leukopenia, neutropenia, peripheral edema, seizures, thrombocytopenia
Teniposide (Vumon)	**I:** 50 mg/5 ml	Hypotension with rapid infusion, diarrhea, nausea, vomiting, mucositis, bone marrow depression, alopecia, anemia, rash, hypersensitivity reaction
Thioguanine	**T:** 40 mg	Anorexia, stomatitis, bone marrow depression, hyperuricemia, nausea, vomiting, diarrhea
Thiotepa (Thioplex)	**I:** 15 mg	Anorexia, nausea, vomiting, mucositis, bone marrow depression, amenorrhea, reduced spermatogenesis, fever, hypersensitivity reactions, pain at injection site, headaches, dizziness, alopecia
Topotecan (Hycamtin)	**I:** 4 mg	Nausea, vomiting, diarrhea, constipation, abdominal pain, stomatitis, anorexia, neutropenia, leukopenia, thrombocytopenia, anemia, alopecia, headaches, dyspnea, paresthesia

(Continued)

Medications

CANCER CHEMOTHERAPEUTIC AGENTS—cont'd

Name	Availability	Side Effects
Toremifene (Fareston)	**T:** 60 mg	Elevated LFTs, nausea, vomiting, constipation, skin discoloration, dermatitis, dizziness, hot flashes, sweating, vaginal discharge or bleeding, ocular changes, cataracts, anxiety
Trastuzumab (Herceptin)	**I:** 440 mg	CHF, S_3 gallop, nausea, vomiting, diarrhea, abdominal pain, anorexia, rash, peripheral edema, back or bone pain, asthenia, headaches, insomnia, dizziness, cough, dyspnea, rhinitis, pharyngitis
Tretinoin (Vesanoid)	**C:** 10 mg	Flushing, nausea, vomiting, diarrhea, constipation, dyspepsia, mucositis, leukocytosis, dry skin/mucous membranes, rash, itching, alopecia, dizziness, anxiety, insomnia, headaches, depression, confusion, intracranial hypertension, agitation, dyspnea, shivering, fever, visual changes, earaches, hearing loss, bone pain, myalgia, arthralgia
Valrubicin (Valstar)	**I:** 200 mg/5 ml	Dysuria, hematuria, urinary frequency/incontinence, red urine, urinary urgency
Vinblastine (Velban)	**I:** 10 mg	Nausea, vomiting, stomatitis, constipation, bone marrow depression, alopecia, peripheral neuropathy, loss of deep tendon reflexes, paresthesias, diarrhea
Vincristine (Oncovin)	**I:** 1 mg, 2 mg, 3 mg	Nausea, vomiting, stomatitis, constipation, pharyngitis, polyuria, bone marrow depression, alopecia, numbness, paresthesias, peripheral neuropathy, loss of deep tendon reflexes, headaches, abdominal pain
Vinorelbine (Navelbine)	**I:** 10 mg, 50 mg	Elevated LFTs, nausea, vomiting, constipation, ileus, anorexia, stomatitis, bone marrow suppression, alopecia, vein discoloration, venous pain, phlebitis, interstitial pulmonary changes, asthenia, fatigue, diarrhea, peripheral neuropathy, loss of deep tendon reflexes

C, Capsules; *CHF,* congestive heart failure; *ECG,* electrocardiogram; *EEG,* electroencephalogram; *GI,* gastrointestinal; *I,* injection; *LFT,* liver function test; *T,* tablets; *UTI,* urinary tract infection.

Corticosteroids

USES

Symptomatic treatment of multiorgan disease/conditions. Rheumatoid arthritis, osteoarthritis, severe psoriasis, ulcerative colitis, lupus erythematosus, anaphylactic shock, status asthmaticus, organ transplant.

ACTION

Suppress migration of polymorphonuclear leukocytes (PML) and reverse increased capillary permeability by their antiinflammatory effect. Suppress immune system by decreasing activity of lymphatic system.

CORTICOSTEROIDS

Name	Availability	Route of Administration	Side Effects
Beclomethasone (Beclovent, Beconase, Vanceril, Vancenase)	**Inhalation, nasal:** 42 mg/spray, 84 mg/spray	Inhalation, intranasal	**I:** Cough, dry mouth/throat, headaches, throat irritation **Nasal:** Headaches, sore throat, sores inside nose
Betamethasone (Celestone, Diprosone)	**I:** 4 mg/ml	IV, intralesional, intra-articular	Nausea, vomiting, increased appetite, weight gain, trouble sleeping
Budesonide (Rhinocort, Pulmicort)	**Nasal:** 32 mg/spray	Intranasal	**Nasal:** Headaches, sore throat, sores inside nose
Cortisone (Cortone)	**T:** 5 mg, 10 mg, 25 mg	PO	Same as betamethasone
Dexamethasone (Decadron)	**T:** 0.5 mg, 1 mg, 4 mg, 6 mg **OS:** 0.5 mg/5 ml **I:** 4 mg/ml	PO, parenteral	Same as betamethasone

(Continued)

CORTICOSTEROIDS—cont'd

Name	Availability	Route of Administration	Side Effects
Fludrocortisone (Florinef)	**T:** 0.1 mg	PO	Same as betamethasone
Flunisolide (AeroBid, Nasalide)	**Inhalation, nasal:** 25 µg/spray	Inhalation, intranasal	Same as beclomethasone
Fluticasone (Flonase, Flovent)	**Inhalation:** 44 µg, 110 µg, 220 mg **Nasal:** 50 mg, 100 µg	Inhalation, intranasal	Same as beclomethasone
Hydrocortisone (Cortef, Solu-Cortef)	**T:** 5 mg, 10 mg, 25 mg **I:** 100 mg, 250 mg, 500 mg, 1 g	PO, parenteral	Same as betamethasone
Methylprednisolone (Solu-Medrol)	**T:** 4 mg **I:** 40 mg, 125 mg, 500 mg, 1 g, 2 g	PO, parenteral	Same as betamethasone
Prednisolone (Prelone)	**T:** 5 mg **OS:** 5 mg/5 ml, 15 mg/5 ml	PO	Same as betamethasone
Prednisone (Deltasone)	**T:** 1 mg, 2.5 mg, 5 mg, 10 mg, 20 mg, 50 mg	PO	Same as betamethasone
Triamcinolone (Azmacort, Kenalog)	**T:** 4 mg, 8 mg **Inhalation:** 100 mg	PO, inhalation	Same as betamethasone **I:** Cough, dry mouth/throat, headaches, throat irritation

I, Injection; *IV,* intravenously; *OS,* oral suspension; *PO,* by mouth; *T,* tablets.

Diuretics

USES

Thiazides: Management of edema resulting from a number of causes (e.g, CHF, hepatic cirrhosis); hypertension either alone or in combination with other antihypertensives.

Loop: Management of edema associated with CHF, cirrhosis of the liver, and renal disease. Furosemide used in treatment of hypertension alone or in combination with other antihypertensives.

Potassium-sparing: Adjunctive treatment with thiazides, loop diuretics in treatment of CHF and hypertension.

ACTION

Thiazides: Act at the cortical diluting segment of nephron, block reabsorption of Na, Cl, and water; promote excretion of Na, Cl, K, and water.

Loop: Act primarily at the thick ascending limb of Henle's loop to inhibit Na, Cl, and water absorption.

Potassium-sparing: Spironolactone blocks aldosterone action on distal nephron (causes K retention, Na excretion). Triamterene, amiloride act on distal nephron, decreasing Na reuptake, reducing K secretion.

DIURETICS

Name	Availability	Dosage Range	Side Effects
Thiazides			
Chlorothiazide (Diuril)	**T:** 250 mg, 500 mg **S:** 250 mg/5 ml **I:** 500 mg	5–20 mg/day	Confusion, fatigue, muscle cramps, upset stomach
Chlorthalidone (Hygroton)	**T:** 15 mg, 25 mg, 50 mg, 100 mg	25–200 mg/day	Same as chlorothiazide
Hydrochlorothiazide (HydroDIURIL)	**T:** 25 mg, 50 mg, 100 mg **C:** 12.5 mg **Solution:** 50 mg/15 ml	25–100 mg/day	Same as chlorothiazide

(Continued)

Medications

DIURETICS—cont'd

Name	Availability	Dosage Range	Side Effects
Thiazides—cont'd			
Indapamide (Lozol)	**T:** 1.25 mg, 2.5 mg	2.5–5 mg/day	Same as chlorothiazide
Metolazone (Diulo, Zaroxolyn)	**T:** 2.5 mg, 5 mg, 10 mg	2.5–10 mg/day	Same as chlorothiazide
Loop			
Bumetanide (Bumex)	**T:** 0.5 mg, 1 mg, 2 mg **I:** 0.25 mg/ml	5–10 mg/day	Orthostatic hypotension
Ethacrynic acid (Edecrin)	**T:** 25 mg, 50 mg **I:** 50 mg vial	50–200 mg/day	Same as bumetanide
Furosemide (Lasix)	**T:** 20 mg, 40 mg, 80 mg **OS:** 10 mg/ml, 40 mg/5 ml **I:** 10 mg/ml	**HTN:** 40–80 mg/day **Edema:** Up to 600 mg/day	Same as bumetanide
Torsemide (Demadex)	**T:** 5 mg, 10 mg, 20 mg, 100 mg **I:** 10 mg/ml	**Edema:** 10–200 mg/day **HTN:** 5–10 mg/day	Constipation, dizziness, headaches, stomach upset
Potassium-Sparing			
Amiloride (Midamor)	**T:** 5 mg	5–20 mg/day	Hyperkalemia
Spironolactone (Aldactone)	**T:** 25 mg, 50 mg, 100 mg	25–100 mg/day	Hyperkalemia, nausea, vomiting, cramps, diarrhea
Triamterene (Dyrenium)	**C:** 50 mg, 100 mg	Up to 300 mg/day	Same as amiloride

C, Capsules; *HTN,* hypertension; *I,* injection; *OS,* oral solution; *S,* suspension; *T,* tablets.

H₂ Antagonists

USES

Short-term treatment of duodenal ulcer (DU), active benign gastric ulcer (GU); maintenance therapy of DU; pathologic hypersecretory conditions (e.g., Zollinger-Ellison syndrome); gastroesophageal reflux disease (GERD); and prevention of upper gastrointestinal bleeding in critically ill patients.

ACTION

Inhibit gastric acid secretion by interfering with histamine at the histamine H_2 receptors in parietal cells. Also inhibit acid secretion caused by gastrin.

H₂ ANTAGONISTS

Name	Availability	Dosage Range	Side Effects
Cimetidine (Tagamet)	T: 200 mg, 300 mg, 400 mg, 800 mg L: 300 mg/5 ml I: 150 mg/ml	**Treatment of DU:** 800 mg/at bedtime, 400 mg 2 times/day or 300 mg 4 times/day **Maintenance of DU:** 400 mg/at bedtime **Treatment of GU:** 800 mg/at bedtime or 300 mg 4 times/day **GERD:** 1600 mg/day **Hypersecretory:** 1200–2400 mg/day	Headaches, fatigue, dizziness, confusion, diarrhea, gynecomastia
Famotidine (Pepcid)	T: 10 mg, 20 mg, 40 mg T (chewable): 10 mg T (DT): 20 mg, 40 mg Gelcap: 10 mg OS: 40 mg/5 ml I: 10 mg/ml	**Treatment of DU:** 40 mg/day **Maintenance of DU:** 20 mg/day **Treatment of GU:** 40 mg/day **GERD:** 40–80 mg/day **Hypersecretory:** 80–640 mg/day	Headaches, dizziness, diarrhea, constipation, abdominal pain, tinnitus

(Continued)

Medications

H₂ ANTAGONISTS—cont'd

Name	Availability	Dosage Range	Side Effects
Nizatidine (Axid)	**T:** 75 mg **C:** 150 mg, 300 mg	**Treatment of DU:** 300 mg/day **Maintenance of DU:** 150 mg/day	Fatigue, urticaria, abdominal pain, constipation, nausea
Ranitidine (Zantac)	**T:** 75 mg, 150 mg, 300 mg **C:** 150 mg, 300 mg **Syrup:** 15 mg/ml **Granules:** 150 mg **I:** 0.5 mg/ml, 25 mg/ml	**Treatment of DU:** 300 mg/day **Maintenance of DU:** 150 mg/day **Treatment of GU:** 300 mg/day **GERD:** 300 mg/day **Hypersecretory:** 0.3–6 g/day	Blurred vision, constipation, nausea, abdominal pain

C, Capsules; *DT*, disintegrating tablets; *DU*, duodenal ulcer; *GERD*, gastroesophageal reflux disease; *GU*, gastric ulcer; *I*, injection; *L*, liquid; *OS*, oral suspension; *T*, tablets.

Human Immunodeficiency Virus (HIV) Infection

USES

Antiretroviral agents are used in the treatment of HIV infection.

ACTION

There are currently four classes of antiretroviral agents used in the treatment of HIV disease: *nucleoside reverse transcriptase inhibitors (NRTIs), nucleotide reverse transcriptase inhibitors (NtRTIs), nonnucleoside reverse transcriptase inhibitors (NNRTIs), and protease inhibitors (PIs).*

ANTIRETROVIRAL AGENTS FOR TREATMENT OF HIV INFECTION

Name	Availability	Dosage Range	Side Effects
Nucleoside Analogues			
Abacavir (Ziagen)	**T:** 300 mg **OS:** 20 mg/ml	**A:** 300 mg 2 times/day	Nausea, vomiting, malaise, rash, fever, headaches, asthenia, fatigue
Didanosine (Videx)	**T:** 25 mg, 50 mg, 100 mg, 150 mg, 200 mg **C:** 125 mg, 200 mg, 250 mg, 400 mg **OS:** 100 mg, 167 mg, 250 mg	**T (>60 kg):** 200 mg 2 times/day; **(<60 kg):** 125 mg 2 times/day **OS (>60 kg):** 250 mg 2 times/day; **(<60 kg):** 167 mg 2 times/day	Peripheral neuropathy, pancreatitis, diarrhea, nausea, vomiting, headaches, insomnia, rash, hepatitis, seizures
Emtricitabine (Emtriva, FTC)	N/A	**A:** 200 mg/day	Hyperpigmentation of palms, soles
Lamivudine (Epivir)	**T:** 100 mg, 150 mg **OS:** 5 mg/ml, 10 mg/ml	**A:** 150 mg 2 times/day **C:** 4 mg/kg 2 times/day	Diarrhea, malaise, fatigue, headaches, nausea, vomiting, abdominal pain, peripheral neuropathy, arthralgia, myalgia, skin rash
Stavudine (Zerit)	**C:** 15 mg, 20 mg, 30 mg, 40 mg **OS:** 1 mg/ml	**A:** 40 mg 2 times/day (20 mg 2 times/day if peripheral neuropathy occurs)	Peripheral neuropathy, anemia, leukopenia, neutropenia
Zalcitabine (Hivid)	**T:** 0.375 mg, 0.75 mg	**A (>60 kg):** 0.75 mg 3 times/day; **(<60 kg):** 0.375 mg 3 times/day	Peripheral neuropathy, stomatitis, granulocytopenia, leukopenia
Zidovudine (Retrovir)	**C:** 100 mg **T:** 300 mg **Syrup:** 50 mg/5 ml, 10 mg/ml	**A:** 500–600 mg/day (100 mg 5 times/day or 300 mg 2 times/day)	Anemia, granulocytopenia, myopathy, nausea, malaise, fatigue, insomnia

(Continued)

Medications

ANTIRETROVIRAL AGENTS FOR TREATMENT OF HIV INFECTION—cont'd

Name	Availability	Dosage Range	Side Effects
Nucleoside Analogues—cont'd			
Zidovudine/lamivudine (AZT/3TC) (Combivir)	C: 300 mg AZT/150 mg 3TC	A: 1 capsule 2 times/day	Bone marrow suppression, peripheral neuropathy, pancreatitis
Zidovudine/lamivudine/ abacavir (AZT/3TC/ABC) (Trizivir)	C: 300 mg AZT/150 mg 3TC/300 mg ABC	A: 1 capsule 2 times/day	Bone marrow suppression, peripheral neuropathy, anaphylactic reaction
Nucleotide Analogues			
Tenofovir (Viread)	T: 300 mg	A: 300 mg/day	Nausea, vomiting, diarrhea
Nonnucleoside Analogues			
Delavirdine (Rescriptor)	T: 100 mg, 200 mg	A: 200 mg 3 times/day for 14 days, then 400 mg 3 times/day	Rash, nausea, headaches, elevations in liver function tests (LFTs)
Efavirenz (Sustiva)	C: 50 mg, 100 mg, 200 mg	A: 600 mg/day C: 200–600 mg/day based on weight	Headaches, dizziness, insomnia, fatigue, rash, nightmares
Nevirapine (Viramune)	T: 200 mg	A: 200 mg/day for 14 days, then 200 mg 2 times/day	Rash, nausea, fatigue, fever, headaches, abnormal LFTs
Protease Inhibitors			
Amprenavir (Agenerase)	C: 50 mg, 150 mg OS: 15 mg/ml	A: 1200 mg 2 times/day C (4–16 yrs, <50 kg): 20 mg/kg	Rash, diarrhea, headaches, nausea, vomiting, numbness, abdominal pain, fatigue

		2 times/day or 15 mg/kg 3 times/day	
Atazanavir (Reyataz)	N/A	A: 400 mg/day	Increased liver function tests, jaundice, scleral icterus
Indinavir (Crixivan)	C: 200 mg, 400 mg	A: 800 mg q8h	Nephrolithiasis, hyperbilirubinemia, abdominal pain, asthenia, fatigue, flank pain, nausea, vomiting, diarrhea, headaches, insomnia, dizziness, altered taste
Lopinavir/ritonavir (Kaletra)	C: 133/33 mg OS: 80/20 mg	A: 400/100 mg/day C (4–12 yrs): 10–13 mg/kg 2 times/day	Diarrhea, nausea, vomiting, abdominal pain, headaches, rash
Nelfinavir (Viracept)	T: 250 mg Oral Powder: 50 mg/g	A: 750 mg q8h C: 20–25 mg/kg q8h	Diarrhea, fatigue, asthenia, headaches, hypertension, decreased ability to concentrate
Ritonavir (Norvir)	C: 100 mg OS: 80 mg/ml	A: Titrate up to 600 mg 2 times/day	Nausea, vomiting, diarrhea, altered taste sensation, fatigue, elevated LFTs and triglyceride levels
Saquinavir (Invirase)	C: 200 mg	A: 600 mg 3 times/day	Diarrhea, elevations in LFTs, hypertriglycerides, cholesterol, abnormal fat accumulation, hyperglycemia
Saquinavir (Fortovase)	C: 200 mg	A: 1200 mg 3 times/day	Diarrhea, elevations in LFTs, hypertriglycerides, cholesterol, abnormal fat accumulation, hyperglycemia

A, Adults; *C,* capsules; *C* (dosage), children; *OS,* oral solution; *T,* tablets.

Medications

Laxatives

USES

Short-term treatment of constipation; colon evacuation before rectal/bowel examination; prevention of straining (e.g., after anorectal surgery, myocardial infarction); to reduce painful elimination (e.g., episiotomy, hemorrhoids, anorectal lesions); modification of effluent from ileostomy, colostomy; prevention of fecal impaction; removal of ingested poisons.

ACTION

Laxatives ease or stimulate defecation. Mechanisms by which this is accomplished include (1) attracting, retaining fluid in colonic contents due to hydrophilic or osmotic properties; (2) acting directly or indirectly on mucosa to decrease absorption of water and NaCl; or (3) increasing intestinal motility, decreasing absorption of water and NaCl by virtue of decreased transit time.

Bulk-forming: Act primarily in small/large intestine. Produce soft stool in 1–3 days.

Lubricants: Promote stool passage by coating the fecal surface with an oil layer that retains fecal fluid and prevents absorption of fecal water by the colon.

Hyperosmotic agents: Act in colon. Produce soft stool in 1–3 days.

Saline: Acts in small/large intestine, colon (sodium phosphate). Produces watery stool in 2–6 hrs (small doses produce semifluid stool in 6–12 hrs).

Stimulants: Act in colon. Produce semifluid stool in 6–12 hrs.

Surfactants: Act in small/large intestine. Produce soft stool in 1–3 days.

LAXATIVES

Name	Onset of Action	Uses
Bulk		
Psyllium (Metamucil, Konsyl)	12–24 hrs up to 3 days	First line for postpartum women; elderly; patients with diverticulosis, irritable bowel syndrome, hemorrhoids. Safe for chronic use
Methylcellulose (Citrucel)	12–24 hrs up to 3 days	First line for postpartum women; elderly; patients with diverticulosis; irritable bowel syndrome, hemorrhoids. Safe for chronic use
Polycarbophil (Fibercon, Mitrolan)	Same as above	Same as methylcellulose
Surfactant		
Docusate sodium (Colace)	1–3 days	Aids in passage of hard, painful feces; prevents straining
Docusate calcium (Surfak)	Same as above	Same as docusate sodium
Docusate potassium (Dialose)	Same as above	Same as docusate sodium
Lubricant		
Mineral oil (Kondremul)	6–8 hrs	Prevents straining
Saline		
Magnesium citrate (Citro-Nesia)	30 min to 3 hrs	Bowel evacuation for colonic procedures/examinations, fecal impaction, hepatic coma

(Continued)

Medications

LAXATIVES—cont'd

Name	Onset of Action	Uses
Saline—cont'd		
Magnesium hydroxide	Same as above	Same as magnesium citrate
Sodium phosphate (Fleets Phospho-Soda)	5–15 min	Same as magnesium citrate
Hyperosmotic		
Glycerin	<30 min	Short-term relief of constipation
Lactulose (Chronulac)	1–3 days	Hepatic comas
Polyethylene glycol-electrolyte solution (GoLYTELY)	30–60 min	Bowel evacuation for colonic procedures/examinations
Stimulant		
Bisacodyl (Dulcolax)	**PO:** 6–12 hrs **Rectal:** 15–60 min	Same as polyethylene glycol-electrolyte solution Acts in 15–60 min.
Casanthranol *(in Peri-Colace)*	6–12 hrs	Same as polyethylene glycol-electrolyte solution
Cascara sagrada	6–12 hrs	Bowel evacuation for colonic procedures/examinations
Castor oil	6–12 hrs	Same as polyethylene glycol-electrolyte solution
Senna (Senokot)	6–12 hrs	Same as polyethylene glycol-electrolyte solution

Nonsteroidal Anti-inflammatory Drugs (NSAIDs)

USES

Provide symptomatic relief from *pain/inflammation* in the treatment of musculoskeletal disorders (e.g., rheumatoid arthritis, osteoarthritis, ankylosing spondylitis); *analgesic* for low to moderate pain; *reduction in fever* (many agents not suited for routine/prolonged therapy because of toxicity).

ACTION

Exact mechanism for antiinflammatory, analgesic, antipyretic effects unknown. Inhibition of enzyme cyclooxygenase, the enzyme responsible for prostaglandin synthesis, appears to be a major mechanism of action. Direct action on hypothalamus heat-regulating center may contribute to antipyretic effect.

NSAIDs

Name	Availability	Dosage Range	Side Effects
Aspirin	**T:** 81 mg, 160 mg, 325 mg **Suppository:** 300 mg, 600 mg	**P (A):** 325–650 mg q4h as needed **C:** Up to 60–80 mg/kg/day **Arthritis:** 3.2–6 g/day **JRA:** 60–110 mg/kg/day **RF (A):** 5–8 g/day **C:** 75–100 mg/kg/day **TIA:** 1300 mg/day **MI:** 81–325 mg/day	GI upset, dizziness, headaches
Celecoxib (Celebrex)	**C:** 100 mg, 200 mg	**OA:** 200 mg/day **RA:** 100–200 mg 2 times/day **FAP:** 400 mg 2 times/day	Diarrhea, back pain, dizziness, heartburn, headaches, nausea, stomach pain

(Continued)

Medications

NSAIDs—cont'd

Name	Availability	Dosage Range	Side Effects
Diclofenac (Voltaren)	**T:** 25 mg, 50 mg, 75 mg, 100 mg	**Arthritis:** 100–200 mg/day	Indigestion, constipation, diarrhea, nausea, headaches, fluid retention, abdominal cramps
Diflunisal (Dolobid)	**T:** 250 mg, 500 mg	**Arthritis:** 0.5–1 g/day **P:** 0.5 g q8–12h	Headaches, abdominal cramps, indigestion, diarrhea, nausea
Etodolac (Lodine)	**T:** 400 mg, 500 mg **T (ER):** 400 mg, 500 mg, 600 mg **C:** 200 mg, 300 mg	**Arthritis:** 600–800 mg/day **P:** 200–400 mg q6–8h	Indigestion, dizziness, headaches, bloated feeling, diarrhea, nausea, weakness, abdominal cramps
Fenoprofen (Nalfon)	**C:** 200 mg, 300 mg **T:** 600 mg	**Arthritis:** 300–600 mg 3–4 times/day **P:** 200 mg q4–6h as needed	Nausea, indigestion, nervousness, constipation, shortness of breath, heartburn
Flurbiprofen (Ansaid)	**T:** 50 mg, 100 mg	**Arthritis:** 200–300 mg/day	Indigestion, nausea, fluid retention, headaches, abdominal cramps, diarrhea
Ibuprofen (Motrin, Advil)	**T:** 100 mg, 200 mg, 400 mg, 600 mg, 800 mg **T (chewable):** 50 mg, 100 mg **C:** 200 mg **S:** 100 mg/5 ml, 100 mg/2.5 ml **Drops:** 40 mg/ml	**Arthritis:** 1.2–3.2 g/day **P:** 400 mg q4–6h as needed **Fever:** 200 mg q4–6h as needed **JA:** 30–40 mg/kg/day	Dizziness, abdominal cramps, stomach pain, heartburn, nausea
Indomethacin (Indocin)	**C:** 25 mg, 50 mg **C (SR):** 75 mg **S:** 25 mg/5 ml **Suppository:** 50 mg	**Arthritis:** 50–200 mg/day **Bursitis/tendinitis:** 75–150 mg/day **GA:** 150 mg/day	Fluid retention, dizziness, headaches, abdominal pain, indigestion, nausea

Ketoprofen (Orudis)	**T:** 12.5 mg **C:** 25 mg, 50 mg, 75 mg **C (ER):** 100 mg, 150 mg, 200 mg	**Arthritis:** 150–300 mg/day **P:** 25–50 mg q6–8h as needed	Headaches, nervousness, abdominal pain, bloated feeling, constipation, diarrhea, nausea
Ketorolac (Toradol)	**T:** 10 mg **I:** 15 mg/ml, 30 mg/ml	**P (PO):** 10 mg q4–6h as needed; **(IM/IV):** 60–120 mg/day	Fluid retention, abdominal pain, diarrhea, dizziness, headaches, nausea
Meloxicam (Mobic)	**C:** 7.5 mg	**Arthritis:** 7.5–15 mg/day	Heartburn, indigestion, nausea, diarrhea, headaches
Nabumetone (Relafen)	**T:** 500 mg, 750 mg	**Arthritis:** 1–2 g/day	Fluid retention, dizziness, headaches, abdominal pain, constipation, diarrhea, nausea
Naproxen (Anaprox, Naprosyn)	**T:** 200 mg, 250 mg, 375 mg, 500 mg **T (CR):** 375 mg **S:** 125 mg/5 ml	**Arthritis:** 250–550 mg/day **P:** 250 mg q6–8h **JA:** 10 mg/kg/day **GA:** 750 mg once, then 250 mg q8h	Tinnitus, fluid retention, shortness of breath, dizziness, drowsiness, headaches, abdominal pain, constipation, heartburn, nausea
Oxaprozin (Daypro)	**C:** 600 mg	**Arthritis:** 600–1800 mg/day	Constipation, diarrhea, nausea, indigestion
Piroxicam (Feldene)	**C:** 10 mg, 20 mg	**Arthritis:** 20 mg/day	Abdominal pain, stomach pain, nausea
Rofecoxib (Vioxx)	**T:** 12.5 mg, 25 mg, 50 mg	**OA:** 12.5–25 mg/day **P:** 25–50 mg/day	Weakness, diarrhea, dizziness, nausea, fluid retention, stomach pain
Sulindac (Clinoril)	**T:** 150 mg, 200 mg	**Arthritis:** 300 mg/day **GA:** 400 mg/day	Dizziness, abdominal pain, constipation, diarrhea, nausea

(Continued)

Medications

NSAIDs—cont'd

Name	Availability	Dosage Range	Side Effects
Tolmetin (Tolectin)	**T:** 200 mg, 600 mg **C:** 400 mg	**Arthritis:** 600–1800 mg/day **JA:** 15–30 mg/kg/day	Fluid retention, dizziness, headaches, weakness, abdominal pain, diarrhea, indigestion, nausea, vomiting
Valdecoxib (Bextra)	**T:** 10 mg, 20 mg	**Arthritis:** 10 mg/day **Primary dysmenorrhea:** 20 mg 2 times/day	Dyspepsia, nausea, headaches

A, Adults; *C (dosage), children; CR,* controlled-release; *ER,* extended-release; *FAP,* familial adenomatous polyposis; *GA,* gouty arthritis; *GI,* gastrointestinal; *I,* injection; *IM,* intramuscularly; *IV,* intravenously; *JA,* juvenile arthritis; *JRA,* juvenile rheumatoid arthritis; *MI,* myocardial infarction; *OA,* osteoarthritis; *P,* pain; *PO,* by mouth; *RA,* rheumatoid arthritis; *RF,* rheumatic fever; *S,* suspension; *T,* tablets; *TIA,* transient ischemic attack.

Nutrition: Enteral

INDICATIONS

Enteral nutrition (EN), also known as *tube feedings,* provides food/nutrients via the gastrointestinal (GI) tract using special formulas, delivery techniques, and equipment. All routes of EN consist of a tube through which liquid formula is infused.

Tube feedings are used in patients with major trauma, burns; those undergoing radiation and/or chemotherapy; patients with liver failure, severe renal impairment, physical or neurologic impairment; preoperatively and postoperatively to promote anabolism; prevention of cachexia, malnutrition.

ROUTES OF ENTERAL NUTRITION DELIVERY

NASOGASTRIC (NG):
INDICATIONS: Most common for short-term feeding in patients unable or unwilling to consume adequate nutrition by mouth. Requires at least a partially functioning GI tract.

ROUTES OF ENTERAL NUTRITION DELIVERY—CONT'D

INITIATING ENTERAL NUTRITION	SELECTION OF FORMULAS

NASODUODENAL (ND), NASOJEJUNAL (NJ):
INDICATIONS: Patients unable or unwilling to consume adequate nutrition by mouth. Requires at least a partially functioning GI tract.

GASTROSTOMY:
INDICATIONS: Patients with esophageal obstruction or impaired swallowing; patients in whom NG, ND, or NJ not feasible; or, when long-term feeding indicated.

JEJUNOSTOMY:
INDICATIONS: Patients with stomach or duodenal obstruction, impaired gastric motility; patients in whom NG, ND, or NJ not feasible or when long-term feeding is indicated.

With continuous feeding, initiation of isotonic (about 300 mOsm/L) or moderately hypertonic feeding (up to 495 mOsm/L) can be given full strength, usually at a slow rate (30–50 ml/hr) and gradually increased (25 ml/hr q6–24h). Formulas with osmolality of >500 mOsm/L are generally started at half strength and gradually increased in rate, then concentration. Tolerance is increased if the rate and concentration are not increased simultaneously.

Protein: Has many important physiologic roles and is the primary source of nitrogen in the body. Provides 4 kcal/g protein.
Carbohydrate (CHO): Provides energy for the body and heat to maintain body temperature. Provides 3.4 kcal/g carbohydrate.
Fat: Provides concentrated source of energy. Referred to as *kilocalorie dense* or *protein sparing.* Provides 9 kcal/g fat.
Electrolytes, vitamins, trace elements: Contained in formulas (not found in specialized products for renal and hepatic insufficiency).

(Continued)

Medications

Nutrition: Enteral—cont'd

COMPLICATIONS

MECHANICAL: Usually associated with some aspect of the feeding tube.

Aspiration pneumonia: Caused by delayed gastric emptying, gastroparesis, gastroesophageal reflux, or decreased gag reflux. May be prevented or treated by reducing infusion rate, using lower fat formula, feeding beyond pylorus, checking residuals, using small-bore feeding tubes, elevating head of bed 30'–45' during and for 30–60 min after intermittent feeding, and regularly checking tube placement.

Esophageal, mucosal, pharyngeal irritation, otitis: Caused by using large-bore NG tube. Prevented by use of small bore whenever possible.

Irritation, leakage at ostomy site: Caused by drainage of digestive juices from site. Prevented by close attention to skin/stoma care.

Tube, lumen obstruction: Caused by thickened formula residue, formation of formula-medication complexes. Prevented by frequently irrigating tube with clear water (also before and after giving formulas/medication), avoiding instilling medication if possible.

GASTROINTESTINAL: Usually associated with formula, rate of delivery, unsanitary handling of solutions or delivery system.

Diarrhea: Caused by low-residue formulas, rapid delivery, use of hyperosmolar formula, hypoalbuminemia, malabsorption, microbial contamination, or rapid GI transit time. Prevented by using fiber-supplemented formulas, decreasing rate of delivery, using dilute formula, and gradually increasing strength.

Cramping, gas, abdominal distention: Caused by nutrient malabsorption, rapid delivery of refrigerated formula. Prevented by delivering formula by continuous methods, giving formulas at room temperature, decreasing rate of delivery.

Nausea, vomiting: Caused by rapid delivery of formula, gastric retention. Prevented by reducing rate of delivery, using dilute formulas, selecting low-fat formulas.

Constipation: Caused by inadequate fluid intake, reduced bulk, inactivity. Prevented by supplementing fluid intake, using fiber-supplemented formula, encouraging ambulation.

METABOLIC: Fluid/electrolyte status should be monitored. Refer to monitoring section. In addition, the very young and very old are at greater risk of developing complications such as dehydration or overhydration.

MONITORING

Daily: Estimate nutrient intake, fluid intake/output, weight of pt, clinical observations.
Weekly: Electrolytes (potassium, sodium, magnesium, calcium, phosphorus), blood glucose, blood urea nitrogen (BUN), creatinine, liver function tests (e.g., SGOT [AST], alkaline phosphatase), 24-hr urea and creatinine excretion, total iron-binding capacity (TIBC) or serum transferrin, triglycerides, cholesterol.
Monthly: Serum albumin.
Other: Urine glucose, acetone (when blood glucose >250), vital signs (temperature, respirations, pulse, blood pressure) q8h.

Nutrition: Parenteral

INDICATIONS

Parenteral nutrition (PN), also known as *total parenteral nutrition* (TPN) or *hyperalimentation* (HAL), provides required nutrients to patients by intravenous (IV) route of administration. The goal of PN is to maintain or restore nutritional status caused by disease, injury, or inability to consume nutrients by other means.

Conditions when patient is unable to use alimentary tract via oral, gastrostomy, or jejunostomy routes. Impaired absorption of protein caused by obstruction, inflammation, or antineoplastic therapy. Bowel rest necessary because of gastrointestinal (GI) surgery or ileus, fistulas, or anastomotic leaks. Conditions with increased metabolic requirements (e.g., burns, infection, trauma). Preserve tissue reserves as in acute renal failure. Inadequate nutrition from tube feeding methods.

COMPONENTS OF PN

Protein: In the form of crystalline amino acids (CAA), primarily used for protein synthesis. Several products are designed to meet specific needs for patients with renal failure (e.g., NephrAmine), liver disease (e.g., HepatAmine), stress/trauma (e.g., Aminosyn HBC), use in neonates and pediatrics (e.g., Aminosyn PF, TrophAmine). Calories: 4 kcal/g protein.
Energy: In the form of dextrose, available in concentrations of 5%–70%. Dextrose <10% may be given

(Continued)

Medications

Nutrition: Parenteral—cont'd

COMPONENTS OF PN—cont'd

peripherally; concentrations >10% must be given centrally. Calories: 3.4 kcal/g dextrose.

IV fat emulsion: Available in the form of 10% or 20% concentrations. Provides a concentrated source of energy/calories (9 kcal/g fat) and is a source of essential fatty acids. May be administered peripherally or centrally.

Electrolytes: Major electrolytes (calcium, magnesium, potassium, sodium; also acetate, chloride, phosphate). Doses of electrolytes are individualized, based on many factors (e.g., kidney and/or liver function, fluid status).

Vitamins: Essential components in maintaining metabolism and cellular function; widely used in PN.

Trace elements: Necessary in long-term PN administration. Trace elements include zinc, copper, chromium, manganese, selenium, molybdenum, and iodine.

Miscellaneous: Additives include insulin, albumin, heparin, and histamine₂ blockers (e.g., cimetidine, ranitidine, famotidine). Other medication may be included, but compatibility for admixture should be checked on an individual basis.

ROUTES OF ADMINISTRATION

PN is administered via either peripheral or central vein.

Peripheral: Usually involves 2–3 L/day of 5%–10% dextrose with 3%–5% amino acid solution along with IV fat emulsion. Electrolytes, vitamins, trace elements are added according to pt needs. Peripheral solutions provide about 2000 kcal/day and 60–90 g protein/day.

Central: Usually uses hypertonic dextrose (concentration range of 15%–35%) and amino acid solution of 3%–7% with IV fat emulsion. Electrolytes, vitamins, trace elements are added according to patient needs. Central solutions provide 2000–4000 kcal/day. Must be given through large central vein with high blood flow, allowing rapid dilution, avoiding phlebitis/thrombosis.

MONITORING

Baseline: Complete blood count (CBC), platelet count, prothrombin time, weight, body length/head circumference (in infants), electrolytes, glucose, BUN, creatinine, uric acid, total protein, cholesterol, triglycerides, bilirubin, alkaline phosphatase, lactate dehydrogenase (LDH), SGOT (AST), albumin, other tests as needed.

Daily: Weight, vital signs (TPR), nutritional intake (kcal, protein, fat), electrolytes (potassium, sodium chloride), glucose (serum, urine), acetone, BUN, osmolarity, other tests as needed.

2-3 times/wk: CBC, coagulation studies (PT, PTT), creatinine, calcium, magnesium, phosphorus, acid-base status, other tests as needed.

Weekly: Nitrogen balance, total protein, albumin, prealbumin, transferrin, liver function tests (SGOT [AST], SGPT [ALT]), alkaline phosphatase, LDH, bilirubin, hemoglobin (Hgb), uric acid, cholesterol, triglycerides, other tests as needed.

COMPLICATIONS

Mechanical: Malfunction in system for IV delivery (e.g., pump failure; problems with lines, tubing, administration sets, catheter). Pneumothorax, catheter misdirection, arterial puncture, bleeding, hematoma formation may occur with catheter placement.

Infectious: Infections (patients often more susceptible to infections), catheter sepsis (e.g., fever, shaking chills, glucose intolerance) where no other site of infection is identified.

Metabolic: Includes hyperglycemia, elevated cholesterol and triglycerides, abnormal liver function tests.

Fluid, electrolyte, acid-base disturbances: May alter potassium, sodium, phosphate, magnesium levels.

Nutritional: Clinical effects seen may be caused by lack of adequate vitamins, trace elements, essential fatty acids.

Medications

Opioid Analgesics

USES

Relief of moderate to severe pain associated with surgical procedures, myocardial infarction, burns, cancer, or other conditions. May be used as an adjunct to anesthesia, either as a preoperative medication or intraoperatively as a supplement to anesthesia. Codeine and hydrocodone have an antitussive effect. Opium tinctures, such as paregoric, are used for severe diarrhea. Methadone relieves severe pain but is used primarily as part of heroin detoxification.

ACTION

Opioids refer to all drugs having actions similar to morphine and to receptors combining with these agents. Major effects are on the central nervous system (produce analgesia, drowsiness, mood changes mental clouding, analgesia without loss of consciousness, nausea and vomiting) and GI tract (decrease HCl secretion; diminish biliary, pancreatic, and intestinal secretions; diminish propulsive peristalsis). Also affect respiration (depressed) and cardiovascular system (peripheral vasodilation, decrease peripheral resistance, inhibit baroreceptor reflexes).

OPIOID ANALGESICS

| Names | Availability | Analgesic Effect | | | Dosage Range |
		Onset (min)	Peak (min)	Duration (hrs)	
Butorphanol (Stadol)	**I:** 1 mg/ml, 2 mg/ml	**IM:** 10–30 **IV:** 2–3	**IM:** 30–60 **IV:** 30	**IM:** 3–4 **IV:** 2–4	**IM:** 1–4 mg q3–4h **IV:** 0.5–2 mg q3–4h
Codeine	**I:** 30 mg, 60 mg **T:** 30 mg, 60 mg	**IM:** 10–30 **PO:** 30–45	**IM:** 30–60 **PO:** 60–120	**IM/PO:** 4–6	**IM/PO (A):** 15–60 mg q4–6h; **(C):** 0.5 mg/kg q4–6h

					IM: 50–100 μg q1–2h
Fentanyl (Sublimaze)	**I:** 50 μg/ml	**IM:** 7–15 **IV:** 1–2	**IM:** 20–30 **IV:** 3–5	**IM:** 1–2 **IV:** 0.5–1	
Hydrocodone	Combination oral	10–30	30–60	4–6	5–10 mg q4–6h
Hydromorphone (Dilaudid)	**T:** 1 mg, 2 mg, 3 mg, 4 mg, 8 mg **S:** 3 mg **I:** 1 mg/ml, 2 mg/ml, 3 mg/ml, 4 mg/ml, 10 mg/ml	**PO:** 30 **IM:** 15 **IV:** 10–15	**PO:** 90–120 **IM:** 30–60 **IV:** 15–30	**PO:** 4–5 **IM:** 4–5 **IV:** 4	**PO:** 1–4 mg q3–6h **IM:** 1–4 mg q3–6h **IV:** 0.5–1 mg q3h **ER:** 3 mg q4–8h
Levorphanol (Levo-Dromoran)	**T:** 2 mg **I:** 2 mg/ml	**PO:** 10–60 **IM:** —	**PO:** 90–120 **IM:** 60	4–5	**PO:** 2–4 mg q4h **IM:** 2–3 mg q4h
Meperidine (Demerol)	**T:** 50 mg, 100 mg **I:** 25 mg/ml, 50 mg/ml, 75 mg/ml, 100 mg/ml	**PO:** 15 **IM:** 10–15 **IV:** 1	**PO:** 60–90 **IM:** 30–60 **IV:** 5–7	2–4	**PO/IM (A):** 50–150 mg q3–4h **(C):** 1–1.8 mg/kg q3–4h **IM/PO:** 2.5–10 mg q3–4h
Methadone (Dolophine)	**T:** 5 mg, 10 mg **OS:** 5 mg/5 ml, 10 mg/5 ml **I:** 10 mg/ml	**PO:** 30–60 **IM:** 10–20 **IV:** —	**PO:** 90–120 **IM:** 60–120 **IV:** 15–30	**PO:** 4–6 **IM:** 4–5 **IV:** 3–4	
Morphine (Roxanol, MS Contin)	**T (ER):** 15 mg, 30 mg, 60 mg, 100 mg, 200 mg **OS:** 10 mg/5 ml, 20 mg/5 ml, 20 mg/ml **I:** 4 mg/ml, 10 mg/ml, 15 mg/ml	**PO:** 30–60 **IM:** 10–30 **IV:** —	**PO:** 90 **IM:** 30–60 **IV:** 20	**PO:** 4 **IM/IV:** 4–5	**PO:** 10–30 mg q4h **IM:** 5–20 mg q4h **IV:** 0.05–0.1 mg/kg q4h
Nalbuphine (Nubain)	**I:** 10 mg/ml, 20 mg/ml	**IM:** 2–15 **IV:** 2–3	**IM:** 60 **IV:** 30	**IM:** 3–6 **IV:** 3–4	**IM/IV:** 10–20 mg q3–6h

(Continued)

Medications

OPIOID ANALGESICS—cont'd

| Names | Availability | Analgesic Effect | | | |
		Onset (min)	Peak (min)	Duration (hrs)	Dosage Range
Oxycodone (Roxicodone)	**T:** 15 mg, 30 mg **OS:** 5 mg/5 ml, 20 mg/ml **T (ER):** 10 mg, 20 mg, 40 mg, 80 mg, 160 mg	30	60	3–4	5–15 mg or 5 ml q4–6h **(ER):** q12h (dose titrated)
Propoxyphene (Darvon)	**T:** 100 mg	15–60	60–120	4–6	**PO:** 100 mg q4–6h

A, Adults; *C,* children; *ER,* extended-release; *I,* injection; *IM,* intramuscularly; *IV,* intravenously; *OS,* oral solution; *PO,* by mouth; *S,* supplement; *T,* tablets.

Opioid Antagonists

USES

Primarily used to reverse respiratory depression induced by narcotic overdosage.

ACTION

Prevents/reverses effects of mu (μ) receptor opioid agonists (e.g., increases respiration, reverses sedative effect).

OPIOID ANTAGONISTS

Name	Availability	Dosage Range	Side Effects
Nalmefene (Revex)	**I:** 100 μg/ml, 1 mg/ml	**IV/IM/SubQ:** Titrated individually	Nausea, vomiting, tachycardia, hypertension
Naloxone (Narcan)	**I:** 0.02 mg/ml, 0.4 mg/ml, 1 mg/ml	**IV/IM/SubQ (A):** 0.4–2 mg May repeat at 2- to 3-min intervals; **(C):** 0.01 mg/kg May give subsequent doses of 0.1 mg/kg	Same as nalmefene
Naltrexone (Depade, ReVia)	**T:** 50 mg	**PO:** 50 mg/day or 100 mg every other day or 150 mg every third day	Abdominal pain, anxiety, diarrhea, tachycardia, increased sweating, loss of appetite, nausea

A, Adults; *C,* (dosage), children; *I,* injection; *T,* tablets.

Sedative-Hypnotics

USES

Treatment of insomnia (e.g., difficulty falling asleep initially, frequent awakening, awakening too early).

ACTION

Sedatives decrease activity, moderate excitement, and have calming effects. Hypnotics produce drowsiness, enhance onset/maintenance of sleep (resembling natural sleep). Benzodiazepines are the most widely used agents (largely replace barbiturates); greater safety, lower incidence of drug dependence.

Medications

SEDATIVE-HYPNOTICS

Name	Availability	Dosage Range	Side Effects
Benzodiazepines			
Estazolam (ProSom)	**T:** 1 mg, 2 mg	**A:** 1–2 mg **E:** 0.5–1 mg	Daytime sedation, memory and psychomotor impairment, tolerance, withdrawal reactions, rebound insomnia, dependence
Flurazepam (Dalmane)	**C:** 15 mg, 30 mg	**A/E:** 15–30 mg	Same as estazolam
Quazepam (Doral)	**T:** 7.5 mg, 15 mg	**A:** 7.5–15 mg **E:** 7.5 mg	Same as estazolam
Temazepam (Restoril)	**C:** 7.5 mg, 15 mg, 30 mg	**A:** 15–30 mg **E:** 7.5–15 mg	Same as estazolam
Triazolam (Halcion)	**T:** 0.125 mg, 0.25 mg	**A:** 0.125–0.25 mg **E:** 0.125 mg	Same as estazolam
Nonbenzodiazepines			
Zaleplon (Sonata)	**C:** 5 mg, 10 mg	**A:** 5–10 mg **E:** 5 mg	Headaches, dizziness, myalgia, somnolence, asthenia, abdominal pain
Zolpidem (Ambien)	**T:** 5 mg, 10 mg	**A:** 10 mg **E:** 5 mg	Dizziness, daytime drowsiness, headaches, confusion, depression, hangover, asthenia

A, Adults; *C,* capsules; *E,* elderly; *T,* tablets.

Sympathomimetics

USES

Stimulation of alpha₁-receptors: Induce vasoconstriction primarily in skin and mucous membranes; nasal decongestion; combine with local anesthetics to delay anesthetic absorption; increases blood pressure in certain hypotensive states; produce mydriasis, facilitating eye exams, ocular surgery.

Stimulation of beta₁-receptors: Treatment of cardiac arrest, heart failure, shock, AV block.

Stimulation of beta₂-receptors: Treatment of asthma.

Stimulation of dopamine receptors: Treatment of shock.

ACTION

The sympathetic nervous system (SNS) is involved in maintaining homeostasis (involved in regulation of heart rate, force of cardiac contractions, blood pressure, bronchial airway tone, carbohydrate, fatty acid metabolism). The SNS is mediated by neurotransmitters (primarily norepinephrine, epinephrine, and dopamine), which act on adrenergic receptors. These receptors include beta₁, beta₂, alpha₁, alpha₂, and dopaminergic receptors. Sympathomimetics differ widely in their actions based on their specificity to affect these receptors.

SYMPATHOMIMETICS

Name	Availability	Receptor Specificity	Uses	Dosage Range
Dobutamine (Dobutrex)	I: 12.5 mg/ml, 500 mg/250 ml	Beta$_1$, beta$_2$, alpha$_1$	Inotropic support in cardiac decompensation	**IV infusion:** 2.5–10 µg/kg/min
Dopamine (Intropin)	I: 40 mg, 80 mg, 160 ml vials, 800 µg/ml, 1600 µg/ml	Beta$_1$, alpha$_1$, dopaminergic	Vasopressor, cardiac stimulant	**Dopaminergic:** 0.5–3 µg/kg/min **Beta$_1$:** 2–10 µg/kg/min **Alpha$_1$:** >10 µg/kg/min
Epinephrine (Adrenalin)	I: 0.1 mg/ml, 1 mg/ml	Beta$_1$, beta$_2$, alpha$_1$	Cardiac arrest, anaphylactic shock	**Vasopressor:** 1–10 µg/min **Cardiac arrest:** 1 mg q3–5min during resuscitation
Norepinephrine (Levophed) **Phenylephrine** (Neo-Synephrine)	I: 1 mg/ml I: 10 mg/ml	Beta$_1$, alpha$_1$ Alpha$_1$	Vasopressor Vasopressor	**IV:** 0.5–1 µg/min up to 2–12 µg/min **IV:** Initially, 10–180 µg/min, then 40–60 µg/min

I, Injection.

Index

Page numbers followed by *f* indicate figures; page numbers followed by *t* indicate tables; page numbers followed by *b* indicate boxes.